Type 2 Diabetes, Pre-Diabetes, and the Metabolic Syndrome

CURRENT CLINICAL PRACTICE

Neil S. Skolnik, Series Editor

For other titles published in this series, go to
www.springer.com/series/7633

TYPE 2 DIABETES, PRE-DIABETES, AND THE METABOLIC SYNDROME

Second Edition

by

RONALD A. CODARIO, MD, FACP

University of Pennsylvania Health System
Clinical Instructor in Medicine
Thomas Jefferson University Hospital
Philadelphia, Pennsylvania
USA

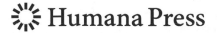
Humana Press

Ronald A. Codario, MD, FACP
Clinical Instructor in Medicine
Thomas Jefferson University Hospital
111 South 11th Street
Philadelphia, PA 19107

Ronald A. Codario, MD, FACP
Diplomate American Board of Internal Medicine
Diplomate American Board of Clinical Lipidology
Diplomate American Board of Vascular Medicine
Clinical Hypertension Specialist (American Society of Hypertension Certified)
Vascular Ultrasound (American Registry of Diagnostic Sonography Certified)

ISBN 978-1-60327-440-1   e-ISBN 978-1-60327-441-8
DOI 10.1007/978-1-60327-441-8
Springer New York Dordrecht Heidelberg London

Printed on acid-free paper

Humana Press is part of Springer Science+Business Media (www.springer.com)

Dedication

This book is dedicated to Rocco Fiorentino, a truly courageous young man and role model for determination, who lost his sight shortly after birth, to his parents Tina and Rocco who have established The Little Rock Foundation bringing joy to the visually impaired and deprived, and to all those who have lost their vision due to diabetes. Hopefully this book will inspire further research and investigation to prevent vision loss and enable many to appreciate this precious gift.

Special appreciation and acknowledgements: To my wife, Celeste and my four children, Ron, Jr., Maria, Christiana and Joseph for their words of encouragement and inspiration.

A special thank you to Noreen and Bill Conroy for transcribing the revisions of this text from my dictation.

Preface

Diabetes has become an ever-increasing problem throughout the world with an estimated 300 million people worldwide to be diagnosed with the disease in the next 10 years and 370 million by 2030. Currently, 240 million people in the world (a prevalence of 5.9%) and 20.8 million people in the United States are currently afflicted (17.2 million with type-2 diabetes), with an additional 5.2 million undiagnosed, and close to 16 million being insulin resistant. More than 9 million women, 8 million men and over 120,000 children less than 18 years of age currently have this disease, while over 20% have the metabolic syndrome.

Type-2 diabetes has escalated to epidemic proportions, with 40% of the American population being at risk for the development of the disease and 1 in 14 currently suffering from this condition. Diabetes is currently the sixth leading cause of death in the United States associated with twice the mortality rate of those without the disease, while the lifetime risk for developing diabetes for individuals born in 2000 is 38.5% for women and 32.8% for men. Women diagnosed with type-2 diabetes at age 40 can expect to lose 14.3 years of life expectancy, while men will lose 11.6 years.

The National Health and Nutrition Examination survey revealed that only 7% of adults with this disease achieved desired goals for lipid, glycemic, and blood pressure control, while almost 60% have A1C's that exceed 7.0%. Close to 95% of individuals with type-2 diabetes in the United States are managed by primary care providers with this disease afflicting approximately 20% of all patients seen in the office setting. The progressive nature of this disorder is not only confined to the deterioration of β cell function, but also the progressive development of severe arteriosclerotic vascular disease. These patients will suffer from their microvascular disease (retinopathy, neuropathy, and nephropathy), but will die from their macrovascular disease including coronary artery disease, complications from peripheral vascular disease, and stroke with many having established micro- and macrovascular complications of the disease at the time of first presentation to their provider.

Increasing obesity, dietary indiscretions, progressive physical inactivity, and advancing age of the population have all contributed to a sharp rise in the disease. In 1992, 2–4% of all newly diagnosed cases of diabetes in children were type 2 diabetics. By 1999, this had risen to 45%. African Americans are more hyperinsulinemic and insulin resistant at puberty with lower resting metabolic rates than white children.

According to statistics published by The American Diabetes Association, 15% of the United States population have either impaired fasting glucose (6.9%), confirmed diabetes (5.9%), or undiagnosed diabetes (2.8%). An alarming 22.7% of Mexican Americans (9.3% confirmed, 4.5% undiagnosed, and 8.9% impaired fasting) and 18.8% of African American non-Hispanics (8.2% confirmed, 3.6% undiagnosed, and 7.0% impaired fasting) are greater than 20 years of age.

The incidence of type-2 diabetes since 1980 has increased by close to 20% with a five-fold increase in children and adolescents since 1994. Each year, over 798,000 new cases are diagnosed in this country alone with close to 180,000 succumbing to the disease and its devastations. Since 1970, this disease has risen 700% in this country alone. According to the Centers for Disease control, 33% of men and 39% of women born in 2000 will develop the disease. The highest lifetime risks are 45% for Hispanic men and 53% for Hispanic women. By the year 2025, nearly 22 million adults in the United States and 300 million worldwide will have diabetes! This disease is the leading cause of end-stage kidney disease and blindness in individuals between 20 and 74 years of age and a major cause of peripheral neuropathy and peripheral vascular disease.

Clearly, diagnosing and managing the type-2 diabetic represents a tremendous challenge to the primary care provider already besieged with managed care issues, medication costs, liability concerns, and health access.

Not to be overlooked is the impact of obesity on metabolic syndrome and diabetes. The phenomenal growth rate of obesity is underscored in the United States, where over 65% of the adult population has a BMI >25, 30% are frankly obese with BMI's >30, and 5.1% fall into the massively obese category with BMI's >40. Canada has the largest growth rate of obesity in children with 16% of those between ages 6 and 19 having a BMI >95 percentile, while among 16 year olds, 30% have elevated BMI's and high normal or elevated systolic blood pressures. Forty-year-old obese nonsmoking males can expect a 5.8-year life expectancy reduction, while their female counterparts can expect a 7.1-year decreased life expectancy.

This book has been designed as a direct result of 10 years of lecturing throughout the country, listening, teaching, and empathizing with fellow primary care practitioners in our ongoing fight with this killer disease. I have designed this as an easy-to-reference state-of-the-art guide to all primary care practitioners, students, care givers, and patients battling the ravages of this ever-increasing epidemic.

This second edition has been substantially revised to include more pathophysiology, the latest in clinical trials, updates on new medications, and an expanded section on Special Populations.

Philadelphia, PA   *Ronald A. Codario, MD, FACP*
May 2010

Series Editor Preface

Type 2 Diabetes, Pre-Diabetes, and the Metabolic Syndrome: *The Primary Care Guide to Diagnosis and Management, Second Edition,* marks an important addition to the literature for primary care clinicians. Like the very well-received first edition published in 2005, this second edition covers concisely and with attention to clinical relevance the full spectrum of insulin resistance and diabetes. Dr. Ronald Codario again emphasizes a practical, no-nonsense approach to understanding the basic pathophysiology of diabetes and the metabolic syndrome, to treatment with oral agents and insulin, and to risk factor management. This edition also includes excellent additional information on pathophysiology, new medications, clinical trials, and special patient populations.

This title will serve as a superb resource for family medicine and internal medicine physicians, physician assistants, nurse practitioners, residents in family medicine and internal medicine, and medical students. Given the explosive growth in these conditions, *Type 2 Diabetes, Pre-Diabetes, and the Metabolic Syndrome: The Primary Care Guide to Diagnosis and Management, Second Edition,* is a timely and invaluable contribution to the field and to this Current Clinical Practice book series. It will provide all readers interested in the topic with a solid understanding of the issues, greatly enhancing patient care for all patients with diabetes, prediabetes, and the metabolic syndrome.

Philadelphia, PA   *Neil S. Skolnik, MD*

Contents

1 Pathophysiology of Type-2 Diabetes

Contents

Key Words: Glucose, Insulin, Type-2 diabetes, Tissue response, Non autoimmune beta cell function, Hepatic glucose production, Islet alpha cell glucagon secretion, Incretins

ETIOLOGY

Appropriate treatment of type-2 diabetes is dependent upon the knowledge of the pathophysiology of the disease, the mechanisms underlying hyperglycemia, and the efficacy of various oral agents and insulins to improve fasting or postprandial hyperglycemia.

Type-2 diabetes is clearly a heterogenous, complex, interrelated disease involving multigenic etiologies. The classical disturbances in this condition as seen in Table 1 are characterized by a combination of insulin resistance and progressive beta cell deterioration resulting in impaired insulin secretion and release, increased hepatic glucose production as the result of enhanced glycogenolysis and gluconeogenesis. The disease demonstrates a wide variance from the predominantly insulin resistant to the predominantly insulin deficient [1].

In the vast majority of type-2 diabetics, no single genetic defect has been elucidated to explain etiology of this process, but results from the combined effects of multigenic heterogeneous and complex and related causes. In a very small percentage of those individuals with monogenic causes of type-2 diabetes, inheritance of two mutant genes from both parents or autosomal inheritance are responsible [2].

From: *Current Clinical Practice: Type 2 Diabetes, Pre-Diabetes, and the Metabolic Syndrome*
Edited by: R.A. Codario, DOI 10.1007/978-1-60327-441-8_1
© Springer Science+Business Media, LLC 2011

Table 1
Classic metabolic disturbances in type 2 diabetes

Increased hepatic gluconeogenesis and glycogenolysis

Impaired insulin secretion

Insulin resistance

From Henry RR. Glucose control and insulin resistance in non-insulin dependent diabetes mellitus. Ann Intern Med 1996;124:97–103

These monogenic causes can effect:

1. Beta cell function as in maturity onset diabetes of youth (MODY) of which six types of different effected genes exist. All these genes except the glucokinase gene, which affects glycolysis, are transcription factors that effect development or gene expression at the beta cell level
2. Insulin gene mutations demonstrating excessive proinsulin and defective insulin molecules with reduced function at the target tissues
3. Insulin receptor mutations of which greater than 50 exist involving both production and function, including Leprechaunism, Rabson–Mendenhall syndrome, and Type A severe insulin resistance syndrome
4. Lipodystrophy with mutations in the LMNA gene and the seipin protein [2]

Despite this genetic heterogenicity a consistent phenotype becomes manifested when the disease condition develops, characterized by:

1. Impaired insulin secretion
2. Insulin resistance
3. Increased hepatic glucose production due to both increased glycogenolysis and gluconeogenesis
4. Impaired incretin release

Recently, significant attention has been devoted to this incretin effect mediated by several gastrointestinal peptides. In humans, the major incretins are glucagon-like peptide-1 (GLP-1) and glucose dependent insulinotropic polypeptide (GIP). Both the GLP-1 and GIP increase glucose dependent and first phase insulin secretion and are rapidly deactivated by dipeptidyl peptidase-4 (DPP-4), but only GLP-1 suppresses glucagon secretion The incretins also have a variety of other systemic effects including appetite suppression by a direct effect on the satiety center, delayed gastric emptying, and an increase in beta cell neogenesis with apoptosis inhibition (animal and in vitro). Both GLP-1 and GIP are released from the intestinal cells in response to nutrient intake with GLP-1 being synthesized from proglucagon in the L cells of the small intestine and GIP in the K cells of the proximal intestinal mucosa [3].

NATURAL HISTORY OF TYPE-2 DIABETES

As seen in Fig. 1, the earliest manifestation of the type-2 diabetes is elevation of postprandial glucose in association with progressive insulin resistance. This results in compensatory islet cell hypertrophy, but eventually insulin production is insufficient to maintain euglycemia. In many instances a loss or delay of early phase insulin release in response to

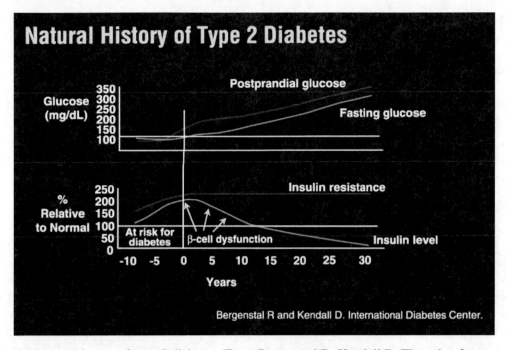

Fig. 1. Natural history of type 2 diabetes (From Bergenstal R, Kendall D. The role of postprandial glucose in type-2 diabetes. Diabetes Endocrinol 2005;7(2)).

a mealtime glucose load will aggravate beta cell deficiency and contribute to the progressive nature of the disorder.

Regulation of postprandial glucose depends upon stimulation of insulin secretion with subsequent suppression of hepatic gluconeogenesis and glycogenolysis. Insulin release subsequently promotes glucose uptake in the muscle and the peripheral tissues. The effect of insulin in suppressing hepatic glucose production and muscle glucose uptake is more potent than the effect of hyperglycemia alone [4].

Fasting glucose levels are dependent upon hepatic glucose production (hepatic glycogenolysis and gluconeogenesis), basal insulin levels, insulin sensitivity, and the level and duration of the previous prandial glucose. Elevated fasting glucose levels due to excessive hepatic glucose production during the sleeping hours (12 Midnight to 8 a.m.) may be responsible for the majority of the increments in day long hyperglycemia [5].

Following a meal or glucose load, elevated glucose levels stimulate insulin release from the beta cell. This secreted insulin binds to the cell surface receptors. Within the receptor site, two extracellular alpha subunits bind to the insulin transmitting a signal to two identical beta subunits via the cell membrane. Type-2 diabetics have either normal or slightly diminished insulin receptor binding affinity. Following the binding process, the beta subunit is phosphorylated, increasing tyrosine kinase activity, and enhancing the phosphorylation of various endogenous protein substrates. This results in a cascading sequence of reactions responsible for the synthesis of RNA, DNA, protein, and intracellular enzymes. Hepatic glucose output is suppressed and glucose uptake by the peripheral tissues, notably skeletal muscle and adipose cells, is subsequently enhanced [6].

Type-2 diabetics demonstrate excessive hepatic glucose production despite significantly elevated insulin levels. The combination of increased hepatic glucose production and fasting hyperinsulinemia illustrates the insulin resistance in these individuals. This is because hepatic glucose production is profoundly reduced with small increases in plasma insulin. In fact, we find across all plasma insulin concentrations, including both pharmacologic and physiologic levels, that the ability of insulin to suppress hepatic glucose production is diminished in type-2 diabetics [7].

One of the most critical effects of insulin is its effects on glucose disposal. As the result of impaired muscle glucose uptake, glucose disposal is significantly reduced resulting in impaired glycogen synthesis, glucose oxidation, and tissue glucose uptake. Glucose transport is rate limiting for overall disposal under most normal physiologic conditions. Of the five types of glucose transporters identified, the GLUT-4 protein is referred to as the insulin sensitive glucose transporter. This transporter is found in high concentrations in adipose cells, skeletal and cardiac muscles and is primarily responsible for glucose uptake and its effects. The GLUT-4 proteins are housed in intracellular vesicles and translocate to the cell surface inserting into the plasma membrane upon insulin stimulation. This causes glucose to enter the cell. Type-2 diabetics usually have normal GLUT-4 levels, but impaired glucose transport. This may indicate that a flaw exists in the insulin influenced translocation of GLUT-4 to the cell surface. This defective signaling pathway between the receptor and the transport stimulation results in insulin resistance in these patients [5].

PATHOPHYSIOLOGY

Type-2 diabetics demonstrate multiple intracellular deficiencies in insulin activity. The most conspicuous being impaired activation of the insulin receptor by stimulating insulin receptor tyrosine phosphorylation. Others include:

1. Impaired ability to phosphorylate and to stimulate the association of IRS-1 (Insulin Receptor Stimulator – 1) with the P85 subunit of PI-3 kinase
2. Impaired phosphorylation of PI-3 kinase
3. Impaired induction of GLUT-4 translocation by PI-3 kinase. Remaining to be elucidated are which defects result from the diabetic state and which actually cause the condition [8]

Hence the impaired ability of endogenous insulin to enhance tissue glucose uptake (primarily in muscle) and suppress hepatic glucose output account for the postprandial rises in plasma glucose that are typical of the diabetic state.

Free fatty acids released from adipose cells due to enhanced lipolysis may also contribute to insulin resistance by inhibiting glucose transport and phosphorylation followed by reduced rates of glucose oxidation and glycogen synthesis, as well as increasing apolipoprotein B secretion and increased hepatic lipase activity. Chronically elevated free fatty acid levels inhibit insulin secretion from the beta cell, and decrease insulin sensitivity in the muscle and the liver [9].

No small wonder then that insulin resistance has been associated with a wide range of clinical maladies including polycystic ovaries, hyperuricemia, acanthosis nigricans, decreased fibrinolytic activity, dyslipidemia, arteriosclerotic vascular disease, obesity, hypertension, and impaired glucose tolerance.

THE NATURAL HISTORY OF TYPE-2 DIABETES

Although both insulin resistance and impaired insulin secretion precede the development of postprandial hyperglycemia and the subsequent type-2 diabetic phenotype, insulin resistance is more prominent in the pre-diabetic state and plays an important role in the pathogenesis of macrovascular disease. Insulin resistance is commonly the earliest manifestation in the development of type-2 diabetes typically originating 5–10 years prior to postprandial glucose levels in the diabetic range (200 mg/dl). As long as the beta cell is able to compensate by increased insulin production, normal glucose tolerance is maintained. Hence not all patients with insulin resistance will develop diabetes [10].

Insulin resistance can be worsened by genetic factors, elevated free fatty acids, hyperglycemia, pregnancy, obesity, sedentary life style, aging, and various medications (i.e., steroids, cis-retinoic acid, estrogens, nicotinic acid, oral contraceptives, phenothiazines, and antipsychotic agents) and is characterized by impaired responses to the physiologic effects of this hormone on glucose, lipid, and protein metabolism as well as affecting vascular endothelial function. The endogenous insulin secreted is inefficiently capable of suppressing hepatic gluconeogensis or stimulating glucose utilization in the muscle and fat [11].

Physicians should be aware that the immune suppressant drug, tacrolimus, can cause an alarming increased incidence in the development of insulin dependent type-2 diabetes in organ transplant patients. Tacrolimus inhibits insulin gene transcription by binding to FKBP-12 (FK506 binding protein-12), which is found in pancreatic beta islet cells. This binding results in inhibition of calcineurin, which activates nuclear transcription factors like nuclear factor activated T cells (NFAT) and cyclic adenosine monophosphate (AMP) response element binding protein (CREB), which are needed for the production of insulin messenger RNA. Calcineurin is a phosphatase whose activity is dependent upon calmodulin and calcium ion [12].

Increases in plasma glucose concentrations by 50–100 mg/dl for as little as 24 h can cause downregulation of the glucose transport system in the muscle (GLUT-4) significantly increasing insulin resistance. With the progression of time, insulin resistance peaks and then plateaus, while increases in plasma insulin compensate to maintain the glycemic state.

Fasting hepatic glucose production is increased in both obese and non-obese diabetics compared to normal individuals and those with impaired glucose tolerance that have not met the criteria for diabetes. It is this increase in hepatic glucose output due to increases in glyogenolysis and gluconeogenesis that result in fasting hyperglycemia in Type-2 diabetics. At some point, usually about 10 years after insulin resistance and hyperinsulinemia develop, postprandial hyperglycemia begins to develop due to beta cell dysfunction and or depletion. This is characterized by a delay in first phase insulin release and blunted second phase output. It is this first phase response that plays an important role in suppression of hepatic glucose production. This progressive deterioration leads to fasting hyperglycemia when insulin levels begin to decline, while insulin resistance remains elevated. The progressive nature of the disease and the progressive lack of glycemic control are due predominately to this ongoing deterioration of beta cell function with subsequent decrease production of insulin [13].

There is a small subset of type-2 diabetics in whom beta cell dysfunction develops with minimal insulin resistance but the progressive hyperglycemia induces subsequent insulin resistance. Essentially all type-2 diabetics with elevation of fasting glucose have deficient insulin secretion. Even those individuals with absolute increases of serum insulin (i.e., higher than normal) have relative insulin deficiency given their levels of hyperglycemia and severity of insulin resistance [14].

Although the triple disturbance of insulin resistance, increased hepatic glucose production and impaired insulin secretion critical to the development of type-2 diabetes have received a great deal of attention in research, and also of compelling interest is the etiologic sequence of events resulting in the diabetic state. Accelerated hepatic gluconeogenesis and glycogenolysis does not seem to exist in the state of impaired glucose tolerance, where insulin resistance and impaired insulin secretion predominate and in fact these two abnormalities precede the onset of hyperglycemia in the diabetic type-2 phenotype. Pre-diabetic individuals have severe insulin resistance, while insulin secretion tends to be normal or increased in the pre-diabetic or impaired glucose tolerant state including first phase insulin responses to intravenous challenges. Hence the type-2 diabetic evolves from the individual with impaired glucose tolerance and insulin resistance. The genetic factors previously mentioned play a key role, but acquired factors are also important including sedentary life style, high fat diets, central visceral obesity, and progressive aging in susceptible individuals [7].

Insulin resistance in the skeletal muscle, vascular endothelium and liver may be promoted by increased levels of inflammatory cytokines like interleukin-6, hs-CRP, and tumor necrosis factor alpha, although several prospective studies have shown an inconsistent relationship between these markers and clinical diabetes except for a large cohort of the Women's Health Initiative Observational Study (WHIOS). Among the 93,676 postmenopausal women aged 50–79 years without cardiovascular disease or diabetes mellitus in the WHIOS, 1,584 women who had developed diabetes during 5.9 years of follow up were matched by ethnicity, age, clinical center, time of blood draw, and duration of follow up to 2,198 study participants without diabetes. In this study, published in the *New England Journal of Medicine* in 2007, hs-CRP and IL-6 levels were significantly associated with diabetes risk regardless of ethnic group. This study provides support for the role of chronic inflammation in the development of type-2 diabetes in women. Interestingly, tumor necrosis alpha by virtue of a direct inhibition of insulin signaling may play an important role in inducing peripheral insulin resistance in obese individuals [15].

Systemic inflammation, indicated by the presence of elevated markers like hs-CRP, TNF-alpha, and IL-6, may also play a pivotal role in the subsequent development of type-2 diabetes. In vitro studies have demonstrated that the downregulation of endothelial nitric oxide synthetase by hs-CRP can induce endothelial dysfunction promoting insulin resistance by generating overproduction of endothelial adhesion molecules, which induces insulin resistance. Obesity related inflammatory and metabolic stress induce insulin resistance by inhibiting insulin receptor activity. In addition, an insulin resistant state may enhance the hepatic production of hs-CRP since insulin has an anti-inflammatory effect while impaired glucose promotes free fatty acid production, resulting in enhanced oxidative stress and elevated levels of hs-CRP [16]. The beneficial effects of anti-inflammatory medication like 3-hydroxy-3-methylglutaryl coenzyme-A inhibitors, angiotensin converting enzyme inhibitors, and proliferator-activated receptor-gamma agonists lend some credence to the role of inflammation in the diabetic state.

However, all obese individuals will not develop diabetes. Despite the strong genetic predisposition, the exact mechanisms for clinical phenotypic differences are still not well known. Research into the role of adipocytokines, secreted from adipose tissue has shed new light on their role in glucose homeostasis.

One such adipokine is adiponectin, a hormone with insulin sensitizing and anti-inflammatory properties secreted by adipocytes. This 244 -amino acid collagen like protein stimulates insulin secretion and fatty acid oxidation while enhancing glucose uptake in skeletal muscle and liver, and suppressing hepatic gluconeogenesis by stimulating various signaling pathways for peroxisome proliferator receptor alpha and 5′AMP activated protein kinase. Hypertrophic adipocytes, seen in obesity, secrete angiogenic and inflammatory factors that inhibit adiponectin secretion with lowered adiponectin levels being associated with enhance risk of type-2 diabetes.

Higher levels of fetuin-A, a hepatic secretory protein inhibits insulin activity and binds to the insulin receptor, with insulin resistance and increased diabetes risk in individuals greater than 70 years of age. The association is independent of inflammatory markers, obesity status, race, gender, and physical activity. Fetuin-A inhibits insulin receptors by binding tyrosine kinase in the insulin receptors of skeletal muscle and adipocytes, resulting in decreased insulin signaling and depressed autophosphorylation rates. It is of interest to note that chromosome 3q27, the metabolic syndrome and diabetes susceptibility locus, houses the human fetuin-A gene [17]. Although blocking fetuin-A binding to the insulin receptor can potentially be a subject of research into the treatment and prevention of various insulin resistant states, fetuin-A knockout mice have demonstrated extensive vascular and soft tissue calcification with lower levels in humans associated with cardiac valvular calcifications and increased mortality following a myocardial infarction. Future research should shed some light into the efficacy of fetuin-A activity inhibition and its utility or futility in glucose metabolism and disease prevention. The body's response to insulin resistance is to enhance the beta cell's secretion of insulin to maintain normal glucose tolerance. The development of type-2 diabetes from the impaired glucose tolerant state occurs as the result of an organized sequence of metabolic events.

Initially, hepatic glyogenolysis and gluconeogenesis increases resulting in enhanced basal hepatic glucose production. This is common in all type-2 diabetics with fasting hyperglycemia. Insulin resistance tends to become more severe and peaks when fasting hyperglycemia develops due to the degree of glycemic load, aging, sedentary life style, obesity, and any other concomitant factors than can effect insulin sensitivity and resistance. Normalization of hepatic glucose production and improvement in insulin resistance can be achieved through antidiabetic treatment resulting in significant amelioration of this particular state. The final sequence of events is a progressive deterioration in beta cell function with subsequent decline in insulin secreting ability [18].

Several factors can be involved in this deterioration, including progressive beta cell exhaustion due to dietary indiscretion, prolonged glucose toxicity along with preprogrammed genetic abnormalities in beta function, all contributing to and resulting in the cumulative loss of function and mass in these pancreatic islet cells By enhancing their secretion of insulin, the pancreatic beta cells can compensate for insulin resistance and can sustain this high output production for many years in some patients who never develop type-2 diabetes. Once insulin secretion begins to fail, glucose levels increase due to a reduction in the inhibitory effects of insulin on glucose release from the liver, enhanced free fatty acid release from the adipocytes, and reduced glucose uptake in the skeletal muscle. This progressive beta cell deterioration results in a worsening of the hyperglycemic state and the subsequent evolution into the type-2 diabetic state [19].

The majority of type-2 diabetics are overweight and hyperinsulinemic at the time of diagnosis. Central obesity is associated with the proliferation of insulin resistant and dysfunctional visceral fat with the obese diabetic demonstrating an enhanced insulin secretory response to hyperglycemia compared to the lean diabetic patient. Obese individuals with increased visceral fat accumulate free fatty acids and triglycerides in the pancreatic beta cells worsening their dysfunction and inducing apoptosis due to intracellular lipotoxicity. The subsequent conversion from the impaired glucose tolerant state to the type-2 diabetic is influenced by concomitant medical conditions, distributions of body fat, degree of obesity, ethnicity, sedentary life style and aging, with a substantial genetic component [20].

Hence, one can see that the type-2 diabetes is at the end of a progressive conglomeration of metabolic defects whose interrelationships directly affect the natural history and progress of the disease [21].

The impaired glucose tolerant state is characterized by mild postprandial hyperglycemia, compensatory hyperinsulinemia, and insulin resistance. Clearly, insulin resistance can be present for many years before an individual becomes diabetic. Even at these stages blood sugar levels do not have to necessarily be elevated.

Understanding the natural history of the disease is important in the early identification of those patients at risk for developing diabetes and developing an effective treatment plan including diet and exercise with weight reduction to prevent or delay the development of the disease. In addition, since insulin resistance is one of the major factors in the prediabetic state and persists in the frankly diabetic individual, improvements in insulin sensitivity with medications like thiazolidinediones and biguanides may be extremely invaluable as first line agents in early treatment. As we will see in a later chapter, the glitazones can be extremely invaluable in not only preserving beta cell function, but also in regenerating beta cell tissue [22].

Early recognition and treatment is of tremendous advantage because macrovascular disease begins with impaired glucose tolerance and microvascular disease begins with diabetic levels of hyperglycemia. Clearly, patients will die from their macrovascular disease, but suffer from their microvascular disease.

Of critical importance is an understanding of how damaging the hyperglycemic state is at the tissue level. Various critical and damaging signaling pathways at the cellular level can be affected due to abnormal glucose tolerance. These damaging pathways can be activated either by the direct toxic effects of the hyperglycemic state, or its metabolic derivatives and their by products, or due to the continuous effects on special signaling pathways at the cellular level caused by the metabolites of glucose.

Several of these pathways have been subsequently characterized. They include:

1. Increased formation of advanced glycation end products
2. Accelerated oxidative stress due to reactive oxygen intermediates
3. Activation of protein kinase C (PKC) isoforms
4. Increases in the polyol pathway flux
5. Enhanced aldose reductase activity
6. Increased flow through the hexosamine pathway, due to the overproduction of superoxide anions induced by the electron transport chain in the mitochondria

Aldose reductase is an enzyme that causes accumulation of sorbitol at the cellular level in various diabetic conditions. Sorbitol accumulation itself directly leads to tissue damage and promotes these complications since excess intracellular sorbitol levels decrease the concentration of various protective organic osmolytes. This is seen in the animal models of cataracts which contain decreased levels of taurine, a potent antioxidant and free-radical scavenger. Interestingly, inhibitors of aldose reductase have been shown to restore levels of protective osmolites and prevent diabetic complications by diminishing sorbitol reduction [22].

In many cellular models progressive elevations of intracellular sorbitol disrupt the signal transduction in related cellular function, and are usually associated with the depletion of protective osmolytes like taurine and myoinositol. It is a deficiency of myoinositol that correlates with the clinical neuropathy responsible for the impaired nerve fiber regeneration and neurologic damage associated with diabetes. Myoinositol deficiencies impair prostaglandin metabolism and nitric oxide synthetase disrupting cyclo-oxygenase pathways, nitric oxide production, and resulting in various defects in the peripheral nerves, the ganglia and the endoneurium. Some have been improved with the addition of prostaglandin E1 analogs and other substances.

Sorbitol accumulation may also destroy pericytes, thereby accelerating retinopathy and neuropathy. The destruction of the pericytes in the nervous tissue and the retina alters the microcirculation resulting in tissue ischemia and increased capillary permeability. This decreases the ability of the tissues to produce vasodilatory nitric oxide, enhancing angiotensin II production, increasing acetylcholine release, and augmenting sympathetic tone. This subsequent diminution in nitric oxide with enhanced polyol pathway flux slows nerve conduction, diminishes blood flow within the endoneurium, and depletes protective intracellular osmolytes [23].

Nitric oxide maintains sodium–potassium ATPase activity critical to nerve metabolism, and impulse transmission, as well as taurine and myoinositol uptake. Hence, disruption in nitric oxide production contributes to the many vascular and metabolic defects in the peripheral nerves, endoneurium, and sympathetic ganglia.

Aldose reductase inhibitors have been shown to prevent many of the microvascular complications of disease in animals and have been shown to preserve nerve conduction velocity. However, they have not shown to be effective in treating or preventing microvascular disease in humans or even in relieving symptoms. Therefore, mere suppression of aldose reductase pathway flux may be inadequate because of the many avenues of hyperglycemic tissue damage.

The modification or the glycation of lipoproteins or proteins by sugars results in the formation of advanced glycation end products. Intracellular and extracellular AGE's are primarily the result of intracellular hyperglycemia. These products are formed by the intracellular oxidation of glucose, fragmentation of phosphate compounds, and the decomposition of glucose derived deoxyfructose lysine adducts (Amadori product), which then react with amino groups from various cellular proteins. This irreversible formation accelerates with aging and with the diabetic state [24].

Impaired cellular function seen in the various diabetic complications result from the cross linkage of proteins and covalent modification by intracellular glucose. This results in abnormal matrix–cell interactions which reduce neurite outgrowth and impair endothelial cell adhesion, decreasing vascular elasticity.

The glycosylated hemoglobin commonly measured to indicate the average blood sugar over a 60 day period of time is the best known example of an advanced glycosylation end product. Enhanced atherogenicity and accelerated atherosclerosis in diabetes is related to the glycosylation of low density lipoproteins, phospholipids, and apolipoprotein B. This subsequently decreases the clearance of LDL and enhances its deposition within the intima of the blood vessels. The formation of intracellular and extracellular advanced glycosylated end products is promoted by intracellular hyperglycemia [25]. These glycosylated end products are irreversibly formed and tend to accumulate with aging as the result of the autoxidation of glucose to form glyoxal in association with fragmentation of various phosphate compounds, which subsequently react with the amino groups of various cellular proteins.

Impaired cellular functioning in diabetes results in alteration of intracellular proteins and abnormal reactions between various matrix components within the cell. This results in false linkages of protein and covalent modification.

A critical sign of extracellular matrix–cell impairment can explain the Dupuytren's contracture found in patients with diabetes and other disorders as a result of adhesive capsulitis along with the stiffening of periarticular structures with impairment in full extension associated with flexion contractures and the "prayer sign" in advanced diabetes.

Advanced glycosylation end products are also responsible for enhanced permeability of the renal glomerular basement membrane, which results in micro and then macroalbuminuria. Inflammatory responses, apoptosis, and mediators of various immune functions are also enhanced by these glycosylation end products which bind to their receptor (RAGE). The binding of advanced glycosylation end products to their receptor sites enhances the expression of pro-inflammatory and pro-coagulant molecules enhancing vascular adhesion and thrombogenesis. This could also explain the impaired wound healing and enhanced susceptibility to infection so prominent in diabetics [26].

Various AGE inhibitors and RAGE blockade substances have been successful in inhibiting many of the detrimental effects of these substances including diminished arterial elasticity, decreased nerve conduction velocity, enhanced urinary albumin excretion, and periodontal inflammation.

The hyperglycemic state induces the formation of harmful free radicals increasing oxidative stress through non-enzymatic reactions as well as enzymatic processes. This oxidative stress results from a chemical imbalance between the reactive nitrogen species known as free radicals and the endogenous cellular defenses against them. The presence of oxidative stress enhances diabetic vascular disease by inhibiting barrier function within the endothelium, promoting leukocytic adhesion and reducing circulating levels of nitric oxide. The subsequent accelerated production of prothrombin by the hyperglycemic state helps to explain diabetic hypercoagulation [27].

Hyperglycemia can produce harmful free radicals and enhanced oxidative stress by both enzymatic and nonenzymatic processes. Free radicals are produced within the mitochondria by oxidative phosphorylation, synthesizing ATP during the process of glucose metabolism and subsequent oxidation. This generates free radicals which can exist independently, containing at least one unpaired electron. These free radicals can then combine with hydrogen, forming a hydroxy radical, contributing to the atherogenic process by initiating lipid peroxidation and subsequent foam cell formation. Unless these free radicals are neutralized by anti-oxidants, they can cause direct cellular damage by oxidation of intracellular mitochondrial DNA, lipids, proteins, and vital cellular structures. Indirectly these radicals can wreak havoc by indirectly activating the signaling pathways that increase the expression of various gene products responsible for the diabetic microvascular complications of retinopathy, nephropathy, and neuropathy.

By diminishing the bioavailable nitric oxide, oxidative stress enhances inflammatory cell adhesion to the endothelial surface, impairing endothelial barrier function and enhancing diabetic and arteriosclerotic vascular disease and endothelial dysfunction [28].

Eating foods high in advanced glycosylation end products and various lipid peroxides enhances a predisposition to postprandial hyperglycemia, impairing endothelial function, increasing lipid peroxidation, and decreasing radical trapping activity. It is not surprising that in diabetic patients increased levels of oxidized LDL and decreased levels of antioxidant vitamins like C and E are present, predisposing these patients to macrovascular disease.

The PKC family is a group of phospholipid dependent protein kinases. These substances mediate various cellular responses to hormones, neurotransmitters, and growth factors subsequently playing a key role in regulating vasodilator release, endothelial activation, and other important cellular functions. The hyperglycemic state increases PKC levels to pathologic ranges increasing the PKC levels directly and enhancing the production of diacylglycerol (DAG) [29].

PKC is a proinflammatory substance which stimulates the release of growth factors like VEGF (vascular endothelial growth factor) which enhances endothelial permeability. The activation of PKC contributes to cardiovascular complications by activating NADPH dependent oxidases, accelerating the production of PAI-1. Inhibitors of PKC have been shown to reverse or prevent impaired angiogenesis in diabetic retinopathy, but the responses seem to vary depending on the patient's genetic background.

PKC activate NF-kappa B (a nuclear transcription factor) that is responsible for signal transduction, thereby exerting proinflammatory effects. The protein kinase family also induces the transcription of various growth factors including:

1. Platelet derived growth factor-beta, which induces vascular wall growth
2. Transforming growth factor, which promotes matrix expansion
3. Endothelin 1, which is a vasoconstrictor
4. VEGF, which increases endothelial permeability and may increase neovascularization

Tissue damage in the diabetic state also involves a shunting of excess intracellular glucose by virtue of the hexosamine pathway [5]. This diverts fructose phosphate from glycolysis to provide substrates for the formation of linked glycoproteins and synthesis of various proteoglycans. Pancreatic beta cells may be especially sensitive to activation of the hexosamine pathway, resulting in increased intracellular hydrogen peroxide levels impairing insulin release, enhancing insulin resistance, and promoting beta cell dysfunction. *N*-acetyl-l-cysteine, an antioxidant has been shown to suppress many of the pathological changes associated with activation of the hexosamine pathway.

The hyperglycemic state is also responsible for the overproduction of superoxide anions by the electron transport system in the mitochondria. This may be the central mechanism that underlies all of the destructive pathways responsible for the diabetic paradigm. This central mechanism has been offered by some as an explanation underlying the mechanism whereby retinopathy may continue to progress long after normoglycemia has been regained. Hyperglycemia can induce mitochondrial DNA mutations due to monocyte adhesion and inhibition of peroxisome proliferator activated receptor activation. The subsequently defective subunits in the electron transport system caused by these mutations may be responsible for increases in the superoxide anion production, continuing to activate tissue damage despite normoglycemic states [28].

Aberrant regulation of the well studied NF-kappa B pathway is associated with arteriosclerosis and diabetes and may be among the initial mechanisms in the tissue damage seen in these states. Bovine endothelial cell data have demonstrated that this pathway regulates numerous genes, including those that express VEGF and RAGE.

When abnormally stimulated, this system can generate an ongoing cycle of dysregulatory metabolic derangements.

Diabetic patients may be prone to enhanced effects of glucosamine on the PAI-1 promoter, subsequently activating PKC isoforms. Hence Type -2 diabetics should be cautioned about using glucosamine because of this potential complication, although its use in diabetic patients has not been shown to induce insulin resistance or insulin sensitivity. Glucosamine is an endogenous amino monosaccharide that is utilized for the biosynthesis of glycosaminoglycans and glycoproteins. One of the most popular dietary supplements, it is synthesized from glucose and present in practically all human tissues with the highest concentrations found in cartilage. Glucosamine can be found in many forms – hydrochloride, sulfate, *N*-acetylglucosamine, or chlorohydrate salt and is approximately 90% absorbed when taken orally. Diabetics should monitor their blood glucose levels when taking this product.

Other kinase pathways in the body enhance insulin resistance, worsening hyperglycemia and related tissue damage and subsequently resulting in a vicious cycle of worsening hyperglycemia and enhanced insulin activity resistance. Inhibition of various detrimental kinase pathways has been shown experimentally to be reversed with use of the antioxidant alpha-lipoic acid. This has been shown in some studies to lower fructosamine levels in patients with type-2 diabetes. It is the subsequent activation of these various detrimental biochemical pathways that is responsible for the cellular damage and the systemic disease characterized by type-2 diabetes [*18*].

SUMMARY

Abnormalities and disruptions of several glucose control mechanisms contribute to the etiology of type-2 diabetes: decreased tissue response and resistance to insulin, impaired insulin production and secretion due to deficient non autoimmune beta cell function, increased hepatic glucose production induced by prolonged islet alpha cell glucagon secretion, and a deficiency in secretion and response to gut hormones called incretins. An appreciation of these pathophysiologic mechanisms and the natural history of the disease are crucial to understanding the therapeutic maneuvers, treatment plans, outcome data, and risk reduction strategies for the diabetic patient.

REFERENCES

1. Tuomi T, Carlsson A, Li H. Clinical and genetic characteristics of type-2 diabetes with and without GAD antibodies. Diabetes 1999;48(1):150–157.
2. Groop LC. Pathogenesis of insulin resistance in type 2 diabetes: a collision between thrifty genes and an affluent environment. Diabetes Obes Metab I Suppl 1999;1:51–57.
3. Gillies Cl. Different strategies for screening and prevention of type-2 diabetes in adults. BMJ 2008; 336(7654):1180–1185.
4. LeRoith D. Beta-cell dysfunction and insulin resistance in type 2 diabetes: role of metabolic and genetic abnormalities. Am J Med 2002;113(suppl 6A):3S–11S.
5. Goldstein BJ. Insulin resistance as the core defect in type 2 diabetes mellitus. Am J Cardiol 2002;90:3G–10G.

6. Haffner SM. The insulin resistance syndrome revisted. Diabetes Care 1996;19:275–277.

7. Grundy SM. Obesity, metabolic syndrome, and coronary atherosclerosis. Circulation 2002;105:2696–2698.

8. Atkinson MA, Maclaren NK. The pathogenesis of insulin-dependent diabetes mellitus. N Engl J Med 1994;331:1428–1436.

9. Budzikowski A. Obesity, diabetes, and hypertension: a growing epidemic. Cardiol Rev 2003;20(9):9–10.

10. Narayan KM, Imperatore G, et al. Targeting people with pre-diabetes. BMJ 2002;325:403–404.

11. Young TK, et al. Type 2 diabetes mellitus in children: prenatal and early infancy risk factors among native Canadians. Arch Pediatr Adolesc Med 2002;156:651–655.

12. Westermark GT, Westermark P. Widespread amyloid deposition in transplanted human pancreatic islets. N Engl J Med 2008;359(9):977–979.

13. Jack L, et al. Aging Americans and diabetes. Geriatrics 2004;59(4):14–17.

14. Sobel BE. Insulin resistance and thrombosis. Am J Cardiol 1999;84(1A):37J–41J.

15. Shepherd PR, Kahn BB. Glucose transporters and insulin action: implications for insulin resistance and diabetes mellitus. N Engl J Med 1999;341:248.

16. Gaede P. Multifactorial intervention and cardiovascular disease in patients with type-2 diabetes. N Engl J Med 2003;348:383.

17. Ix J, Wassel C, Kanaya A. Fetuin-A and incident diabetes mellitus in older persons. JAMA 2008;300(2):182–188.

18. Sinha R, et al. Prevalence of impaired glucose tolerance among children and adolescents with marked obesity. N Engl J Med 2002;346:802–810.

19. Leahy JL, Bonner-Weir S. Beta cell dysfunction induced by chronic hyperglycemia: current ideas on mechanism of impaired glucose induced insulin secretion. Diabetes Care 1992;15:442.

20. Ferrannini E. Insulin resistance versus insulin deficiency in non-insulin dependent diabetes mellitus: problems and prospects. Endocr Rev 1998;19:477.

21. Fagan TC, Deedwaqnia PC. The cardiovascular dysmetabolic syndrome. Am J Med 1998;105(suppl 1A):77S–82S.

22. Cubeddu LX, Hoffmann IS. Insulin resistance and upper normal glucose levels in hypertension: a review. J Hum Hypertens 2002;16(suppl 1):S52–S55.

23. Seely BL, Olefsky JM, Insulin Resistance. David E Mohier, ed. Wiley & Sons Ltd. Publisher 1993;187–252.

24. Deedwania PC. Mechanism of the deadly quartet. Can J Cardiol 2000;16(suppl E):17E–20E.

25. Consensus Report of the American Diabetes Association. Diabetes Care 1998; 21:310–314.

26. Rose G. High risk and population strategies of prevention: ethical considerations. Ann Med 1989; 21:409–413.

27. Narayan KM, et al. Lifetime risk for diabetes mellitus in the United States. JAMA 2003;290(14):1884–1890.

28. Harris M. Undiagnosed type 2 diabetes: clinical and public health issues. Diabetes Care 1993;16:643.

29. United Kingdom Prospective Diabetes Study (UKPDS) Group. Intensive blood glucose control with sulfonylureas or insulin compared with conventional treatment and risk of complications in patients with type 2 diabetes (UKPDS 33). Lancet 1998;352:837–853.

SUPPLEMENTARY READINGS

American Diabetes Association. Diagnosis and classification of diabetes mellitus. Diabetes Care 2010;33 (suppl 1):S62–S69.

Boden G. Pathogenesis of type 2 diabetes: insulin resistance. Endocrinol Metab Clin North Am 2001;30:801–815.

Centers for Disease Control and Prevention. 2007 national diabetes fact sheet. http//www.cdc.gov/diabetes/pubs/factsheet07.htm

Diabetes Control and Complications Trial Research Group. The effect of intensive treatment of diabetes on the development and progression of long term complications in insulin-dependent diabetes mellitus. N Engl J Med 1993;329:977–986.

Desai J, Geiss L, Muktar Q, et al. Public health surveillance of diabetes in the United States. J Public Health Manag Pract 2003;Suppl:S44–S51.

Grimble RF. Inflammatory status and insulin resistance. Curr Opin Clin Nutr Metab Care 2002;5:551–559.

Kahn BB. Gluocse transport: pivotal step in insulin action. Diabetes 1996;45:1644–1654.

Marshall JA, Bessesen DH. Dietary fat and the development of type 2 diabetes. Diabetes Care 2002;25:620–622.

Patel P, Macerollo A. Diabetes mellitus: diagnosis and screening. Am Fam Physician 2010;81(7):863–870.

2   Guidelines and Classifications

Key Words: Type-1 diabetes, Insulin dependent diabetes, Type-2 diabetes, Non-insulin dependent diabetes, Screening, Diet, Medications, Gestational diabetes, Malnutrition-associated diabetes

CLASSES OF DIABETES

The American Diabetes Association lists five classes within the group of disorders that represent the diabetic syndrome. These include:

1. Type-1 diabetes
2. Type-2 diabetes
3. Diabetes associated with contributing clinical states, diseases, drugs and/or chemicals
4. Gestational diabetes
5. Malnutrition-associated diabetes [1]

TYPE-1 DIABETES (INSULIN DEPENDENT DIABETES)

This autoimmune disease is the result of genetic environmental triggers. These patients demonstrate CD8 cell infiltration of the islet cells that are likely involved with subsequent beta cell destruction. A long prodrome is usually present from genetic pre-disposition to

From: *Current Clinical Practice: Type 2 Diabetes, Pre-Diabetes, and the Metabolic Syndrome*
Edited by: R.A. Codario, DOI 10.1007/978-1-60327-441-8_2
© Springer Science+Business Media, LLC 2011

onset of disease. These patients may demonstrate various antibodies to islet antigens including insulin, glutamic acid decarboxylase (GAD), and tyrosine phosphatase 1A-2. Hence, a combination of markers rather than a single test should be used for predictive and diagnostic testing to enhance sensitivity without losing specificity.

A curious form of autoimmune diabetes is found in autoimmune polyglandular syndrome – Type I. This results from a mutation of the autoimmune regulator gene (AIRE) resulting in a wide array of endocrine disturbances [2].

The environmental trigger in development of type-1 diabetes in genetically susceptible individuals is believed to be the Coxsackie virus. This may be due to the antigenic similarity between the virus and the antigen in islet cell tissue. This is referred to as molecular mimicry.

Type-1 diabetics are either totally or almost totally devoid of insulin due to beta cell immunological destruction. Insulin is necessary to prevent hyperglycemia, which can be profound, as well as life threatening ketoacidosis. Although most of these patients are lean and under the age of 20, this condition can develop at any age.

Latent autoimmune diabetes in adults (LADA) is a slower onset form of type-1 diabetes. These people can often be diagnosed as type-2 diabetics. These patients can be identified by antibodies to GAD, low C-peptide levels (a by-product of insulin degradation), low endogenous insulin production with antibodies to insulin islet cells. These individuals usually do not show the usual manifestations of the metabolic syndrome and progress to insulin dependency faster than type-2 diabetics, but longer than the classical Type I diabetics. Approximately 10% of type-2 diabetics may actually have LADA and hence are actually type-1's [3].

The risk of developing type-1 diabetes in first degree relatives of type-1 probands can be 5–7% for North American white populations compared to less than 1% without a family history and 0.12% in the general population. These patients require lifetime daily therapy with exogenous insulin to prevent the severe complications of ketoacidosis, lactic acidosis, and metabolic decompensation [4].

TYPE-2 DIABETES (NON-INSULIN DEPENDENT DIABETES)

Type-2 diabetes or non-insulin diabetes is responsible for about 90–95% of all diagnosed diabetics in the United States with a special predilection for African Americans, Native Americans, Hispanics, and Pacific Islanders. Ninety percent of these diabetics have a family history of the disease with identical twins showing 60–90% occurrence rate. Although these patients may become ketonemic, they do not become ketoacidotic due to the diabetes. These individuals are frequently overweight with close to 90% being obese, especially central obesity.

About 13.3% or 32 million African Americans compared to 13.1 million or 8.7% of whites have diabetes, which is currently the sixth leading cause of death in the United States resulting in $92 billion in direct cost and $40 billion in premature mortality, work loss, and disability.

Race and gender have been linked to socioeconomic status encompassing occupation, income, education, and socioeconomic equality by the MacArthur Foundation Research Network in Socioeconomic Status and Health [5]. These various factors have a significant impact on access to medical care, health related behaviors, perceived discrimination, and social support leading to adverse health outcomes with community based interventions addressing poverty as a determinant of health, shown to be highly beneficial. African Americans have one of the highest rates of diagnosed diabetes among all races with an incidence of 11.9%. From 1980 to 1994 the prevalence of diagnosed diabetes was three times high in blacks compared to whites (33 vs. 11%). By 2050 diabetes will increase in black by 275%! Hispanics have a lifetime risk of one in two at birth and one in three residual risk at 60 years of age, being 1.7 times more likely to have diabetes compared to whites, and with the prevalence of diabetes among Hispanics increasing more rapidly than among whites or blacks [6]. The prevalence of diabetes in South Asians is about 19% while Pima Indians have the highest rate of diabetes in the world with a prevalence of 41% in women and 34% in men. While 60% of Pima Indians between 34–64 years of age are diabetic, the etiology of the higher rates in these ethnic groups is certainly multifactorial with genetic predisposition and obesity being the major factors. Fifty percent of Pima Indians are obese compared to 47% of African American women [7]. Genetic factors like the Thr394Thr polymorphism of the peroxisome proliferator-activated receptor (PPAR) coactivator-1 alpha gene is found in South Asians. The Pro12Ala polymorphism of the PPAR-gamma gene, protective in whites, does not appear to have the same protective effect in South Asians [8].

One of the major demographic changes within the USA in the next 20 years will be the dramatic 34% increase in those individuals over 65 years of age! In the year 2000, 35 million Americans were 65 or over. By 2030 this number will double to over 70 million due to the baby boomer population after World War II. More than half of all Americans will be over 40 by this time, experiencing the normal increases in aged related hypertension, hearing deficiencies, arthritis, cardiovascular diseases, and diabetes [9].

According to the Centers for Disease Control, one fifth of those individuals currently over 60 years of age have diabetes, with two thirds of the entire international diabetic population being greater than 60 years old by 2025, especially those with minority populations at risk for the disease [10].

In addition, the risks, complications, and disabilities of the disease – both macrovascular and microvascular are more severe among older adults. Declining cognitive functioning, decreased health care accessibility, and diminished financial resources add to the geriatric diabetic dilemma.

In order to respond to this overwhelming challenge a coordination of efforts from medical and public health initiatives and partnerships, enhanced patient provider and caretaker communication, patient education, and financial assistance are critical to enhance the health, quality of life, and functional independence of this growing segment of the population. Clearly, the key to controlling this explosion in the incidence of type-2 diabetes rests in prevention and must be initiated for all women who have had gestational diabetes which occurs in 5–9% of pregnancies in the USA and continues to increase in prevalence. Approximately 70% of women with gestational diabetes will develop overt type-2 diabetes within 5 years. Data now suggest that this rate can be sharply reduced with lifestyle modification and pharmacological intervention with thiazolidinediones [11]. At a minimum, all women with previous gestational diabetes should be on a diet and exercise with blood glucoses levels monitored on a regular basis.

Primary prevention strategies which delay or halt the development of the disease in all patients begins with therapeutic lifestyle changes with increased physical activity and weight reduction. Patients enrolled in weight reduction programs can significantly improve their cardiovascular disease risk factors with a 10% weight loss over a 26-week period with 1–2% A1-C reduction. However, this approach alone will not maintain glycemic control within 1 year in most patients necessitating pharmacotherapy to achieve euglycemia. Secondary prevention interventions seek to prevent complications of the disease in those already diagnosed, focusing on blood pressure, lipid and glycemic control. Tertiary prevention centers on control of the microvascular (nephrophathy, neuropathy, and retinopathy) and macrovascular complications (stroke, myocardial infarction, and peripheral vascular disease). Established elements of quality diabetes care include regular eye, dental, and foot exams along with A1-C testing [12].

Regrettably, ethnic and racial minorities are less likely to have annual dilated ophthalmological and dental exams, twice yearly A1-C testing, and self monitored blood glucose measurements; lower extremity amputations, end stage renal disease, and hospitalizations for uncontrolled diabetes are higher among ethnic and racial minorities. The causes of these disparities are, indeed, multifactorial and include patient factors (poor compliance, biological and genetic factors, patient preferences, refusal of treatment, economic restraints, lack of health care insurance and access), physician factors (stereotyping and bias, managed care, and formulary restrictions), and healthy system factors (linguistic and cultural challenges, cost, coverage for testing and medication). The Institute of Medicine in 2003 related disparities in healthcare to primary care provider time constraints, cost containment considerations, communication and cultural bias, stereotyping, access barriers, and the legal, regulatory, and policy milieu of the multiple and varied health systems [13].

Empowered to implement public health initiatives for all Americans with diabetes, the Division of Diabetes Translation has been coordinating findings from scientific research into public health and clinical practice guidelines. This is accomplished with a combined effort from research institutions, health care organizations, health care providers, universities, community based organizations, and distinct controlled diabetes prevention and control programs [14].

Their initiatives include articles on the following topics:

1. Guidelines for the treatment of diabetes in the geriatric population
2. The roles of collaborative care and psychosocial interventions to improve successful diabetes management among the aging
3. Implementation of guidelines for the treatment of diabetes in the elderly
4. Diabetes prevention

Efforts by this organization serve to underscore the critical need for combined multidisciplinary approaches addressing an increasing population at need.

At the other end of the spectrum, age of onset of type-2 diabetes is decreasing rapidly and has reached epidemic proportions in adolescents and young adults. Examples of progression from impaired glucose tolerance (IGT) to type-2 diabetes are abounding in the medical literature especially with the Pima Indians, the Nauruan Islanders, and Mexican Americans. Progression is clearly related to weight gain which is related to dietary indiscretion. Increased weight leads to increased insulin resistance and increased insulin secretion. Life style changes have been shown to have a dramatic effect on achieving weight loss, improving insulin sensitivity, and even preventing type-2 diabetes as we will see in the upcoming chapters [9].

Type-2 diabetes is most often diagnosed after the age of 30; however we are beginning to notice individuals at a younger age being diagnosed with this condition with increasing frequency, especially in African American and Hispanic adolescents. Indeed, increases in both obesity and type-2 diabetes represent worldwide twin epidemics.

It is clear that obesity is the driving force in the increased etiology of type-2 diabetes in childhood. Obesity enhances insulin resistance by increasing fatty acid flow from the fat depots in the viscera to insulin sensitive tissues. Fatty acids compete with glucose for substrate utilization. In addition lipid depots in muscle and liver may also increase insulin resistance. This occurs when the translocation of the glucose transport 4 to the cell membrane is delayed due to insulin receptor defects in glucose utilization.

Patients that are insulin resistant or predisposed to the development of diabetes have larger adipocytes that are poorly capable of storing triglycerides. These smaller adipocytes may also be the source for the production of adiponectin, which improves insulin sensitivity while the larger adipocytes produce resistin, interleukin-6, and TNF-alpha which impair insulin sensitivity.

Known risk factors for type-2 diabetes in children and adolescents are:

1. Low physical activity
2. High calorie diets, especially those with trans fatty acids and saturated fats
3. Small size for gestational age as a newborn
4. Positive family history in first or second degree relative
5. High risk ethnic group – i.e., Hispanic, African-American, Pacific Islander
6. Increased insulin resistance [15]

The intrauterine environment during fetal development may significantly affect glucose metabolism. Intrauterine malnutrition may affect the number and function of beta cells impairing insulin secretion in adulthood. There also has been an increased risk of type-2 diabetes and insulin resistance for children with mothers who had gestational diabetes. Maternal hyperglycemia can stimulate fetal hyperinsulinemia resulting in increased lipogenesis. A recent report in the *Journal of the American Medical Association (JAMA)* indicated that the introduction of cereal before the third month or after the seventh month of life can increase by fivefold the child's risk of developing type-2 diabetes, while the addition of gluten based supplements to the diet of an at risk infant before the age of three months can increase diabetic risk fourfold [16].

Most offspring of mothers with type-1 diabetes exhibited characteristics that put them at great risk of developing type-2 diabetes. This association was independent of a genetic predisposition [17]. Clearly more study will be necessary to see whether this will be the case.

Occasionally, the patient may present to the physician with classic symptoms of polyphagia, polydipsia, weight loss, polyuria, but usually complains of more subtle symptoms like fatigue, lightheadedness, dizziness, vertigo, recurrent fungal infections, impaired wound healing, sexual dysfunction, or even gustatory sweating.

Unfortunately, the diagnosis of type-2 diabetes is often made many years after the condition begins with insulin resistance and postprandial hyperglycemia. Hence the early catastrophic macrovascular effects become well established by the time the diagnosis is made [18].

DIABETES ASSOCIATED WITH OTHER RISK FACTORS

Type-2 diabetes can also be associated with other clinical states, drugs, and chemicals:

1. Genetic syndromes – Huntington's chorea, muscular dystrophy, and lipodystrophic diseases
2. Pancreatic diseases – chronic pancreatitis, pancreatectomy states, hemochromatosis, and cystic fibrosis
3. Endocrinopathies – primary aldosteronism, Cushing syndrome, acromegaly, pheochromocytoma, glucagonoma, and polycystic ovaries
4. Drugs – thiazide diuretics, beta-blockers, glucocorticoids, phenytoin, nicotinic acid, catecholamines, tacrolimus, estrogen and progesterone preparations, antidepressant medications, especially clozapine, olanzapine and risperidone [18]
5. Chemicals – Tetrachlorodibenzoparadioxin (TCDD)

Usually in these conditions treatment of the underlying condition or elimination of the offending drug enhances glycemic control although some chemicals may cause permanent alterations and establishment of the diabetic state.

U.S. regulators have proposed that six anti-psychotic medications can increase the risk of IGT and diabetes. These medications are:

1. Zyprexa (olanzapine)
2. Risperdal (risperidone)
3. Clozaril (clozapine)
4. Seroquel (quetiapine)
5. Geodon (ziprasidone)
6. Abilify (aripiprazol)

Recent studies, involving almost 20,000 schizophrenic patients across the USA, showed that patients taking Risperdal had an increase in diabetes of 49% and Zyprexa 27%, while patients taking Seroquel had 3.34 times as many cases of diabetes as those on older anti-psychotic medication. It is important to consider that schizophrenic patients have a greater tendency to be overweight and weight gain can increase the risk for type-2 diabetes [19].

In a recent study in the *Journal of Clinical Pharmacology*, diabetic patients with psychoses had a 3% higher risk of developing diabetes within one month of starting olanzapine and a 42.6% increase risk within 12 months of treatment, compared to controls. Hence management of patients with psychoses should routinely include body weight and blood glucose monitoring with advice to promote exercise and minimize weight gain [20].

Certain drugs that possess anticholinergic properties may have a direct effect on pancreatic islet beta cells impacting insulin secretion via the muscarinic M3 receptors which innervate these cells. These effects can have an effect on those patients with mental disorders and are overweight, dislipidemic, or diabetic. Many of the atypical antipsychotic medications function as M3 receptor antagonists, inhibiting insulin secretion by the beta cells by binding to these M3 receptors in the pancreas [21].

In order to maintain euglycemia, a balance must exist between the effects of hyperglycemic hormones like growth hormone corticosteroids, epinephrine and glucagon, and the hypoglycemic hormones like insulin. Insulin secretion is increased by parasympathetic stimulation with vagus nerve fibers exerting control over the endocrine and exocrine function of the pancreas by connecting with the intra-pancreatic ganglia.

Intra-pancreatic nerve terminals release acetylcholine, the principal parasympathetic neurotransmitter during feeding and subsequently bind to the M3 receptors in the beta cell resulting in an increase in nutrient-induced insulin secretion during feeding. Insulin secreting cells have been found to contain high concentrations of enzymes involved in the degradation of acetylcholine (acetylcholinesterase) and its synthesis (acetylcholine transferase). Reports of severe hypoglycemia and even with ketoacidosis following treatment with atypical antipsychotics have fostered further research into the effects of these agents on insulin secretion.

Transgenic mice with either an overexpression of the pancreatic M3 receptors or an absence of those receptors have been noted to produce opposite effects on insulin secretion, with marked decreases in insulin secretion and subsequent glucose intolerance in the absence of beta cell M3 receptors and lower glucose levels and overproduction of insulin with an overexpression of these receptors. Both olanzapine and clozapine have been demonstrated to block muscarinic receptor activation with high affinity subsequently decreasing insulin secretion, with 10–100 nanomoles per liter significantly impairing cholinergic mediated insulin secretion due to a direct effect on the pancreatic beta cells. These effects were not seen with ziprasidone, risperidone, haloperidol, and thiothixene which demonstrate low M3 receptor affinity. The hyperglycemic effects of olanzapine and clozapine can occur even in the absence of weight gain, and hence the choice of an antipsychotic medication can have significant effects on glucose metabolism. Other antipsychotics exhibiting high M3 receptor binding affinity with subsequent increased capacity for inducing glucose intolerance are chlorpromazine and thioridazine [22].

A 2004 consensus development conference made recommendations concerning the therapeutic use of first generation and second generation antipsychotics, thus highlighting increased risk of developing diabetes in patients treated with olanzapine and clozapine endorsing a family history for diabetes, dyslipidemia, hypertension, obesity, and cardiovascular disease at baseline followed by regular monthly measurements of waist circumference, weight and blood pressure along with baseline and quarterly measurements of fasting plasma glucose and lipid profiles [23].

In addition, the effect of weight gain caused by anti-depressives is a well recognized troublesome side effect. High binding affinities for the M3 receptors have also included antidepressives like amitriptyline, doxepin, imipramine, mirtazepine, phenelzine, tranylcypromine, and paroxetine, demonstrating increased propensity for weight gain. Whereas, sertraline, fluoxetine, venlafaxine, and bupropion have demonstrated lower binding affinities for the M3 receptors and have decreased risk for causing significant weight gain with long term use.

Weight gain induced by psychotropic agents should be kept in mind when initiating therapy because of the increased risk of metabolic syndrome, diabetes, hypertension, and their subsequent complications. Within the anti-depressant class, desipramine, nortriptyline, paroxetine, and protriptyline have the capacity for inducing mild weight gain with the potential change of 1–5 pounds in 1 year; while in the antipsychotic class, fluphenazine, haloperidol, paliperidone, and perphenazine may also induce mild weight gain, while the anti-seizure mood stabilizer medication carbamazepine may induce more increased weight gain of 6–10 pounds [24].

Moderate to severe weight gain of 11–15 pounds has been seen with the mood stabilizer lithium and valproate, with severe weight gain of greater than 15 pounds per year seen with clozapine and olanzapine. The antidepressants bupropion and fluoxetine along with the antiseizure medicine topiramate have been associated with weight loss up to 5 pounds in 1 year with some patients responding with even greater weight reductions.

Weight gain in early treatment of psychotrophic drugs may be a harbinger of future weight increases and can be a problem in those patients who are overweight prior to treatment. Depression, of course, is a known risk factor for obesity, diabetes, and metabolic syndrome with their joint occurrence being even more common than the predicted prevalence rate for the various individual conditions.

The weight gain induced by many of these agents is usually the result of appetite stimulation and clinicians should be aware of the risk versus benefits when selecting psychotrophic agents, avoiding those drugs that may induce weight gain in patients with metabolic syndrome, glucose intolerance, or obesity unless clinical mental health circumstances dictate otherwise. Among older individuals with diabetes, risk for hospitalization due to hyperglycemia can be significantly increased with initiation of antipsychotic medication and increased further with continued use.

This therapeutic decision is critical since patients may display significant clinical inertia, resisting treatment due to feelings of guilt over an inability to adhere to therapeutic life style changes or achieve weight reduction, resulting in depression, poor self esteem, and other mental health disorders. The DAWN study (The Diabetes Attitudes Wishes and Needs) demonstrated that 41% of diabetic patients had poor psychological well being with only 12% stating that they received any psychological support in the previous 5 years [25].

For those individuals at risk for developing diabetes, fasting blood glucose should be measured within 4 months of starting an anti-psychotic medication and at regular intervals (at least yearly) if weight gain develops. The physician should be alert for the symptoms of diabetes, like fatigue, polyuria, and polydipsia.

One of the more curious, recent associations has been exposure to the herbicide, Agent Orange and its contaminant, tetrachlorodibenzoparadioxin or TCDD, with the subsequent development of type-2 diabetes – a relationship now recognized by the Veterans Administration. Agent Orange was a mixture of two herbicides – 2,4,5-T (trichlorophenoxyacetic acid) and 2,4-D (dichlorophenoxyacetic acid). Both of these herbicides, especially 2,4,5-T, contained a contaminant, as a by-product of their manufacturing, called TCDD. The substance is a very potent chemical inducer, affecting the production of various enzyme and coenzyme systems within the body [26].

TCDD or "dioxin" has been implicated as a cause of birth defects; impaired immune function; gastrointestinal disturbances including hemorrhaging; porphyrin disturbances, especially porphyria cutanea tarda; acute and subacute central and peripheral neuropathies; skin disturbances like chloracne; and various malignancies including soft tissue sarcoma, Hodgkin's and non Hodgkin's lymphoma, multiple myeloma, prostate cancer, chronic lymphocytic leukemia, nasopharyngeal carcinoma, liver, lung, tracheal, bronchial and gastrointestinal carcinomas; lipid disturbances; and type-2 diabetes [27].

The VA's decision regarding service connection was prompted by a report in November 2000 cited in Disabled American Veteran magazine issued by the National Academy of Sciences Institute of Medicine that found "limited, suggestive evidence of a link between type-2 diabetes and Agent Orange and other herbicides used in Vietnam."

According to current statistics from the Veterans Administration, 9% of the 2.3 million Vietnam veterans, still alive, have type-2 diabetes with 16% of those currently hospitalized having the disease.

Documentation of the type-2 phenotype must be demonstrated with C-peptide levels and absence of anti-islet cell, anti-glutamic acid decarboxylase (GAD), and anti-insulin antibodies.

Steroid therapy can often unmask diabetic tendencies or aggravate glycemic control. Steroids vary according to their mineralocorticoid and glucocorticoid potency. Dexamethasone is the most potent glucocorticoid, followed by methylprednisolone, prednisone, and hydrocortisone. The order is reversed for their mineralocorticoid potencies. Steroids exert their glycemic effects by aggravating insulin resistance.

Thiazide diuretics, by inhibiting insulin output from the pancreas, can worsen hyperglycemia, especially with higher doses, which can induce hypokalemia inhibiting insulin output from the pancreas.

DIAGNOSING DIABETES

The following are the criteria for diagnosing diabetes in the clinical setting (Table 1):

1. Fasting glucose equal to or greater than 126 mg/dL (7.0 mmol/L) or
2. Glucose concentration 2 h after the administration of 75 g oral glucose load equal to or greater than 200 mg/dL (11.1 mmol/L) or
3. Random glucose equal to or greater than 200 mg/dL or
4. Hemoglobin A1-C equal to or greater than 6.5%

The criteria for impaired fasting glucose (IFG) include a fasting glucose concentration on two occasions equal to or greater than 100 mg/dL and less than 126 mg/dL (5.6–6.9 mmol/L).

The criteria for IGT include postprandial sugars or two 75 g oral glucose tolerance test values greater than 140 mg/dL or less than 200 mg/dL (7.8–11.0 mmol/L).

IGT is not defined by clinical signs and symptoms, but strictly by plasma glucose levels alone. This state has also been referred to as chemical diabetes, borderline diabetes or

Table 1
Criteria for the diagnosis of diabetes [34]

1. Symptoms of diabetes and a random plasma glucose 200 mg/dL (11.1 mmol/L)

Or

2. Fasting plasma glucose >125 mg/dL (7 mmol/L)

Or

3. 2 h postprandial glucose 200 mg/dL

Tolerance test with 75 g anhydrous glucose

Or

4. A1-C ≥6.5%

Impaired fasting glucose (IFG) is >100 mg/dL (5.5 mmol/L) and <126 mg/dL (7.0 mmol/L)

Impaired glucose tolerance (IGT) is postprandial glucose >140 mg/dL

(7.8 mmol/L) and <200 mg/dL (11.1 mmol/L)

pre-diabetes. Although these patients do not yet have the microvascular complications of diabetes mellitus, they are at risk for and begin to develop macrovascular complications due to arteriosclerotic deposition secondary to the hyperglycemic state and are at significant risk for developing diabetes, especially when associated with concomitant risk factors of hypertension, body mass index greater than 25 kg/m^2, sedentary life style, dyslipidemia (especially increased small, dense LDL and increased triglycerides), history of gestational diabetes, polycystic ovaries and associated ethnicity (African American, Latin American, Native American, and Asian-Pacific Islanders) [28].

In the USA alone, close to 15 million adults (40–74 years of age) have IGT and close to ten million have IFG.

Curiously, minimal overlap between the two impaired states exist with only 16 % of individuals possessing both IFG and IGT, while 23% have IFG alone and 60% having IGT alone. Individuals with IGT have a 3.6–8.7% per year chance of developing diabetes [29]. These individuals frequently have the metabolic syndrome which will be discussed in detail in a later chapter.

SCREENING RECOMMENDATIONS [14]

Strongly Recommended
Greater than 45 years of age with BMI >25 kg/m^2
Recommended
Less than 45 years of age with BMI >25 kg with one of the following risk factors:
Family history of diabetes (i.e., parents or sibling with diabetes)
Physical inactivity
At risk ethnic group (African Americans, Hispanic Americans, Native Americans, Asian Americans, and Pacific Islanders)
IFT and/or IGT
History of gestational diabetes or delivery of high birth-weight infant (>9 pounds)
Polycystic ovary syndrome
Arteriosclerotic vascular disease
Hypertension
HDL <35 mg/dL
Triglycerides >150 mg/dL (Table 2)

Fasting glucose has been used for many years as the sole screening test for diabetes, but strong consideration must be given to using the postprandial glucose test preferably (75 g glucose tolerance test) to identify the more than 30% of patients who will be missed by screening with just fasting levels alone, affording the opportunity of earlier detection since the postprandial glucose or 2 h oral glucose tolerance test is often elevated before fasting glucose elevations. The fructosamine measures the average blood glucose over a 2-week period of time, whereas the hemoglobin A1-C measures the average glucose over a 60–90 day period of time.

Various assays measure the hemoglobin A1-C (glycated hemoglobin, GHb), but they do not reflect the glucose level at the time the blood sample is tested. Hence these measurements are more efficacious in guiding glycemic control on a long term basis rather than a day to day basis. The process of glycation (glycosylation) refers to a protein/carbohydrate linkage. This process is irreversible and occurs as plasma combines with the hemoglobin

Table 2
Patients to be tested for diabetes [43]

All adults over age 45

First degree relatives of an individual with type-2 diabetes

Body mass index >25 kg/m^2

Delivery of a baby greater than 9 pounds

Patients diagnosed with gestational diabetes

Hypertension

HDL <40 mg/dL in men or <50 mg/dL in women

Triglycerides greater than 150 mg/dL

Increased small, dense LDL

Members of a high risk ethnic population (e.g., African American, Latino, Native American, Asian American, Pacific Islander)

Those with impaired glucose tolerance or impaired fasting glucose

Conditions associated with insulin resistance (e.g., polycystic ovary syndrome or acanthosis nigricans)

A1-C ≥5.9% or fasting glucose >99 mg/dL

component of red blood cells. These assays reflect average blood glucose concentration over a 2–3 month period of time because the life span of the red cells is approximately 120 days. Therefore the amount of the circulating glucose concentration to which the red cell is exposed will affect the amount of the glycosylated hemoglobin [30].

In addition to its oxygen carrying capacity, hemoglobin molecules allow the red cells to facilitate the flow of glucose into and out of the red cell. Muscle and liver cells possess insulin controlled gated mechanisms, regulating the influx and efflux of glucose.

This is not the case with the red cell. The value of the A1-C is given as a percentage to indicate what percent of the A1-C molecules are linked to glucose. A variety of terms have been used to describe this test. These include: the glycosylated hemoglobin, the GHbs, and the glycohemoglobin. Even the nomenclature has been changed recently to just A1-C instead of HbA1-C.

The process of glycosylation refers to the linkage of a molecule to a glycosyl group. This process can by facilitated by coenzymes. When accomplished nonenzymatically, the process is referred to as glycation. Glucose links itself to hemoglobin nonenzymatically.

Ketoamine reactions between free amino groups on the alpha and beta chain of the hemoglobin molecule and glucose result in glycated forms of hemoglobin. Only glycation of the N-terminal valine of the beta chain provides a negative charge sufficient enough to allow charge dependent separation, collectively referred to as hemoglobin A1 of which the major form is hemoglobin A1-C, where the carbohydrate is glucose. Four to six percent of total hemoglobin is in this form. Other hemoglobin A1 species include fructose 1,6 diphosphate (HbA1a1) and glucose-6 phosphate (HbA1a2). The A1-C can be measured by immunoassays, boronate affinity chromatography, cation exchange chromatography, and electrophoresis. Some laboratories may still measure all of the HbA1 glycohemoglobins and report a GHbs. Although the A1-C measures the average glucose over an 80–120 day period of time (2–3 months), it is weighted to more recent (previous month) readings.

It is important to understand that there are certain conditions that can interfere with the accuracy of the hemoglobin A1-C result. Falsely low concentrations can be present in those conditions that decrease the life of the red blood cell such as sickle-cell trait, excessive bleeding (particularly on a chronic basis), therapeutic phlebotomies, hemolytic anemias, and hemoglobinopathies (hemoglobins C, D, and S). Falsely high concentrations are likely in situations that increase the life span of the red blood cell. This can be seen specifically in splenectomy states. Other conditions associated with a falsely elevated hemoglobin A1-C when a cation exchange chromatography assay is used include persistence of fetal hemoglobin, uremia, high concentrations of ethanol, and high aspirin doses (greater than 10 g per day). Physicians should be aware that if an immunoassay is used to measure A1-C, a falsely *low* estimate of A1-C can occur with fetal hemoglobin, since the assay will not recognize the gamma globin terminus of hemoglobin F, but only the beta globin terminus [31].

Regular monitoring of glycosylated hemoglobin is critical to follow the patient's progress and can be correlated with microvascular outcomes. The hemoglobin A1-C represents a sum of the fasting blood sugar and the postprandial sugars. Many individuals can present with elevated hemoglobin A1-C's with normal fastings indicating that the patient is having postprandial excursions to a significant degree [19].

Other proteins, however, are glycated and can be measured as an indicator of glycemic control. Fructosamine, formed by nonenzymatic glycosylation of serum proteins (largely albumin), can be measured in patients with gestational diabetes. Serum proteins (albumin) have a shorter half life (17–20 days) compared to hemoglobin (50 days). Hence measurement of serum fructosamine represents a shorter amount of average glucose control (2–3 weeks). Since serum albumin has a half life of 14–21 days, fructosamine units (micromoles per liter) can be correlated with levels of hemoglobin A1-C with a fructosamine of 320 µmol/L equivalent to an 8% hemoglobin A1-C, while 250 µmol of fructosamine is equivalent to a hemoglobin A1-C of 10. Reductions in serum albumin that can occur with liver disease or nephrotic syndrome may lower the fructosamine level.

Since the prevalence rate of type-2 diabetes increases dramatically with age, screening becomes an important part of the primary care physician's surveillance for this condition. For every diagnosed case of type-2 diabetes, 0.6 cases are undiagnosed according to NHANES-2 data. Glucose intolerance increases from approximately 9% at age 20–44 years to 42% at age 65–74 years. Since the macrovascular complications of this disease develop with glucose tolerance it is hoped that significant mortality and morbidity can be prevented with more aggressive early detection [32].

Recent data from the Diabetes Epidemiology: Collaborative analysis of Diagnostic criteria in Europe (DECODE) trial indicate that as many as one-third of diabetics can be missed by simply using a fasting blood sugar since postprandial glucose elevations precede the development of fasting hyperglycemia [33]. Therefore, the following patient types should be considered for diabetic screening with postprandial sugars:

1. Individuals who are equal to or greater than 140% of ideal body weight
2. Patients who have previously been identified as having impaired fasting or glucose tolerance
3. Those individuals who are Hispanic, African American or other ethnic groups predisposed to diabetes

4. Individuals with hypertension and hyperlipidemia particularly those with elevated triglycerides, low HDL, and a preponderance of small dense LDL
5. Women with large birth-weight babies equal to or greater than 9 pounds [34]

Strong clinical evidence exists that diet and exercise can be significantly effective in reducing the risk of progression of impaired glucose tolerant (IGT) states to the development of diabetes. Seven major clinical trials have yielded important data about the efficacy of diets and medication in these conditions.

EFFICACY OF DIETS AND MEDICATIONS

1. The Diabetes Prevention Program
2. The Finnish Diabetes Prevention Study
3. STOP-NIDDM Study
4. Da Qing IGT and Diabetes Study
5. TRIPOD Study
6. The DREAM Study
7. The XENDOS Trial

Let's look at each study individually to judge their merits and importance.

The Diabetes Prevention Study – This involved 3,234 patients with BMI's greater than 24 kg/m^2 IGT. There were three groups for assignment: placebo, metformin (850 mg BID), or intensive lifestyle changes. The lifestyle modifications included dietary instruction, 150 min of exercise weekly, and a calorie restricted, low fat diet. These patients were followed for an average of 2.8 years and the study demonstrated a 58% relative risk reduction in progression to diabetes with diet and exercise compared to a 31 % relative risk reduction with metformin. Lifestyle changes in those individuals 60 years of age and older reduced their risk by 71%. The number needed to treat was 7 for 3 years, for lifestyle modification, and 14 for metformin in this landmark trial. The metformin seemed to be more effective in the younger patients with higher BMI's and higher fasting glucose levels than patients greater than 60 years of age, who showed the least benefit with the drug [35].

The Finnish Diabetes Prevention Study – In this trial, 522 patients with a mean BMI of 31 kg/m^2 and IGT were evaluated. A control group was compared to a lifestyle changes group with the same exercise as the Diabetes Prevention Study with similar fat and calorie restricted diets, with a fiber intake of at least 15 g/1,000 calories. Once again, a 58% relative risk reduction was seen after 4 years, while the number needed to treat was 22 for 1 year and 5 for 5 years with this study. The cumulative incidence of diabetes was 23% in the control group and 11% in the interventional group with a p value of <0.001. The ability of patients to achieve their exercise and dietary goals was correlated with a small absolute weight loss [36].

The STOP-NIDDM Study evaluated 1,429 patients with IGT and a mean BMI of 31 kg/m^2. Here, acarbose (Precose) reduced the risk of progression by 24% with the number need to treat of 10 for 3.3 years. Interestingly, this risk reduction was lost when acarbose was discontinued at the termination of the study.

The DaQing IGT and Diabetes Study was conducted in China with 577 cohorts with IGT and BMI's of 25.8 kg/m^2. The patients were assigned to four groups: diet alone, diet plus exercise, exercise alone, and control. The patients were followed for 6 years and showed a 46% relative risk reduction in the exercise group, 42% in the combined group, and 31% in the diet group compared to the control.

The numbers needed to treat to were: 14 for 6 years (exercise), 16 for 6 years (exercise and diet), and 17 for 6 years (diet alone) The incidence of diabetes was 46% in the diet and exercise group, 41% in the exercise-only group, 44% in the diet-only group, and 68% in the control group [37].

The TRIPOD Study evaluated 236 Hispanic women with gestational diabetes and mean BMI's of 30 kg/m^2. This trial used troglitazone, 400 mg daily and demonstrated a 55% relative risk reduction of diabetes with the number need to treat of 15 for 2.5 years. The 121 women on placebo developed diabetes at a rate of 12% yearly, compared with 5% among the 114 who received troglitazone. In addition, lowered plasma insulin levels were found in 89% of individuals on troglitazone. The decreased secretory demands on the beta cells by reduction in insulin resistance not only delayed the development of diabetes, but preserved beta cell function [35].

An interesting sidelight of this study occurred with the removal of troglitazone from the market. This necessitated reapproval for use of a different glitazone (pioglitazone).

In an analysis of the 84 still non-diabetic women 8 months after the study, medications had to be stopped. The rate of progression to type-2 diabetes was 21% in the placebo group and 3% in the troglitazone group, for a 92% risk reduction. This would not have been seen if the glitazone has simply been masking the disease.

The DREAM (Diabetes Reduction Assessment with Ramipril and Rosiglitazone Medication) study evaluated the effects of ramipril and rosiglitazone on the progression to type-2 diabetes from IGT. Those IGT individuals treated with rosiglitazone had a reduction of the composite outcome of death or diabetes of 60%, albeit with an increased risk of congestive heart failure in the thiazolidinedione treated group along with an increased weight gain of 2.2 kg [38].

The role of thiazolidinediones (glitazones) in preventing diabetes and beta cell regeneration will be discussed in a later chapter.

The Xenical in the Prevention of Diabetes in Obese Subjects (XENDOS) trial demonstrated a 37% reduction in the risk of developing diabetes among non diabetics over a 4-year period of time when compared to placebo with the use of 120 mg of orlistat before each meal. In this study 21% of the participants were IGT, while 79% were normal. Overall there was a greater degree of weight loss with orlistat (5.8 kg) compared to placebo (3.0 kg) [39].

Clearly these trials have demonstrated the important role of lifestyle changes including both diet and exercise in altering the progression of glycemic tolerance. Further discussion on the importance of these studies in outcome reduction for cardiovascular disease will be discussed in a later chapter on glycemic control.

GESTATIONAL DIABETES

Gestational diabetes most often develops between the 24th–28th weeks of pregnancy in 2–5% of cases and usually disappears with the termination of the condition. Gestational diabetes is more common in older, obese, or diabetic prone ethnic groups and those with a positive family history. Eighty to ninety-four percent of women with gestational diabetes will return to normal following delivery. Hispanic females and Native Americans are especially prone to developing diabetes following an episode of gestational hyperglycemia with the occurrence rate being as high as 50% within 5 years of pregnancy termination. The others will have a 30–40% chance of developing diabetes in 10–20 years [40].

A diagnosis of gestational diabetes is established with a 50 g oral glucose tolerance load followed by a 1 h glucose determination. If the plasma glucose is greater than 139 mg/dL then a 100-g 3-h glucose tolerance test in the fasting state is required. Normals for the 100-g test are as follows:

1. Fasting – 105 mg/dL
2. 1 h – 190 mg/dL
3. 2 h – 165 mg/dL
4. 3 h – 145 mg/dL

If any two of the four glucose values are exceeded, the patient has gestational diabetes [19].

Type-2 diabetes is increasing in incidence in children and adolescents. Beginning at age ten or with the onset of puberty, children, who are considered at high risk should be screened for type-2 diabetes.

MALNUTRITION ASSOCIATED DIABETES

Diabetes associated with malnutrition usually presents in young individuals between the ages of 10–40. These patients do not get diabetic ketoacidosis, but require insulin for glycemic control.

The American Diabetes Association has directed that the following patients should be tested for diabetes:

1. All adults over age 45
2. First degree relatives of an individual with diabetes
3. A body mass index greater than 27 or 20% above ideal weight
4. Waist greater than 35 inches in women or 40 inches in men
5. Delivery of a baby greater than 9 pounds
6. Hypertension
7. IGT, (fasting or postprandial)
8. HDL less than 40 mg/dL in men or 50 mg/dL in women
9. Triglyceride levels greater than 150 mg/dL especially in association with increased small, dense LDL (10) High risk ethnic groups: African American, Native American, Asian, or Hispanic [41]

Three different approaches can be used for glucose testing in order to diagnose diabetes:

1. Oral glucose tolerance test
2. Random plasma glucose measurements
3. Fasting plasma glucose measurements
4. Hemoglobin A1-C

The fasting plasma glucose test is the most popular choice and is currently used to diagnose approximately 90% of all individuals with type-2 diabetes. However, it is important to understand that postprandial hyperglycemia will precede fasting hyperglycemia and should be strongly considered to screen patients, particularly those at risk.

An oral glucose tolerance test can serve this purpose by giving excellent postprandial data and can also be used to concomitantly measure insulin levels to ascertain the patient's insulin sensitivity. It is recommended that, regardless of the type of test used, laboratory values that are abnormal should be documented at least twice to avoid missed diagnoses by laboratory errors, unless the values are extremely high or associated with classic symptoms.

The American Diabetes Association and the European Association for the Study of Diabetes and the International Diabetes federation have recommended the A1-C as the preferred test for diagnosing diabetes [42].

It is only with a high index of suspicion and comprehensive examination that patients at risk can be identified and the risk of macrovascular diseases be reduced [18].

REFERENCES

1. Olson DE, Norms SL. Overview3 of AGS guidelines for the treatment of diabetes mellitus in geriatric populations. *Geriatrics* 2004;59:18–25.
2. Herold KC. Anti-CD3 monoclonal antibody in new onset type-1 diabetes mellitus. *N Engl J Med* 2002;346:1692.
3. Atkinson MA, Eisenbarth GS: Type-1 diabetes: new perspectives on disease pathogenesis and treatment. *Lancet* 2001;358:221.
4. Pietropaolo M, Le Roth D. Pathogenesis of diabetes: our current understanding. *Clin Cornerstone* 2001;4L:1–16.
5. Agency for Healthcare Research and Quality. 2007 National Healthcare Disparities Report (NHDR), Agency for Healthcare Research and Quality, Rockville, MD, 2008.
6. Schmidt MI, Duncan BB, Bang H. Identifying individuals at high risk for diabetes. *Diabetes Care* 2005;28:2013–2018.
7. Griffin SJ, Little PS, Hales CN. Diabetes risk score: towards earlier detection of type-2 diabetes in general practice. *Diabetes Metab Res Rev* 2000;16:164–171.
8. Kanaya AM, Wassel Fyr CL, de Rekeneire N. Predicting the development of diabetes in older adults. *Diabetes Care* 2005;28:404–408.
9. Ramlo-Halsted BA, Edelman SV. The natural history of type 2 diabetes. Implications for clinical practice. *Prim Care* 1999;26:771–789.
10. Cowie CC, Rust KF, Byrd-Holt DD, Eberhardt MS. Prevalence of diabetes and impaired fasting glucose in adults in the U.S. population. National Health and Nutrition Examination Survey. 1999–2002. *Diabetes Care* 2006;29:1263–1268.
11. Yki-Jarvinen H. Thiazolidinediones. *N Engl J Med* 2004;351:1106.
12. Wellcome Trust Case Control Consortium. Genome wide association study of 14,000 cases of seven common diseases and 3000 shared controls. *Nature* 2007;447:661–678.
13. Zeggini E, Scott LJ, Saxena R, Voigt BF, Marchini JL. Meta-analysis of genome wide association data and large scale replication identifies additional susceptibility loci of type-2 diabetes. *Nat Genet* 2008;40:638–645.
14. Engelgau MM, et al. Screening for type 2 diabetes. *Diabetes Care* 2000;23:1563–1580.
15. American Diabetes Association. Screening for type 2 diabetes. *Diabetes Care* 2003;26(Suppl 1): S21–S24.
16. Rolka DB, Natayan KM, et al. Performance of recommended screening tests for undiagnosed diabetes and dysglycemia. *Diabetes Care* 2001;24:1899–1903.
17. Van Hoeck M, Dehghan A, Witteman JC, van Duijn CM. Predicting type-2 diabetes based on polymorphisms from genome wide association studies: a population based Study. *Diabetes* 2008;57:3122–3128.
18. American Diabetes Association. Position Statement: Standards of Medical Care for Patients with Diabetes Mellitus. American Diabetes Association. *Diabetes Care* 2003;7–27.
19. American Association of Clinical Endocrinologists. Medical guidelines of the management of diabetes mellitus: The AACE system of intensive diabetes self management. 2002 update. *Endocr Pract* 2002;8(Suppl 1):40–82.
20. Brown AF, Mangione CM, Saliba D, et al. Guidelines for improving the care off the older person with diabetes mellitus. *J Am Geriatr Soc* 2003;51(5 Suppl Guidelines):S265–S280.

21. Lyssenko V, Jonsson A, Almgren P, Pulizzi N, Isomaa B. Clinical risk factors, DNA variants, and the development of type-2 diabetes. *N Engl J Med* 2008;359:2220–2232.
22. Harris R. Screening adults for type 2 diabetes. *Ann Intern Med* 2003;138:215.
23. Gennuth S. Expert Committee on the Diagnosis and Classification of Diabetes Mellitus. *Diabetes Care* 2003;26:3160.
24. Franz MJ. Evidence based nutrition principles and recommendations for the treatment and prevention of diabetes and related complications. *Diabetes Care* 2002;25:148.
25. Alberti G. The DAWN study. *Pract Diabetes Int* 2002;19:22–24.
26. Codario R, et al. The Vietnam experience, an overview of the health problems associated with Vietnam service. The Pennsylvania Department of Health, Harrisburg, PA, 1989 3–19.
27. Codario R. et al. Toxic Herbicide Exposure, The Physician's Resource. The Pennsylvania Department of Health, Harrisburg, PA 1984, 2–28.
28. Unwin N, Shaw J, et al. Impaired glucose tolerance and impaired fasting glycemia: the current status on definition and intervention. *Diabet Med* 2002;19:708–723.
29. Gregg EW, Caldwell BL, Cheng YJ, Cowie CC. Trends in the prevalence and ratio of diagnosed to undiagnosed diabetes according to obesity levels in the U.S. *Diabetes Care* 2004;27:2806–2812.
30. Davidson MB. The case for screening for type 2 diabetes in selected populations. *BMJ USA* 2001;1:297–298.
31. Selvin E, Marinopaoulos S, Berkenblit G. Meta-analysis: glycosylated hemoglobin and cardiovascular disease in diabetes mellitus. *Ann Int Med* 2004;141:421–431.
32. Genuth S, Alberti KG, Bennett P, Puse J, Defronzo R, Kahn R, et al. Follow up report on the diagnosis of diabetes mellitus. *Diabetes Care* 2003;26:3160–3167.
33. The European Diabetes Epidemiology group (DECODE). Glucose tolerance and cardiovascular mortality; comparison of fasting and two hour diagnostic criteria. *Arch Int Med* 2001;161:397–405.
34. American Diabetes Association. Standards of medical care in diabetes. *Diabetes Care* 2004;27(Suppl 1): S15–S35.
35. Kanaya M, Narayan KM. Prevention of type 2 diabetes: data from recent trials. *Prim Care* 2003; 30:511–526.
36. Saaristo T, Peltonen M, Keinanen-Kiukaanniemi S, Vanhala M. National type-2 diabetes prevention programme in Finland. *Int J Circumpolar Health*. 2007;66:101–112.
37. Pan XR, Li GW, Hu YH, Wang JX, Yang WY. Effects of diet and exercise in preventing NIDDM in people with impaired glucose tolerance. The Da Qing IGT and Diabetes Study. *Diabetes Care* 1997;20:537–544.
38. The DREAM Investigators. The effect of rosiglitazone on the frequency of diabetes in patients with impaired glucose tolerance or impaired fasting glucose. *Lancet* 2006;368:1096–1105.
39. Torgerson JS, Hauptman J, Bodrin MN, Sjostrom. XENical in the prevention of diabetes in obese subjects study. *Diabetes Care* 2004;27:155–161.
40. Mudaliar S, Henry RR. New oral therapies for type-2 diabetes mellitus: the glitazones or insulin sensitizers. *Ann Rev Med* 2001;52:239–257.
41. U.S. Preventive Services Task Force. Screening for type-2 diabetes mellitus in adults: recommendations and rationale. *Ann Intern Med* 2003;138:212–214.
42. American Diabetes Association. Standards of care for diabetes mellitus. *Diabetes Care* 2009;32:1327–1234.
43. American Diabetes Association. Standards of medical care for patients with diabetes Mellitus. *Diabetes Care* 2002;25(Suppl 1):S33–S49.

SUPPLEMENTARY READINGS

European Diabetes Policy Group 1999. A desktop guide to type 2 diabetes mellitus. *Diabet Med* 1999; 16(9):716–730.
Greco P, Eisenberg J. Changing physicians' practices. *New Engl J Med* 1993;329(17):1271–1273.
Joint National Committee. The sixth report of the Joint National Committee on prevention, detection, evaluation and treatment of high blood pressure. *Arch Intern Med* 1997;157(21):2413–2446.
Lorber D. Revised clinical practice recommendations. *Practical Diabetology* 2001;3:36–38.

Rao S, et al. Impaired glucose tolerance and impaired fasting glucose. *Am Fam Phys* 2004;69(8):1961–1968.

The Expert Committee on the Diagnosis and Classification of Diabetes Mellitus. Report of the Expert Committee on the Diagnosis and Classification of Diabetes Mellitus. *Diabetes Care* 2003;26(Suppl 1): S5–S20.

Wagner E, Austin B, Von Korff M. Improving outcomes in chronic illness. *Manag Care Q* 1996;4(2):12–25.

3 Exercise

Contents

Key Words: Precautions, Sedentary lifestyle, Exercise, Stress echocardiography, Stress testing

INTRODUCTION

Sedentary life style and obesity represent independent risk factors for the pathogenesis of impaired glucose tolerance and ultimately the diabetic paradigm [1]. As seen in Table 1, regular aerobic exercise has been shown to delay or even present the subsequent development of type-2 diabetes by directly improving insulin sensitivity, with favorable effects on metabolic control and cardiovascular risk factors, glycemic control, lipids and hypertension. Patients with type-2 diabetes should exercise 2.5 h weekly according to the American Heart Association [2]. This should be meted out to a minimum of 30 min of physical activity for at least 5 days a week.

The Diabetes Prevention Program trial was a multicentered study designed to determine the role of medication (metformin) and/or diet and exercise in preventing or delaying the development of type-2 diabetes in 3,234 individuals having impaired glucose tolerance with a mean age of 50 years and a BMI of 34 kg per meter. Randomization involved three groups; placebo, metformin (titrated to 1,700 mg per day), and intensive exercise/nutrition counseling. The intensive exercise group incorporated an exercise program of over 15 min weekly with supervision. The cohorts were followed for up to 2.8 years. The diet and exercise group demonstrated a 58% relative reduction in the progression to diabetes

From: *Current Clinical Practice: Type 2 Diabetes, Pre-Diabetes, and the Metabolic Syndrome*
Edited by: R.A. Codario, DOI 10.1007/978-1-60327-441-8_3
© Springer Science+Business Media, LLC 2011

Table 1
**Atherosclerotic risk factors in diabetes modi-
fied by regular exercise**

Hyperglycemia

Hyperinsulinemia

Hypertension

Low HDL

Obesity

Stress

Coagulability

Young [35]

compared with a 31% reduction in the metformin group. Mean weight loss in the intensive group was 6% of initial body weight [3].

Rinstrum, Erickson, and Tuomilehto demonstrated an identical 58% reduction in 522 adults with a mean age of 55 and BMI's of 31 kg per m². The ability to prevent progression to the diabetic state was correlated with the following parameters:

1. The ability to achieve 5% weight reduction
2. Reduction of total and saturated fat intake
3. Increased fiber intake to greater than 15 g
4. A minimum of 150 min per week of exercise [4]

Therefore, life style modification remains the cornerstone of the approach in preventing or delaying diabetes. Patients that are impaired glucose tolerant should be counseled in weight reduction and exercise with follow-up counseling being critical for success. Regular aerobic exercise reduces hyperglycemia by effecting adenosine monophosphate which has a direct effect on improving insulin sensitivity at the cellular level.

Diabetics who exercise regularly can reduce the dosage and even the need for insulin and oral agents while decreasing LDL cholesterol, triglycerides, and blood pressure in association with increasing HDL. Consistent aerobic activity improves overall survival and decreases heart rate and the risk of sudden death. Increased total working capacity and maximal oxygen uptake, muscle strength, and joint flexibility observed with enhanced exercise as well increases in lean body mass, improves psychological well being and stress reduction among the other advantages. However, important risks can be associated with exercise as well.

It is crucial to remember that patients on secretagogues and/or insulin can experience an increased risk of hypoglycemia with enhanced physical activity. The doses of these agents may need to be reduced when the patient begins an aggressive exercise program.

Due to the increased incidence of peripheral vascular disease and peripheral neuropathy, diabetics may increase their risk of traumatizing foot with enhanced activity. Autonomic neuropathy may increase the risk of silent ischemic events.

While ill-advised or non-supervised exercise may increase the risk of a cardiovascular event, weight lifting or anaerobic activity may increase the risk of hemorrhage with diabetic proliferative retinopathy.

We should strongly urge our patients to self monitor their blood glucoses before and after exercising to determine their glycemic state and medication requirements, while encouraging them to improve their activity status whenever possible.

Whatever the physical activity, patients must enjoy the experience or they will soon abandon it. Curiously, primary care physicians in a recent survey seemed reluctant to advice and counsel patients on physical activity. Only 34% of patients reported being counseled about exercise with their last physician visit.

Physician characteristics associated with encouraging physical activity among patients were:

1. Over 35 years of age
2. Knowledge of the benefits of exercise
3. Being a primary care provider [5]

Walsh and his colleagues reported only 12% of the surveyed physicians were familiar with the Surgeon General's recommendation to exercise 30 min or more with moderate physical activity on most days of the week [6]. To overcome barriers to physician counseling for physical activity, the following recommendations are given by Cardinal et al.:

1. Brief sessions (1–3 min) are usually very effective.
2. Be supportive of the patient's efforts while referring to individuals with specialized training in physical activity and counseling.
3. Provide the patients with easily understood written material supporting and listing the benefits of physical therapy [7].

Physicians should attempt to improve their own counseling effectiveness by increasing their knowledge of basic exercise and physical activity guidelines and principals listed in Table 2. Physician advice and support for patients remain crucial to their adaptation to a life style change. Physicians must recognize that it is important to put these principals into practice, sharing your own experience with exercise with your patients, and encouraging them to match their own efforts in staying in shape [8].

Sharing experiences with patients helps them realize that these life style changes are possible and effective. More importantly, patients realize that their physician shares in the same problems and experiences that they do.

Both the American Diabetes Association in their clinical practice recommendations and the American College of Sports Medicine endorse exercise and appropriate endurance of resistant straining as major therapeutic modalities for type-2 diabetics. Resistant training causes muscles to contract, building tone, mass and strength. This can be accomplished with standing weights, machines, rubber tubing, bands and calisthenics [9].

Boule et al. found that exercise reduced A-1C levels by .066% in a meta-analysis of 14 trials. When appropriately prescribed and supervised, resistance training can have beneficial effects in cardiovascular function, strength and endurance [10].

The American Diabetes Association recommends moderate weight training using repetitions and light weights at least twice weekly consisting of at one set of 8–10 exercises to benefit the larger muscles of the upper and lower body. Preferably the weight intensity should be set at 30–50% of maximum strength with 12–15 repetitions [11].

Machines are preferable to free weights because of their wide availability and ease of use, isolating certain muscle groups, and reducing the likelihood of injury due to faulty lifting technique.

Table 2
General guidelines for exercise training in diabetes

(1) Warm up and cool down of 5–10 min each

Judicious use of stretching, calisthenics and low level aerobic exercise like walking or cycling

(2) Types of exercise

(a) Aerobic – walking, cycling, swimming and rowing

(b) Resistance – weight lifting with machines rather than free weights for safety and ease of use

(3) Intensity

(a) Aerobic exercise at 55–79% of maximum heart rate for those with multiple risk factors and 55 to 60% of maximum heart rate for those with low level of fitness

(b) Resistance training – 8 to 10 exercises at 30–50% with one repetition maximumMinimum of 1 set of 12 to 15 repitions with workload increasing when 15 repitions can be done without difficulty

(4) Duration

(a) Aerobic exercise for 30–45 min (i.e., treadmill walking at the desired target heart rate for 30 min)

(b) Resistance training – 20 min for each set of exercises

(5) Frequency

(a) Aerobic exercise should be done 3–4 times weekly

(b) Resistance exercise should be done at least twice weekly

N.B. Exercise stress testing should be performed before any patient embarks on a structured program of exercise
Stewart [*36*]

Diastolic dysfunction is the most common abnormality in the diabetic heart characterized by prolonged relaxation, increased deceleration time, and reduced compliance. These diastolic changes usually precede systolic dysfunction. Tirumhi reported a diastolic dysfunction prevalence of 32% in type-2 diabetics with normal systolic function. Exercise training may improve diastolic function by enhancing early diastolic filling and increasing maximal oxygen uptake [*12*].

Randomized trials of exercise training are needed to confirm the expected improvement in diastolic function suggested mostly by animal data.

By increasing blood flow to active muscles, endothelium derived nitric oxide is stimulated with exercise, enhancing smooth muscle relaxation, and vasodilatation. Exercise improvements in brachial artery relaxation and forearm blood flow were demonstrated in patients with type-2 diabetes completing an 8 week program of aerobic exercise. The endothelium plays a critical role in regulating vasomotor tone, fibrinolysis, and thrombosis as well as vascular smooth muscle proliferation.

Diabetes and insulin resistance enhances arterial stiffness due to degeneration of the media in the artery with increased collagen and calcium deposition along with smooth muscle proliferation. All these effects are mediated by angiotensin II secreted at the tissue level.

Elevated glucose, insulin, and triglyceride levels enhance this process probably due to changes in the interstitial collagen mediated by glycation induced cross linking.

These structural changes reduce arterial compliance, increase systolic blood pressure, and accelerate arteriosclerosis. Although some limited trials have suggested a reduction in arterial stiffness with exercise, more randomized studies are necessary to clarify the benefits since evidence supporting this view is limited at the present time.

Both the Arteriosclerosis Risk in Community and the Woman's Health Study reported that inflammatory markers like interleukin 6 and C-reactive protein along with endothelial dysfunction predicted the development of type-2 diabetes. These were independent of smoking, exercise, alcohol use, and body mass index. Hence we can understand that the tissue insult in diabetes takes place at the cellular level with these inflammatory markers indicating cell injury [13].

Higher self reported physical activity was associated with decreased inflammatory markers in a study of 5,888 men and women. C-reactive protein levels were reduced by 9 months of distance running and not with sedentary controls. This suggested improvement in inflammation when associated with reductions in various clinical markers. This available data indicates that further research is warranted to evaluate these effects [14].

Mourier et al. demonstrated that type-2 diabetics who performed high intensity aerobic exercise three times weekly for a 2 month period of time were able to increase both insulin sensitivity and aerobic capacity despite little change in body weight. Interestingly there was a concomitant loss of visceral and subcutaneous abdominal fat. Visceral fat loss was better correlated with improved insulin sensitivity. This data suggests an important effect at the adipocyte level may be associated with exercise to modify risk factors in arteriosclerotic cardiovascular disease [15].

GUIDELINES FOR EXERCISE

The manifest benefit of exercise in type-2 diabetes for both glycemic and blood pressure controls should be followed soon by research confirming reduction in cardiovascular endpoints as well. These benefits need to be accompanied by certain guidelines for proper management. The American Diabetes Association Guidelines are listed in the Handbook of Exercise in Diabetes [16].

As the result of the increased cardiovascular risk in diabetics, exercise stress testing is vital to identifying blood pressure responses, arrhythmias, heart rate responses, and risk stratification in these patients. Ideally patients need to burn a minimum of 1,000 total calories weekly with aerobic exercising while participating in resistance training. This should be achieved with a minimum of three sessions weekly with aerobic exercising gradually increasing to 45 min per maximum benefit. Each session should be preceded by a warm-up period and conclude with deceleration activities to allow for gradual transition from the higher demands of the accelerated phase of the workout [17].

The intensity of the aerobic workout can be monitored by tracking the pulse with a monitor. Target heart rates vary from 60 to 90% of the maximum with slight lower rates of 55–79% for those with autonomic neuropathy, hypertensive responses, obesity, and deconditioning. The maximum heart rate is 220 minus the age. The use of beta-blockers and exercise stress test findings of ischemia can have a bearing on the maximum desirable heart rate. Interestingly beta-blockers usually do not prevent the training effects on muscle strength and aerobic capacities.

PRECAUTIONS

Stress testing is imperative before embarking on an exercise program. Blood pressure should be controlled and guided by the response to exercise testing. Self monitoring of blood glucose is particularly important in these patients taking insulin. Although exercise does not normally aggravate diabetic neuropathy and may even reduce or delay the risk of ophthalmic complications, straining as seen in heavy resistance training should be avoided by those with proliferative retinopathy due to the increase risk of vitreous hemorrhage and retinal detachment. It is not known whether patients who have undergone laser procedures can tolerate more aggressive resistance activity [18].

EFFECTS AND TIMING OF EXERCISE

Common misconceptions about exercise include [19]:

Morning vs. Evening Exercise

1. Research has shown that exercise before bedtime can alter sleep patterns for deconditioned but not fit people, but regular exercise actually helps normalize sleep quality over a longer period of time. There is no evidence to support the thought that morning exercise boosts the metabolic rate better than evening exercise.

Exercise and Appetite

2. In general, exercise neither stimulates nor suppresses appetite. In uncontrolled diabetics or those with impaired glucose tolerance, by enhancing insulin activity, particularly in the postprandial period, glycemic excursions are reduced and these excursions can play a role in stimulating appetite. For those with postprandial hyperglycemia, a brisk walk 1–2 h after eating can enhance glycemic control. In fact, exercising in a fasting state may result in increased eating after the workout, and hence these individuals would be better advised to pursue the postprandial exercise approach.

Exercise and Weight Loss

3. Exercise is more important in maintaining muscle tone and strength, but dieting results in weight loss. Studies comparing the effects of exercise to diet for weight loss have shown that dieting results in more robust weight reduction. Exercise can be associated with an increase in muscle mass and muscle is heavier than fat. Hence resistance training is usually associated with gaining more muscle than aerobic activity.

Duration vs. Intensity

4. Research has shown that it is the duration not the intensity of the workout that correlates best with glycemic control and reductions in insulin resistance. Therefore have your patients choose an activity that they enjoy and one that is convenient for them to perform. The more that exercise becomes a chore and a job the more likely it will become a bore and a flop. Patients should exercise for 30–35 min four to five times weekly for maximum benefit.

Stress Testing

It is critical to determine if the diabetic patient is a candidate for exercise from a cardiovascular point of view. Noninvasive cardiac testing, including the electrocardiogram, exercise electrocardiography, echocardiography, and radionucleotide testing can be invaluable to asses severe clinical questions. These include:

1. Is ventricular function normal?
2. Does the patient have diastolic dysfunction?
3. Does the patient have significant valvular disease?
4. Does the patient have coronary artery disease?
5. What is the patient's exercise tolerance?
6. What are the blood pressure responses to exercise?
7. Does the patient develop an arrhythmia with exercise?

An understanding of the performance characteristics of these tests can guide the physician in evaluating the patient's performance on these tests [20].

1. Exercise tolerance – The ability of the patient to complete at least 6 min or more of a standard Bruce Protocol is indicative of normal work capacity and performance. Estimated functional capacity norms in metabolic equivalents (METS) are stratified by age and gender. The test begins with the treadmill set at low speed 1.7 miles per hour at a 10% incline with increases in speed and incline angle every 3 min. Exercise duration correlates with functional capacity and is the strongest prognostic variable in men, women, and the elderly while also providing risk stratification in those with known coronary artery disease. A 50–59 year old woman who can exercise at 8 METS has average functional capacity, placing her at low risk for overall mortality. This concept was explored in the CASS (The Coronary Artery Surgery Study) trial by analyzing 30 different variables in 4,083 patients with symptomatic coronary artery disease. In this trial, survival was 100% in 4 years for those who were able to exercise for 12 min or more [21].
2. Pressure/peak rate product (the double product). The tests could be inconclusive if the patient does not perform enough cardiac work to induce ischemia. This is determined by multiplying the peak heart rate sustained by the peak systolic pressure. Tests with a double product of 18,000 are indicative of a satisfactory work performance. Failure to raise the heart rate or a drop in blood pressure with a failure to achieve the work double product may indicate an underlying cardiac abnormality. Exercise hypertension occurs if the systolic blood pressure is greater than 190 and may predict future hypertension in normotensive individuals. Although a study from the Mayo clinic indicated that exercise induced hypertension was significantly associated with cardiovascular events during a mean follow up of 7.7 years, another from the Cleveland Clinic did not show this association. However, an increase in systolic blood pressure in the early post-exercise recovery period has been shown to be a marker of underlying coronary artery disease. Exercise hypotension is systolic blood pressure that is lower with exercise than at rest. This indicates an inability of the cardiac output to increase with exercise and is associated with left ventricular systolic dysfunction and/or severe coronary artery disease (triple vessel or left main coronary artery). The heart rate should normally increase during exercise greater than 80% of expected or 62% in patients with beta blocker therapy.
3. Symptoms during the testing with ECG changes. Symptoms of dyspnea, chest discomfort, or fatigue during the test with associated electrocardiographic changes are more consistent with coronary artery disease.
4. Heart rate recovery after exercise –This is defined as the rate after 1 min of peak exercise. Abnormal is 12 beats per minute or less after a 1 min recovery period in the upright position, or 18 beats per minute at 1 min supine, or a difference of 22 beats per minute after 2 min of recovery for standard exercise testing. Abnormalities in the return of heart rates to normal following exercise have been associated with up to a sixfold increased

risk of death over a 6 year period in men and women, regardless of age and those with and without known coronary artery disease [22].

5. ST segment depression – The greater the degree of ST depression, the more likely that the patient has coronary artery disease. Depressions of 2 mm or greater, lasting at least 0.08 s are significant

6. Ventricular ectopy – When these increase in frequency with exercise, concern for an underlying myocardial ischemic process is raised. When ventricular ectopy improves with exercise a more benign process can be predicted. Sustained ventricular tachycardia or ventricular fibrillation are, of course, life threatening. Ventricular tachycardia, arising from the right ventricular outflow tract, can occur in healthy young adults.

7. Chronotropic index – This represents the percentage of heart rate reserve that is used during exercise. The patient's resting heart rate is subtracted from his/her peak heart rate. Next subtract the patient's age and resting heart rate from 220. Then divide the result of the first calculation by the result of the second calculation. A value of 0.8 or less has been shown in long term studies to increase the relative risk of death fourfold [23].

T and U wave inversions can be associated with associated left ventricular hypertrophy, rather in addition to ischemia with the latter being more commonly associated with hypokalemia.

TYPES OF STRESS TESTS

Stress echocardiography is effective in demonstrating the effects of exercise and regional wall motion in addition to valvular incompetence. Four views are routinely evaluated, parasternal long, parasternal short, apical 4-chamber, and apical 2-chamber with the rest and exercise images juxtaposed. New or significant wall motion abnormalities suggest myocardial ischemia. In this technique, images are compared at rest and within 1–2 min of exercise. This can provide helpful information on both the location and the amount of myocardial tissue in jeopardy as well as evaluating left ventricular and cardiac functioning [24].

Nuclear perfusion testing and radionucleotide imaging assess myocardial perfusion and are performed with a variety of different tracers and various techniques. Most laboratories currently use the SPECT or single photon emitted computed tomography which can literally reconstruct anatomic slices of myocardial tissue. This technique is invaluable in assessing regional cardiac blood flow.

As with the echocardiography, images are produced following exercise or pharmacological intervention and compared with resting images. The pharmacological agents used work in different ways.

Adenosine and dipyridamole increase blood flow to non-arteriosclerotic vessels unmasking stenoses in other arteries with their vasodilatory action. These agents should not be used if an individual has asthma or severe obstructive lung disease, since bronchospasm can be worsened.

Dobutamine is a positive inotropic agent, inducing ischemia by increasing cardiac work load. This agent should be avoided in individuals with ventricular or atrial arrhythmias since it can accelerate ventricular and atrial ectopys and heart rate.

Two major types of radionucleotide isotopes are normally used; to assess myocardial perfusion and viability: thallium 201 and Tc 99 m (sestamibi, teboroxime, or tetrofosmin). Thallium redistributes to areas of ischemia quickly while sestamibi permits imaging several areas after injection. The single photon emitted computed tomography SPECT technique is superior to planar imaging. Reversible defects are evidence of myocardial ischemia, while fixed defects represent previous infarction and areas of old scarring [20].

Occasionally apparent perfusion defects can be caused by artifact (breast tissue or diaphragmatic attenuation). This defect commonly occurs in only one view in the inferior or apical area due to imaging defects between the heart and the scanning camera.

Exercise and pharmacologic stress testing demonstrate equal sensitivities with both nuclear and stress echocardiography for detecting coronary artery disease and ischemia, the echocardiogram evaluating wall motion, while the isotopic scan evaluating perfusion.

It is important to understand and determine the patient's tolerance for exercise by these stress testing techniques prior to advising a patient on his capabilities. Stress testing can also provide a valuable insight into the patient's hypertensive blood pressure response, heart rate variability, and recovery times, which can be critical in advising patients as to their maximum duration of exercise.

Any abnormalities in perfusion should be treated aggressively in the diabetic patient who already is at significant risk for a myocardial event. Reversible defects on thallium imaging, significant ST segment depressions, and hypomotility on stress echocardiography should warrant more aggressive evaluation in the diabetic patient.

In some diabetic patients, the presence of electrocardiographic abnormalities makes exercise ECG inappropriate. Radionucleotide or echocardiographic imaging technology would be the test of choice when the amount and the location of jeopardized myocardium is an important consideration [25].

In general, imaging is not only superior to and provides more clinical information that exercise ECG alone, but can improve outcomes by indentifying patients at risk with comparable cost effectiveness. Stress echocardiography has higher specificity, but radionucleotide imaging has greater sensitivity, with stress echocardiography being more cost effective.

The Duke treadmill score can provide an additional method of evaluating the patient who has received an exercise ECG. The treadmill score is the exercise time minus ($5 \times$ ST elevation in millimeters) minus ($4 \times$ exercise angina) where $0 =$ no angina; $1 =$ nonlimiting angina; and $2 =$ exercise limiting angina. Low risk is a score of $5 +$ or higher, moderate risk is -10 to $+4$; and high risk is -11 or lower [26].

The indications for radionucleotide perfusion or echocardiographic imaging and not exercise electrocardiography are:

1. Complete left bundle branch block
2. Paced ventricular rhythm
3. Wolff–Parkinson–White preexcitation syndrome or other conduction abnormalities
4. Patients with greater than 1 mm of ST segment depression at rest
5. Patients with angina who have undergone bypass surgery or stenting in whom ischemic localization, myocardial viability, or severity of obstructive lesions is desired

The standard echocardiogram can give the clinician invaluable information in managing the diabetic and the hypertensive patient. Quantification of valvular regurgitation and assessment of valvular stenosis and incompetence can be of value in determining appropriate therapy for hypertension [27].

Assessment of diastolic function by measuring the isovolumetric relaxation time, the deceleration time, the E/A ratios and the transmitral gradients can help determine the degree of diastolic impairment and serve as a baseline for therapeutic endeavors.

These are defined as follows:

1. The isovolumetric relaxation time is the time interval between closure of the aortic valve and the opening of the mitral valve.
2. The deceleration time represents the interval between the peak of the E wave and the return of early diastolic flow velocity to base line.
3. The E wave represents the rapid filling phase of left ventricular diastole. The A wave represents atrial systole.

Caution must be observed, however, with a normal stress test in the diabetic patient with identification of those at low risk still remains challenging. Interestingly diabetics with normal stress tests still have greater than double the likelihood of cardiac death or myocardial infarction compared to nondiabetics with normal stress images. This may be related to the presence of diffuse, small vessel disease, which can cause false normal test results and if the patient is unable to exercise, the pharmacologic stress test will not be able to assess functional capacity – an important parameter in prognostic assessment. Autopsy data reveal that up to 75% of diabetics greater than 65 years of age have silent coronary artery disease. The Detection of Ischemia in Asymptomatic Diabetics (DIAD) prospective study of 1,123 adults aged 50–75 years revealed that 22% had abnormal nuclear stress tests and 12% of the total participants had moderate or large perfusion defects, while another trial from the Mayo clinic reported 58% with abnormal scans with high risk results in 18%. The DIAD trial demonstrated that screening with radionucleotide perfusion imaging did not reduce coronary heart disease events. Those individuals with moderate or large perfusion defects had higher event rates of 2.4% per year compared to those with small or no defects who had an event rate of 0.4% yearly [28].

The issue of screening asymptomatic diabetic patients remains a source of controversy, although the ADA does not recommend routine screening of all asymptomatic patients. Clearly, the greater the number of associated cardiac risk factors present in any given patient, the greater the likelihood that an asymptomatic patient will have coronary artery disease, particularly if the patient has autonomic neuropathy or some evidence of other vascular (femoral, carotid, and renal) or peripheral arterial disease.

Another important factor to consider is the concept that diabetics less than 65 years of age seem to have a 1–2 year warranty period with the younger group with normal scans showing a 6 month hard event rate of 0.9% compared to 3% in those greater than 65.

Hence, the timer period for repeating a stress test may well be shorter for those asymptomatic individuals greater than 65. In addition, the benefit of revascularization once the disease is detected is controversial and largely unproven with aggressive risk factor modification and medical therapy addressing lipid, hypertensive, and glycemic control with aspirin and angiotensin converting enzyme inhibitors an alternative approach.

For those diabetics with an abnormal scan, management depends upon ischemia severity. Revascularization should be a strong consideration in those with multivessel disease and moderate to severe ischemia although percutaneous intervention (if indicated) should also be considered. More data comparing surgical revascularization with percutaneous intervention in diabetics is needed.

The MiSAD trial (Milan Study on Atherosclerosis and Diabetes) explored the prognosis of those with mild to moderate ischemia on stress testing. This trial reported that asymptomatic diabetic patients with abnormal stress testing had more aggressive risk factor management with a smaller number of events than those with normal testing. Faglia reported on the results of revascularization in asymptomatic diabetic patients with abnormal scans and noted a significantly lower rate of cardiac events after 53 months [29].

Larger trials need to be done to confirm whether detecting and aggressively treating asymptomatic diabetics with invasive (revascularization or percutaneous) or medical treatment improves prognosis and reduces events.

Exercise can be an important therapeutic modality for a variety of patients with diabetes. For many patients 20–30 min of walking three times weekly can be an important step in increasing exercise activity. Post exercise enhancement of glucose metabolism as a result of increased insulin sensitivity may last for several hours or even days.

Studies have shown that better glycemic control results from the additive effect of repeated exercise sessions and are not related to overall physical fitness, consistently improving insulin sensitivity and carbohydrate metabolism in addition to reducing baroreflex sensitivity and heart rate variability in type-2 diabetics. This was directly related to the duration and not the intensity of exercise, with 30–60 min per session three to four times a week being associated with a decrease of hemoglobin A1-C of 10–20% with improvements greatest in those patients that were most insulin resistant. This is a strong evidence for the impact of exercise on insulin resistance [14]. A review in the Archives of Internal Medicine indicated that a combination of 90 min of aerobic and 60 min of resistance exercise three times weekly represented the best strategy to improve functional limitations and insulin resistance in otherwise sedentary and obese older adults [30].

This improved insulin sensitivity correlates with lowered cardiovascular risk. Weight loss combined with exercise and diet therapy significantly decreases intra-abdominal fat and is associated with a better sense of well being, better mood, and higher self esteem. The matter in which exercise is attempted is strictly based on patient preference.

In general, the aerobic exercises such as swimming and walking are preferred. Resistance training, although beneficial, can be somewhat hazardous in patients with orthopedic or vascular problems although properly designed resistance programs can be shown to be beneficial. Light weight repetitions are very effective and can be used extremely well to maintain tone.

Exercise intensity should be limited so that systolic blood pressure does not exceed 180 mmHg with a maximum heart rate being 220 minus the patient's age. For those patients who are taking insulin, care should be taken to insure the coincidence of peak insulin absorption with exercise activities.

Ideally, weekly exercise causes an expenditure of 700–2,000 calories. Make sure the patient consumes sufficient fluid frequently during the exercise period to compensate for sweat loss and other insensible fluid losses. Quantitative measurements of progress can be helpful further for those patients who are extremely goal oriented, but not necessarily mandatory. Patients should choose those activities that are appropriate for their general physical condition and life style and start slow working up gradually [31].

Other types of activity include biking and stationary cycling, aerobic water exercises, and swimming in addition to walking in a moderate pace (3–5 miles per hour). Diabetic patients should always be encouraged to carry identification and monitor blood glucose levels pre and post exercise. In addition to constantly being aware of the signs and symptoms of hypoglycemia during subsequent workouts diabetics should carry appropriate, readily available carbohydrate sources to treat hypoglycemia.

Since most individuals with type-2 diabetes are overweight and are in poor cardiovascular health, prior to initiating an exercise program the focus should be on low intensity exercises that are easy to initiate and maintain provided the patient has successfully completed a stress test evaluation.

Appropriate energy economy represents a balance between the expenditure and energy intake. Hence a cornerstone in maintaining helpful weight and an adjunct in losing weight remains an expenditure of energy through subsequent physical activity. One needs to put the number of calories expended during exercise into perspective and it is more valuable for weight maintenance rather than weight loss.

Clearly, low cardiorespiratory fitness increases mortality. A study in *JAMA* in 2003 from the Coronary Artery Risk Development in Young Adults (CARDIA) group indicated that poor fitness in young adults' increases risk, while enhancing the development of cardiovascular risk factors and obesity and that improving fitness can improve the risks [32].

The participants in this study were young white and black men and women (ages 18–30) who completed treadmill testing and then were followed from 1985–2001. Glucose, lipids, and blood pressures were measured while physical activity was assessed by interview and self reporting. Outcome measurements included hypercholesterolemia, metabolic syndrome, hypertension, and type-2 diabetes.

The 15 year incidence rates per 1,000 patient years were as follows: [33]

1. Diabetes – 2.8
2. Metabolic Syndrome – 10.2
3. Hypercholesterolemia – 11.7
4. Hypertension – 13.0

Patients with low fitness (<20th percentile) were three to six times more likely to develop diabetes, hypertension, and the metabolic syndrome than patients with higher fitness (>60th percentile). Adjustment for body mass index lowered the strength of the associations. Those patients who improved their fitness over 7 years reduced their risk of diabetes and the metabolic syndrome.

These results are similar to others where maximum oxygen uptake was used to measure fitness rather than treadmill testing time. Nonetheless it does underscore the fact that suboptimal physical activity and fitness increases risk for cardiovascular disease, diabetes, lipid disorders, and metabolic syndrome.

Exercise has been shown to be of benefit in diabetics because:

1. Regular aerobic exercise has been shown to reduce the dosage or need for insulin or oral hyperglycemic agents.
2. It reduces cardiovascular risk factors by lowering triglyceride, blood pressure, and LDL cholesterol.
3. It improves glycemic control by increasing tissue sensitivity to insulin.
4. It raises HDL levels.
5. It improves collateral blood flow in patients with ischemic arterial disease.
6. It decreases heart rate at rest while increasing maximal oxygen uptake in total working capacity.
7. It decreases central obesity and waist to hip ratio.

8. It improves muscle strength and joint flexibility.
9. It serves as an important adjunct to weight reduction program in decreasing obesity, and accelerating and enhancing weight loss.

Exercise training is widely regarded as crucial in the management of type-2 diabetes by having a beneficial effect on surrogate markers of inflammation, lipid disorders, and glycemia. It is hoped and expected that these benefits will result in more favorable cardiovascular and metabolic outcomes. Future research efforts should be targeting physical fitness and incorporating exercise into medical practices, workplaces, and community fitness centers [*34*].

SUMMARY

Adherence to exercise is a very important predictor of subsequent success for patients in any type of weight reduction or behavior modification program. Although the thrust of biomedical research and development has been involved with more enticing gene mapping and identification, it is clear that exercise therapy can be extremely valuable, practical, and more readily available. It is important to appreciate that type-2 diabetics contemplating an exercise program should consult with their primary providers to assess risk profiles and physical condition keeping in mind the potential cardiac risks, foot problems, microvascular disease, and hypoglycemia that can complicate increased physical activity.

REFERENCES

1. Thompson PD: Additional steps for cardiovascular health. N Engl J Med. 2002; 347:755–756.
2. American Diabetes Association. Physical activity/exercise and diabetes mellitus. Diabetes Care 2004; 27(suppl 1):S58.
3. Krishna B, Richard B: Physical activity and type 2 diabetes. Phys Sportsmed. 2004; 32:1.
4. Zinman B, Ruderman N, et al.: Physical activity, exercise and diabetes mellitus. Diabetes Care 2003; 26(suppl 1):S73–S77.
5. Pierce NS: Diabetes and exercise. Br J Sports Med. 1999; 33(3):161–172.
6. Walsh JM, Swangard DM, Davis T, McPhee SJ: Exercise counseling by primary care physicians in the era of managed care. Am J Prev Med. 1999; 16:307–313.
7. Cardinal B, Levy S, John D, Cardinal M: Counseling patients for physical activity. Am J Med Sports 2002; 4:364–371.
8. American Diabetes Association. Physical activity, exercise and diabetes mellitus. Diabetes Care 2003; 26(suppl 1)S73–S77.
9. Tanasescu M, Leitzmann MF, Rimm EB, Hu FB: Physical activity in relation to cardiovascular disease and total mortality among men with type-2 diabetes. Circulation 2003; 107:2435–2439.
10. Boule NG, Haddad E, Kenny GP, Wells GA, Signal RJ: Effects of exercise on glycemic control and body mass in type-2 diabetes mellitus. JAMA 2001; 286:1218–1227.
11. Boule NG, Haddad E, Kenny GP, et al.: Effects of exercise on glycemic control and body mass in type 2 diabetes mellitus: a meta-analysis of controlled clinical trials. JAMA 2001; 286(10):1218–1237.
12. Schneider SH, Amorosa LF, Khachaduria AK, et al.: Studies on the mechanism of improved glucose control during regular exercise in type 2 diabetes. Diabetologia 1984; 26(5):355–360.
13. Hendrickson EJ: Invited review: effects of acute exercise and exercise training on insulin resistance. J Appl Physiol. 2002; 93:788–796.
14. Henriksen EJ: Invited review: effects of acute exercise and exercise training on insulin resistance. J Appl Physiol. 2002; 93:788–796.
15. Mourier A, Gautier JF, De Kerviler E: Mobilization of visceral adipose tissue related to the improvement in insulin sensitivity in response to physidal training in NIDDM. Diabetes Care 1997; 20:385–391.

16. Loimaala A, Huikuri HV, Koobi T, Rinne M: Exercise training improves baroreflex sensitivity in type-2 diabetes. Diabetes 2003; 52:1837–1842.
17. Maiorana A, et al.: The effect of combined aerobic and resistance exercise training on vascular function in type 2 diabetes. J AM Coll Cardiol. 2001; 38:860–866.
18. Lim J, et al.: Exercise training: an essential lifestyle intervention for prevention and management of type 2 diabetes mellitus. Am J Med Sports 2003; 5:341–347.
19. Borghouts LB, KEizer HA: Exercise and insulin sensitivity: a review. Int J Sports Med. 2000; 21:1–12.
20. Lipinski M, Froelicher V et al.: Comparison of treadmill scores with physician estimates of diagnosis and prognosis in patients with coronary artery disease. AM Heart J. 2002; 143:650–658.
21. Killip T, Passamani E, Davis K: Coronary artery surgery study (CASS). Circulation 1985;72:102–109.
22. Marrero D: Initiation and maintenance of exercise in patients with diabetes. *Handbook of Exercise in Diabetes*. Alexandria: American Diabetes Association, 2002, 289–310.
23. Albright A, Franz M, Hornsby G, Kriska A: American College of Sports Medicine position stand: exercise and type-2 diabetes. Med Sci Sports Exerc. 2000; 32:1345–1360.
24. Vanhees L, Fagard R, et al.: Prognostic significance of peak exercise capacity in patients with coronary artery disease. J Am Coll Cardiol. 1994; 23:358–363.
25. Myers J, Prakash M, et al.: Exercise capacity and mortality among men referred for cardiac rehabilitation. Circulation 2001; 104:2996–3007.
26. Pate RR, Pratt M, Blair SN, Haskell WL: Physical activity and public health. JAMA 1995; 273:402–407.
27. Shephard RJ, Blaady GJ: Exercise as cardiovascular therapy. Circulation 1999; 99(7):963–972.
28. Wackers FJ, Young LH, Inzucchi SE: Detection of silent myocardial ischemia in asymptomatic diabetic patients: the DIAD study. Diabetes Care 2004; 27:1954–1961.
29. Faglia E, Favales F, Calia P, Paliari F, Segalini G: Cardiac events in 735 type-2 diabetic patients who underwent screening for unknown asymptomatic coronary artery disease. The Milan Study on Atherosclerosis and Diabetes (MiSAD). Diabetes Care 2002; 25(11):2032–2036.
30. Lee CD, Sui X, Blair S: Combined effects of cardiorespiratory fitness, not smoking, and normal waist girth on morbidity and mortality in men. Arch Intern Med. 2009; 169(22):2096–2101.
31. Chipkin SR, Klugh SA, et al.: Exercise and diabetes. Cardiol Clin. 2001; 19(3):489–505.
32. Carnethon MR, Gidding SS, Nehgme R, Sidney S, Jacobs DR, Liu K: Cardiorespiratory fitness in young adulthood and the development of cardiovascular disease risk factors. JAMA 2003; 290:3092–3100.
33. Willey KA, Singh MA: Battling insulin resistance in elderly obese people with type 2 diabetes: bring on the heavyweights. Diabetes Care. 2003; 26:1580–1588.
34. American Diabetes Association. Diabetes mellitus and exercise. Diabetes Care 2000; 23(suppl 1) S50–S54.
35. Young J: Exercise: missing link in diabetes management. Am J Med Sports 2001; 3:28–35.
36. Stewart K: Exercise training and the cardiovascular consequences of type 2 diabetes and hypertension. JAMA 2002; 288(13):1622–1630.

SUPPLEMENTARY READINGS

Froelicher V: Exercise testing in the new millennium. Prim Care 2001; 28:1–4.
Pan X, Li G, Hu Y, et al.: Effects of diet and exercise in preventing NIDDM in people with impaired glucose tolerance: The Da Qing IGT and Diabetes Study. Diabetes Care 1997; 20:537–544.
Petrella RJ, Koval JJ, Cunningham DA, Paterson DH: Can primary care doctors prescribe exercise to improve fitness? Am J Prev Med. 2003; 24:316–322.
Schneider SH, Ruderman NB: Exercise and NIDDM (technical review). Diabetes Care 1994; 17:924–937.
Shue P, Froelicher VF: EXTRA: an expert system for exercise test reporting. J Non-Invasive Test. 1998; II-4:21–27.
Wasserman DH, Zinman B: Exercise in individuals with IDDM (technical review). Diabetes Care 1994; 17:924–937.
Williamson DF, Thompson TJ, Thun M, et al.: Intentional weight loss and mortality among overweight individuals with diabetes. Diabetes Care 2000; 23:1499–1504.

4 Nutrition

CONTENTS

Key Words: Carbohydrates, Proteins, Fats, Minerals, Vitamins, Dietary Supplements

INTRODUCTION

Dietary management and control is crucial to any diabetic therapeutic strategy to normalize plasma glucose, reduce postprandial excursions, reduce obesity, and regulate lipid and protein metabolism and homeostasis. Unfortunately, because of poor patient compliance, lack of self control, inadequate patient education, and the ease of obtaining fast foods, dietary management for type-2 diabetes is only partially successful [1].

In order to be completely successful, patient education is critical and the diet must be adjusted according to the needs and preferences of each individual. Quite often, preprinted guidelines with no personal direction or disregard for ethnic preferences are often fruitless. Most physicians do not have the time or even the expertise to structure such customized dietary instruction for each patient. Hence certified diabetic educators, dietitians, and other properly trained physician extenders can be invaluable in counseling diabetic patients.

Medical nutrition therapy represents an important therapeutic lifestyle change that should be designed to prevent and reduce the risk of micro and macrovascular complications of the disease by improving lipid and blood pressure levels and enhance glycemic control.

This can be especially challenging today with the various family and ethnic preferences, food aversions, intolerances and allergies, and hectic lifestyles that are more conducive to fast food dining than home cooked meals. These goals can be achieved by providing adequate caloric intake to reach and maintain normal body weight in adults and normal

From: *Current Clinical Practice: Type 2 Diabetes, Pre-Diabetes, and the Metabolic Syndrome*
Edited by: R.A. Codario, DOI 10.1007/978-1-60327-441-8_4
© Springer Science+Business Media, LLC 2011

Table 1
Nutrition recommendations for diabetics

Carbohydrates

Total amount of carbohydrate in the diet is more important than the source or type

Low fat milk, fruits, whole grains, and vegetables should be included as dietary carbohydrate sources

Sucrose and sucrose containing foods do not need to be restricted and can be substituted for other carbohydrate sources

Non nutritive sweeteners are safe when consumed within the acceptable daily intake levels established by the Food and Drug Administration

Protein

Ingested protein does not increase plasma glucose concentrations

Ingested protein is just as potent a stimulant of insulin secretion as carbohydrate

Fat

Less than 7% of energy intake should be in the form of saturated fat

Dietary cholesterol intake should be less than 200 mg/day

From Franz [45]

development in adolescence and balancing intake, activity, and medical therapies to normalize fasting glucose and minimize postprandial excursions.

Some general recommendations, as seen in Table 1, should be followed in an attempt to achieve these goals. Consensus guidelines recommend a diet consisting of 12–15% of calories as protein, 50–60% as carbohydrates, and 30% as fat with reduction of saturated fats and trans fatty acids to less than 7% (even eliminated completely if possible) emphasizing monosaturated and polyunsaturated fatty acids [2]. Any sustained weight loss is beneficial in diabetic management, but long-term compliance is more likely if the caloric restriction is not too severe. In general, 20 kcal/kg of ideal body weight allows for gradual weight reduction, while regular exercise enhances the feeling of well being, improves insulin sensitivity, and enhances glycemic control.

DIABETES AND CARBOHYDRATES [3]

Carbohydrates in the diet include monosaccharides and disaccharides, the starches and the indigestible carbohydrates like cellulose, pectins, gums, and psyllium. The American Diabetes Association recommends the following terms: sugars, starch and fiber, while terms like simple sugars, complex carbohydrates, and fast acting carbohydrates should be avoided since they are not well defined.

Carbohydrates in the form of whole grains, fruits, vegetables, legumes, and low fat milk are recommended. Normally the diet contains 45–55% of total calories as carbohydrates. The minimal amount of carbohydrate needed for the brain to function is 130 g daily as is set by the Food and Nutrition Board of the National Academy's Institute of Medicine in their Dietary Reference Intakes in 2002. Most people exceed this amount with median ranges of 200–300 g daily for men and 180–230 g daily for women [4].

Carbohydrates, like monosaturates do not have significant effects on cholesterol, however, they can have significant effects on lipoprotein metabolism. This is because high carbohydrate diets stimulate the synthesis of very low density lipoprotein (VLDL), triglycerides, and subsequently can raise serum triglyceride levels. This usually effects the high density lipoprotein (HDL) in a reciprocal fashion with decreased levels. Removal of fats from the diet and replacement with carbohydrates reduces LDL levels despite the HDL lowering effects.

Many patients consider the benefits of a low carbohydrate (20–60 g daily) or low glycemic index diet for improved glycemic control. The concept of the glycemic index considers the effects of various foods on postprandial glucose, appreciating the fact that some foods have different effects on blood glucose despite the same carbohydrate content. Hence, a diet based on low glycemic index foods would result in lower A1C levels with less glucose excursions. The glycemic index is the area of blood glucose plotted on a graph generated over a 3-h period time following the ingestion of a food containing 50 g of carbohydrate compared with the area plotted after giving a similar quantity of reference food. The reference point for the index is white bread or pure glucose, which is given an arbitrary rating of 100, with low glycemic indices below 56 and high greater than 69. White bread is preferred to glucose because it less of a tendency to show gastric emptying due to high tonicity which often happens with a glucose solution. The higher the index, the more rapidly the serum glucose rises within 2 h of eating as carbohydrate is released into the blood and the more rapid the insulin response. This rapid insulin response has the capacity to induce reactive hypoglycemia with appetite stimulation and subsequent increased caloric intake – a phenomenon that can often be seen in individuals who consume diets high in carbohydrates and low in fats. The subsequent hyperinsulinemia induced by high glycemic index diets has been implicated in increasing cardiovascular risk in patients with the metabolic syndrome.

There are some drawbacks to the concept of the glycemic index, however. The index is not listed on food labels and variations occur for the same food depending on the reference source. In addition, the index is unknown for many food and pertains to foods eaten individually, while most people are consuming several foods simultaneously (i.e., stew, chili, etc.). In addition, portion sizes are not taken into consideration with this index, with the quantity of food containing 50 g often not representative of a service size. This can result in the overestimation or underestimation of the effect on blood glucose. The index can be significantly affected by how the various foods are prepared, with steaming, baking, frying, and grilling resulting in different glycemic indices.

A meta-analysis of randomized controlled clinical trials indicated a decrease of 0.43% in A1C levels with low glycemic index diets. These diets have also been noted to increase HDL, and lower serum triglycerides, high sensitivity C-reactive protein, and plasminogen activator inhibitor 1 (PAI-1), while reducing overall cardiovascular events. However, more long term data is necessary to confirm this concept since most studies reported have an average of 10 weeks in duration [5].

Diets that contain less than 20 g of carbohydrates (i.e., The Atkins Diet) often allow unrestricted intake of fat and protein. These may reduce the A1C and improve insulin sensitivity and triglycerides short term, but may increase cardiac risk long-term due to the increased fat ingestion. In addition, these diets may lack fiber, minerals vitamins, and other nutrients that are essential for well balanced nutrition. Although the ADA has approved these low carbohydrate diets for weight loss in diabetic patients, providers are urged to monitor protein intake in patients with nephropathy, lipid profiles, and kidney function and advise patients not to remain on these diets longer than 1 year. It is important to appreciate that since mealtime insulin needs may decrease significantly, on low carbohydrate diets, particularly patients taking insulin and or secretagogues, proper counseling concerning hypoglycemia is indicated.

Another concept is that of the glycemic load, which provides a measurement of the glycemic response to food servings. The glycemic load is equal to the glycemic index multiplied by the number of grams of carbohydrate in the serving. High glycemic loads are greater than 19, and low glycemic loads are less than 11. This is an interesting concept when we consider certain foods like spaghetti, which has a low glycemic index of 42; however, its glycemic load is high at 20 due to the number of carbohydrates per serving (about 48 g). On the other hand, whole wheat bread, with a high glycemic index of 73 has a low glycemic load of ten with only about 14 g per serving.

Some general guidelines for nutritious eating utilizing both the glycemic index and load concepts are: (1) avoid beverages and foods with added sugar or caloric sweeteners, especially high fructose corn syrup, (2) substitute whole grains for refined foods (3) eat plenty of vegetables several times weekly including legumes, green leafy vegetables, orange and starchy vegetables (4) drink three cups of low fat or fat free milk or the equivalent in yogurt daily (5) incorporate fresh fruits into the daily dietary routine – especially those with lower glycemic loads.

Fiber, indigestible carbohydrates in the diet, is a particularly important component of reducing risk in diabetics with 25–50 g required daily, this can be best obtained through diets rich in whole grain cereals, fruits, vegetables, legumes, and brown rice instead of white rice, pasta and bread

Fiber can be described as soluble or non soluble. Soluble fibers include psyllium, certain gums and pectins. Beta-glycan, a gum derivative, is the predominant soluble fiber in beans and oat bran. Higher intakes of soluble fiber can lower serum cholesterol by as much as 3–5%. Some examples of soluble fiber include: oatmeal, oat bran, nuts, seeds, apples, pears, blueberries, strawberries, and legumes (beans, peas, and lentils).

The insoluble fiber in the diet is mainly cellulose as found in wheat bran. Cellulose increases bulk in the stools and aids in promoting regularity. The intake of increased amounts of insoluble fiber can decrease the risk of developing diverticulosis. Examples of insoluble fiber include: carrots, cucumbers, zucchini, celery, brown rice, barley, apple and pear skins, couscous and whole wheat breads.

Cereal fibers have been generally shown to have little, if any, metabolic effects except for barley and oat fiber, with increases in wheat fiber of up to 20 g daily having no significant effect on A1C or other chronic disease biomarkers in patients with type-2 diabetes.

A randomized clinical trial published in *JAMA* in 2008 compared the effects of a high cereal fiber to a low glycemic index diet in 210 participants with type-2 diabetes over a 6-month period. In this study, the low glycemic index diet produced lower A1C levels (0.33% difference) compared to the fiber diet. In addition, the lower glycemic index diet reduced the risk for coronary artery disease. This is of interest since the US Food and Drug Administration (FDA) recognizes A1C reductions greater than 0.3% as clinically meaningful when evaluating therapies for diabetes treatment [6].

The effects of a plant based low carbohydrate or Eco-Atkins diet compared to a high carbohydrate-low fat diet were studied in 47 individuals and published in the *Archives of Internal Medicine* in June, 2009. This demonstrated similar body weight reductions to an

Atkins-like diet, but significantly reduced LDL levels compared to low carbohydrate diets with animal derived fats and protein. This study also showed a reduction in apolipoprotein B as well as reduced apo-B/apo A1 ratios [7].

High carbohydrate vegetarian diets like the Ornish regimen have also been associated with reduced LDL concentrations and weight loss with reduced progression of coronary artery disease, while the inclusion of soy and nuts has also been shown to increase HDL concentrations when incorporated as part of low fat diets. This is important to keep in mind since diets based on impressively low fat intake can lower HDL in addition to LDL.

Various factors can effect glycemic excursions with food intake including the type of sugar (lactose, fructose, sucrose, and glucose), type of cooking and food processing, type of starch (amylose and amylopectin), food components (lectins, tannins, and phytates), the levels of preprandial and postprandial glucoses, and the degree of insulin resistance.

Studies lasting 2–12 weeks comparing high vs. low glycemic diets showed no consistent improvements in A1C, fructosamine, or insulin levels with mixed nonconsistent effects on lipids. This is somewhat surprising since low glycemic diets can reduce postprandial sugars. Thus far no clear trend in beneficial outcomes has been shown with various glycemic index diets. The ADA concludes that the total amount carbohydrate in meals and or snacks is more important than the source (starch vs. sugar) or glycemic index [8]. Nonetheless, some patients subjectively feel better when eating foods with a lower glycemic index like beans, lentels, and yogurt as opposed to higher glycemic index foods like bread, white rice, pasta, potatoes, yams, sweet corn, and honey.

In general, low carbohydrate diets have more favorable effects on insulin resistance, serum triglycerides, HDL levels, and LDL particle distribution improving metabolic risk factors. Although preliminary data supports favorable effects on glycemic control and inflammation, further studies are necessary to determine whether or not these effects are diet or specifically low carbohydrate related. Low carbohydrate diets are not recommended by the ADA endorsing a diet in which 45–65% of total calories are in the form of carbohydrates with low glycemic index foods like barley, oats, whole grains, legumes, and fruits replacing refined carbohydrates like white bread and potatoes.

A significant volume of information does support the effectiveness of a high fiber, low fat, and low carbohydrate diet in the prevention and treatment of diabetes. Hence choosing carbohydrates from the lower end of the glycemic scale seems to be advisable at this point. High fiber diets are associated with improved ability to handle blood sugar. Dietary fibers can slow the rate of food progression through the intestine, hence attenuating postprandial glucose excursions. This is in distinction to lower fiber meals that are absorbed quickly into the blood and may cause a surge in hyperglycemia.

Water retaining fibers such as oat, bran, and guergum contain mucilaginous compounds that reduce the rate of glucose absorption and slow gastric emptying. Fiber containing foods like whole grains, fruits, and vegetables should be encouraged in type-2 diabetics providing vitamins, minerals, and essential nutrients. Large amounts of fiber can have a positive impact on glucose and lipids and promote regularity. Current recommendations are for at least 38 g of fiber for men and 25 g for women if less than 50 years of age. Soluble fiber reduces total and LDL cholesterol especially if accompanied by a diet low in saturated fat, trans fatty acids, and cholesterol. In a meta-analysis of 67 controlled trials, soluble fiber had a small effect on total and LDL cholesterol without dietary fat restriction. The ADA does not recommend that type-2 diabetics consume more fiber than other individuals.

Isocaloric amounts of starch and sucrose have equal effects on glycemia according to the latest available evidence from clinical trials. Hence sucrose intake need not be restricted in diabetics and can be substituted for other carbohydrate sources in the context of a healthy diet. Fructose causes less glycemic excursions than sucrose but can increase the VLDL and triglycerides. Hence the use of fructose for sweetening is not recommended although diabetics need not avoid naturally occurring fructose in vegetables, fruits, and other foods.

Sugar alcohols (sorbitol, xylitol, and mannitol) have a lower postprandial glucose response than sucrose, fructose, and glucose and are generally safe, but may cause diarrhea. The FDA has approved four nonnutritive sweeteners; saccharin, aspartame, acesulfame potassium (Sunett), and sucralose. On a gram for gram basis these substances are much sweeter than sucrose with no calories. Saccharin has been implicated as a carcinogen in rats with an increased incidence of bladder cancer in male rats fed large amounts. These have not been reproduced in humans. The American Diabetes Association considers them safe when consumed within acceptable daily levels established by the FDA.

Fructose, sorbitol, mannitol, and xylitol are nutritive sweeteners and should be reserved for those who are at an ideal body weight with normal lipids and acceptable glycemic control. There is no evidence at present to support claims that resistant starch (corn starch or high amylose corn starch) can affect postprandial glucose, prevent hyperglycemia, and reduce A1C levels.

Many Americans consume large amounts of alcohol with estimates of the average intake being 5% of total calories. Although there is recent data about cardioprotection of some wines, one must keep in mind that alcohol intake can raise serum triglyceride levels by stimulating the production of VLDL – triglycerides in the liver.

DIABETES AND PROTEIN [9]

Since protein is more satiating than fats or carbohydrates, high protein diets are popular for weight loss usually associated with lower blood pressures and lower glycosylated hemoglobin in diabetic patients.

Protein intake accounts for 15–20% of average daily intake and does not appear to vary in diabetics. The effects of protein on appetite suppression, long term weight loss, and regulation of energy intake has not been widely studied. Essential amino acids should be supplied in the diet to allow for protein synthesis.

The proteins with the most essential amino acids are found in eggs, fish, poultry, lean meats, and dairy products. In general, protein will stimulate insulin to the same degree as carbohydrate. When diabetes is controlled, ingested protein will not increase plasma glucose, since this ingested protein will not appear in the general circulation.

Curiously, a recent review done at the Veterans Affairs Medical Center in Minneapolis at the University of Minnesota evaluated the change in blood glucose over 8 h in men consuming 50 g of beef or water. During the 8 h after the beef was ingested, the glucose increased by an average 3 mg/dl in the first hour and then decreased similar to the water ingesters. In general, the glucose produced from protein is likely stored in the liver as glycogen as long as an adequate amount of insulin is present [10].

In cases of insulin deficiency gluconeogenesis can be stimulated when protein intake does not exceed 20% of the total daily consumption. There is no increased risk of diabetic nephropathy; although long-term consumption of greater than this amount has not been studied, the ADA recommends avoiding such excess protein intake. The safety and long term efficacy of low carbohydrate, high protein diets remains unknown and is not been widely studied although these diets can produce short term weight loss and improve glycemic control.

There is no evidence to support the fact that protein can slow the absorption of carbohydrate. When equal amounts of protein and glucose are ingested, the peak glucose response was the same as the same amount of glucose ingested alone. The glycemic response to the carbohydrate content of the meal determines peak glucose response.

Protein plus carbohydrates works just as well as carbohydrates alone to prevent hypoglycemia, with a 15-g carbohydrate snack before or after exercise usually being sufficient to avoid an attack of hypoglycemia.

Diabetic women tend to lose more on high protein diets with greater fat loss compared to diabetic women on a low protein diet with no differences noted in men [11]. A 12-month follow-up study by Samaha and others noted that 54 patients with type-2 diabetes showed a statistically significant improvement in A1C (0.7%) with a low carbohydrate, low fat, and high protein diet [12].

DIABETES AND FATS [13]

Since the essential component of the diabetic paradigm is atherogenesis, it is critically important for diabetics to limit their intake of dietary cholesterol, saturated fat, and trans fatty acids. These remain important determinates of the plasma LDL cholesterol.

Unsaturated fatty acids in the diet are in the form of monounsaturated and polyunsaturated fats. Monounsaturated fats have a single double bond in their long carbon chain while polyunsaturated fats have two or more double bonds.

Some of the common unsaturated fats in the diet are:

1. Omega-9 (oleic acid).
2. Omega-6 (linoleic acid).
3. Omega-3 (linolenic, eicosapentaenoic acid, and docosahexaenoic acid).

Linolenic acid is most often found in commonly consumed foods. Linoleic acid is an 18 carbon fatty acid with two double bonds. One of these double bonds is located six carbon atoms from the terminal carbon atom, hence the 6-omega fatty acid designation.

Linolenic acid has a double bond in the omega-3 position, 18 carbon atoms, and three overall double bonds.

Oleic acid is an 18 carbon containing compound with one double bond in the omega-9 position.

The omega-6 polyunsaturated fats (linoleic acid) for many years were perceived to have cholesterol lowering effects Linoleic acid has been reported to lower the serum total cholesterol level about half as much as saturated fatty acids raise these levels with subsequent reduction in the LDL cholesterol as well. This concept has not been proven with experimentation, however. Postulated mechanisms include:

1. Promoting excretion of cholesterol from the body, reducing body stores of cholesterol
2. Reduction of the cholesterol carrying capacity of LDL
3. Redistribution of cholesterol between serum and tissues
4. Increase in the number of LDL receptors

Dietary sources of linoleic acids are:

1. Safflower oil
2. Sunflower seed oil
3. Soybean oil
4. Corn oil

The omega-3 fatty acids found in fish like EPA (eicosapentaenoic acid) and DHA (docosahexaenoic acid) lower serum triglycerides by inhibiting the synthesis of triglycerides.

The ADA is much more judicious in their recommendation of intake of polyunsaturated and monounsaturated fats. In general, however, research shows that low fat diets are usually associated with modest weight loss that can be maintained as long as the diet is continued. This is not nearly as substantial as the weight loss that can be derived for restriction of carbohydrate intake.

Both the American Heart Association and the American Diabetes Association suggest at least two servings of fish per week [14]. Omega-3 fatty acids can have a triglyceride lowering effect, but the question always arises about the PCB and TCCD concentration of the omega-3 fatty acids, particularly farm raised fish, due to these contaminants in the feeding. Omega-3 fatty acids represent a family of polyunsaturated fatty acids that can be found naturally in plants (alpha-linolenic acid) and fish (as docosahexaenoic acid, DHA, and eicosapentaenoic acid, EPA) [15].

Increasing amounts of clinical data supports the benefit of omega-3 fatty acid ingestion from a pathophysiologic point of view. The omega-3 fatty acids induce the peroxisome proliferator activated receptor (PPAR) alpha system benefiting and lowering triglyceride levels subsequently raising HDL. Populations with a high intake of omega-3 fatty acids, such as the Inuit Eskimos, have been shown to have significantly low rates of cardiovascular disease. The Western Electric Study, with 30 years of follow-up data, demonstrated that men who ingested at least 35 g of fish per day had a decreased mortality from coronary heart disease and a decreased risk of sudden death from myocardial infarction [16].

In the Nurses Health Study, higher consumption of fish and omega-3 fatty acids was also associated with significant benefit [17]. The Diet and Reinfarction Trial studied 2,033 Welsh men who had an acute myocardial infarction. When given a diet containing 1.5 g of fish oil for 2 years, a 29% reduction in total mortality and 33% reduction in coronary mortality was demonstrated [18].

In the GISSI trial, 11,324 patients who had taken omega-3 fatty acid supplementation showed a significant reduction in all cause mortality after only 3 months of supplementation and the risk of sudden death was significantly reduced after only 4 months. Omega-3 fatty acids exert their cardioprotective effects in several pleiotrophic mechanisms [19]. They have consistently been shown to decrease platelet aggregation, improve endothelial function, reduce blood pressure, lower serum triglycerides, and enhance antiarrhythmic benefits. It may well be that the antiarrhythmic effects play an important role in reduction of sudden cardiac death, with the omega-3 fatty acids being shown to reduce heart rate variability, and subsequently reduce ventricular arrhythmia.

The best available current evidence with omega-3 fatty acids in diabetics suggest that these substances have either no effect on insulin sensitivity or might actually improve it slightly. A recent meta-analysis of placebo controlled trials show that doses of 3–18 g/day of fish oil had no effect on glucose control for approximately 12 weeks. These patients demonstrated a significant decrease in triglyceride and also an increase in LDL of 8.1 mg/dl. In this study there was no significant effect in glycosylated hemoglobin or HDL.

Additional studies have targeted the effects of omega-3 supplementation on vascular function showing that these substances can have a beneficial effect on lipid peroxidation, and antienzymatic and antioxidant enzyme activity [20].

In the Nurses Health Study, over 5,000 women with type-2 diabetes and increase risk for cardiovascular disease showed that a higher consumption of fish was associated with a significantly lower total mortality. In these particular patients there was reduced platelet aggregation, improved endothelial function, lower triglycerides, and antiarrhythmic effects [21].

Approximately, 4 g of omega-3 fatty acids can reduce serum triglycerides by 35%, increasing LDL cholesterol by 5–10%, and increasing HDL cholesterol 1–3%. Various meta-analyses demonstrate that the effects on triglycerides are most significant in patients with triglyceride levels greater than 177 mg/dl. The triglyceride lowering effects, however, have not been as potent as with niacin or fibrates [22].

The American Heart Association recommends 1 g daily of omega-3 fatty acids for a cardioprotective effect and 2–4 g a day of EPA plus DHA for patients with elevated triglycerides.

It is curious to note that the preparation method for the fish seems to be relevant to the reduction of ischemic heart disease. Lower risk is not obtained with consumption of fried fish or fish sandwiches, but rather broiled or baked fish. Frying seems to increase the omega-6 to omega-3 ratio and lipid oxidation, blunting any expected benefit.

It is the fatty fish such as tuna, mackerel, salmon, herring, and sardines that have the highest concentration of marine omega-3 polyunsaturated fats. Due to the concern of high doses of pollutants and methylmercury, the FDA recommends that children, pregnant women, and nursing mothers limit their fish intake avoiding those species that may be high in mercury. Mercury levels can be found to be elevated in shark, swordfish, mackerel, and tuna.

The current recommendation is that all patients with diabetes and high risk for cardiovascular disease consume more fish in their diet, particularly those with higher omega-3 fatty acid concentration. Due to concerns of polychlorinated biphenyls and TCDD contamination, it is recommended that the skin be removed from the fish prior to cooking with further clinical trials necessary to elucidate the ultimate long term effect of this supplementation.

Polyunsaturated fats have not been extensively studied in diabetics. These fats appear to lower LDL cholesterol, but not as well as monounsaturated fats. The American Heart Association recommends a fat intake equal to or less than 30% of the total whereas the dietary reference intakes and the National Cholesterol Education Program recommend ranges for the percentage of total fat consumption. The National Cholesterol Education Program recommendation for total fat is in the range of 25–35% of total energy intake, but makes the recommendation that trans fatty acids and saturated fats should be kept as low as possible [23].

Fat intake should clearly be individualized with monounsaturated fat and carbohydrates providing 60–70% of total energy intake. For example, low saturated fat diets (supplying less than 10% of energy) along with high carbohydrate intake increased postprandial glucose levels, insulin, triglycerides, and decreased HDL when compared to isocaloric high monounsaturated fat diets. However, high monounsaturated fat diets have not been shown to lower hemoglobin A1C values or have a beneficial effect on fasting plasma glucose. Hence these high monounsaturated fat diets may result in weight gain and increased energy intake in an uncontrolled setting.

An important concept to keep in mind is that nutritional therapy recommendations depend upon the metabolic profile and the need to lose weight. Saturated fat content along with its percentage of carbohydrates and monounsaturated fat should take into consideration culture and ethnic preferences.

It is important to keep the trans fatty acid and saturated fat content as low as possible when consuming a nutritionally adequate diet because neither of these substances has been shown to be of beneficial effect in preventing arteriosclerotic vascular disease and in fact have been shown to accelerate atherogenesis. Further, the polyunsaturated and monounsaturated fats reduce plasma cholesterol concentrations when they replace these fatty acids in the diet. Patients must ingest two types of polyunsaturated fatty acids, alpha-linolenic acid (an omega-3 fatty acid), and linolenic acid (an omega-6 fatty acid). The body is unable to synthesize these otherwise [24].

Dietary cholesterol has no role in preventing chronic disease and can enhance atherogenesis. Hence, intake should be as minimal as possible. The NCEP guidelines recommend an intake of less than 200 mg/day. There is evidence to suggest that diabetics are more sensitive to risks from increased dietary cholesterol intake with higher dietary cholesterol intake associated with an increased risk of coronary disease.

It is important for diabetics to be counseled about the importance of consuming adequate amounts minerals and vitamins from natural food sources, and to be aware of the potential toxic effect of mega doses of vitamin and mineral supplements. Interest in the antioxidant vitamins in people with diabetes has increased with the knowledge that diabetes may be a state of increased oxidative stress.

As of the present time, mega doses of dietary antioxidants like selenium, beta-carotene, vitamin E, and vitamin C have not demonstrated cardioprotection in diabetics and even in some clinical trials, such as the HOPE trial, have actually been shown to be inferior to certain medications particularly ACE inhibitors [25].

Oxidation is the removal of electrons from a molecule. This process can cause tissue damage by modifying lipids, proteins, and nucleic acids, leading to various diseases like arteriosclerosis and cancers.

Antioxidants significantly retard or inhibit this destructive oxidative process. Certain antioxidants are endogenous like ferritin, transferrin, and urate, while others are acquired.

Exogenous oxidants, like vitamins, E, A, and C, by counteracting oxidative damage, have stimulated research into their effects.

There have been various observation studies that report benefits from these vitamins. The problems with observational studies are:

1. Usually the people enrolled in these studies are non smokers, health conscious, exercise regularly, and limit fat intake.
2. These trials rely heavily on subjective data that is self reported and depends on 24 h recall.
3. Various diets and even supplements contain a variety of substances, making it irksome at times to sort out what specific nutrient is beneficial.
4. More often than not, when a double blinded randomized, placebo controlled trial is designed to prove the efficacy of these supplements, the beneficial effects are not demonstrated.

Some studies of merit are: [26]

1. The Iowa Women's Health Study – this evaluated the intake of various antioxidants vitamins found in foods and supplements to their relationship to coronary artery disease and overall mortality. This study evaluated close to 35,000 post-menopausal women (aged 55–69) with no history of cardiovascular disease for 7 years. Intake of vitamins A, E, and C were estimated by questionnaires and then correlated with plasma levels of beta carotene and vitamin E (alpha tocopherol). A high intake of vitamin E and not vitamin A or vitamin C protected against death from coronary artery disease [27].

2. The Rotterdam Study – This evaluated the relationship between dietary intake of beta carotene, vitamin C, and vitamin E in 4,800 people aged 55–95 with no history of myocardial infarction. This study demonstrated that beta carotene and not vitamin E or C was protective against myocardial infarction [28].

3. The Established Population for Epidemiologic Studies of the Elderly (EPESE) followed over 11,000 people aged 67–105 for 8–9 years to evaluate the effects of vitamins E and C on overall mortality and risk of death from coronary artery disease [29]. Here, vitamin E was associated with a reduced mortality due to coronary artery disease.

4. The Nurses' Health Study – This evaluated over 87,000 female nurses aged 34–59 with no cardiovascular disease or cancer, demonstrating that vitamin E supplementation for more than 2 years decreased the risk of coronary heart disease [30].

5. The Scottish Heart Health Study – This trial involved over 4,000 men and 3,800 women aged 40–59 with no history of heart disease to determine the effects of dietary and supplemental intake of vitamin C, beta carotene, and vitamin E on coronary artery disease. Vitamin E conferred no benefit here, although vitamin C and beta carotene reduced coronary artery disease events in men only [31].

6. The Finnish Study – This evaluated over 5,100 Finnish men and women aged 30–69 free of coronary disease and followed for 14 years to evaluate the effects of dietary beta carotene, vitamin C, and vitamin E on coronary mortality. Here, vitamin E conferred protection to both men and women with beta carotene and vitamin C conferring benefit in women only [32].

7. NHANES I – This evaluated over 11,300 US adults aged 25–74 for all cause mortality and cardiovascular disease with regard to intake of vitamin C. This showed a benefit from vitamin C in men, but not in women [33].

Although we can see that these studies showed some benefit from antioxidant use, especially vitamin E, the results were inconsistent. This data is to be contrasted with studies like the Heart Protection Study, the Primary Prevention Project, and the GISSI (Gruppo Italiano per lo Studio della Sopr11vivenza nell'Infarto Miocardico) study, which demonstrated no benefit from vitamin E. Data from the HATS (HDL Atherosclerosis Treatment Study) evaluated 160 men under age 63 and women under age 70 with established coronary artery disease and showed that vitamin E seemed to diminish the beneficial effect of simvastatin and niacin by blunting the HDL-2 elevations seen with niacin [34].

Both the Alpha Tocopherol Beta Carotene Cancer Prevention Study and the Beta Carotene and Retinal Efficacy trial showed that patients taking supplemental beta carotene had a statistically higher incidence of lung cancers and increased mortality compared to placebo [35].

The Cambridge Heart Antioxidant Study (CHAOS) evaluated over 2,000 patients with angiographically proven coronary artery disease. They received either 400 or 800 IU of vitamin E and although the number of cardiovascular deaths was not reduced, there were fewer nonfatal myocardial infarctions in those taking vitamin E [36].

The role of folate supplementation to lower homocysteine levels and subsequently reduce cardiovascular events is still not clear. However, the role of folate in preventing birth defects is widely accepted. Serum homocysteine levels are elevated in folate deficiency as well as B12, B6 deficiencies, renal insufficiency, hypovolemia, hypothyroidism, psoriasis, and inherited metabolic defects.

In obtaining homocysteine levels it is prudent to obtain methylmalonic acid levels, since 96% of B12 deficiency is associated with hyperhomocysteinemia and 98% of B12 deficiencies are associated with elevated methylmalonic acids levels.

Hyperhomocysteinemia is considered by many to be an independent risk factor for cardiovasucular disease and mortality, especially in women and diabetics. This topic will be discussed in greater detail in the chapter on risk reduction.

The intake of vitamins B1, B6, and B12 has not been established to be of benefit in the treatment of diabetic neuropathy and cannot be recommended based on clinical evidence.

The prevention of osteoporosis is important in older patients, particularly in female diabetics with a recommendation of 1,500 mg of elemental calcium daily. This amount can be reduced to 1,000 mg daily with concurrent bisphosphonate therapy.

Currently, a beneficial effect of nicotinamide to preserve beta cell mass in newly diagnosed type-1 diabetics is under investigation. Deficiencies of zinc and chromium may aggravate carbohydrate intolerance and benefits have recently been reported on glycemic control with chromium supplementation. There are, however, other studies raising the question of any benefit from chromium intake. Hence the benefit of chromium ingestion in the diabetic remains to be determined [36].

Interest in chromium was reported in the 1950s when Walter Mertz at the United States Department of Agriculture (USDA) published data indicating a benefit of chromium picolinate in lowering blood glucose [37].

Low chromium levels have been associated with impaired glucose tolerance and the beneficial effects have been thought by many to apply only to deficiency states. Chromium levels tend to decline with aging despite playing a role in regulating insulin dependent reactions, including glucose uptake, glucose storage, and glucose oxidation.

The USDA sponsored a study of 180 patients in China in 1997 showing that 200 μg of chromium picolinate daily lowered A1C from 8.5 to 7.5 and to 6.5% in those taking 1,000 μg. Cefalu found that 100 μg of chromium picolinate vs. placebo resulted in significant improvements in insulin sensitivity in both 4 and 8 month studies in obese, non diabetic, insulin resistant individuals, and not the placebo group [38].

Cefalu and others contend that chromium exerts stronger effects in obese vs. lean individuals based on rat models. Lydic and others also report benefit of chromium supplementation in polycystic ovary syndrome using the 100 μg dose [39].

Chromium appears to be well tolerated with no associated adverse effects reported in the CADRE summit reports at the 100 μg doses with no significant drug interactions.

The human body cannot synthesize chromium so it must be supplied through foods or supplements. Foods that contain chromium include apples, coffee, mushrooms, green beans, broccoli, bananas, wine, tea, cheese, brewer's yeast, and whole grain wheat bread.

Chromium picolinate has the highest bioavailabilty of the supplements available.

Chromium appears to exert its effects at the cellular level by influencing phosphorylation of tyrosine kinase. It may do so by both inhibiting protein tyrosine phosphatase and directly enhancing tyrosine phosphorylation, along with GLUT-4 activity, enhancing glucose uptake and metabolism in skeletal muscle [40].

A number of other nutritional supplements have been touted as beneficial in managing insulin resistance these include:

1. Omega-3 fatty acids – Daily intake of 1,500–4,000 mg of eicosapentaenoic acid (EPA) and 1,000–2,000 mg of docosahexaenoic acid (DHA) have been shown to improve insulin sensitivity in skeletal muscle, reducing fasting glucose, and improving lipids.
2. Magnesium – daily intake of 200–400 mg has been reported by some to improve insulin receptor function and glucose transport.
3. Vanadium – This element has been reported to be an insulin signal enhancer, increasing movement of GLUT-4 to the surface of the cell when given in doses of 15–50 mg.
4. l-arginine – This has been reported to improve insulin sensitivity and stimulate nitric oxide production at 200 mg daily which can enhance endothelial functioning.
5. Alpha Lipoic Acid – This has been shown to be of some benefit in managing diabetic peripheral neuropathy and enhancing insulin sensitivity. This natural coenzyme reduces oxidative stress and has a significant body of data to support its use – particularly in diabetic neuropathy. Some evidence indicates that this botanical may block the activation of NF-kappa B, a stress activated and redox sensitive transcription factor. When given intravenously, it has been shown to increase insulin sensitivity with oral administration of 1,200 mg daily showing reductions in fructosamine levels in a 12-week study by 15% in 15 patients. Recommended dose is 600–1,800 mg daily in divided doses.
6. Selenium – A randomized clinical trial published in the *Annals of Internal Medicine* by Severio Stranges and others tested the efficacy of selenium supplementation (200 µg daily) in preventing type-2 diabetes. This was based on animal data indicating that supplementation of this antioxidant may exert beneficial effects on glucose metabolism and may even delay or prevent the disease and its complications. This clinical trial, however, not only found that selenium supplementation did not prevent type-2 diabetes, but may increase risk for the disease [41].

Further clinical investigation and trials need to be done to determine any official recommendations or endorsements by the ADA for any of these supplements.

Reports of the hypoglycemic effects of sodium salicylate on older diabetic patients have existed for decades. With recent data indicating an important role for inflammation in the pathogenesis of type 2 diabetes and the role of the transcription nuclear factor kappa-B, agents like sodium salicylate, which inhibits this nuclear factor have received more attention in achieving glycemic control. The TINSAL-T2D (Targeting Inflammation using Salsalate in type-2 Diabetes) trial evaluated the efficacy of this generic product in a small cohort of 81 patients who showed that salsalte lowered A1C by 0.5% from baseline over 14 weeks. The small cohort size and short treatment period requires further study before any recommendations can be made [42].

While herbal medicines have been touted they cannot compete with standard pharmaceuticals for type-2 diabetes. Interestingly metformin was originally derived from *Galega officinalis* (Goat's Rue) [43]. Some herbals of note include:

1. Panax Ginseng – When taken 30–40 min prior to a meal, 1–3 g of Panax ginseng can slow absorption and digestion of carbohydrates. An aqueous extract of ginseng root has

been shown to produce hypoglycemia in diabetic animals and glucose loaded healthy animals by inducing glucose transporter production in the liver, increasing polypeptide interaction with adrenergic receptors, and enhancing insulin biosynthesis. Polysaccharides in ginseng have also been shown to enhance tissue glucose uptake and decrease hepatic gluconeogenesis. In a placebo controlled 8 week clinical study, 200 mg of ginseng resulted in decreased blood glucose and glycated hemoglobin compared to placebo. Diabetic patients should use ginseng with caution due to increased risk of central nervous system (CNS) effects including difficulty concentrating, insomnia, manic-like symptoms, tremulousness, and hypoglycemic effects. In addition, this herb can inhibit warfarin, decrease the potency of the loop diuretics, falsely elevate digoxin serum assays or directly increase digoxin levels, and increase plasma levels of nifedipine by inhibiting its metabolism. The usual dose is 100–200 mg daily.

2. Gurmar (*Gymnema sylvestre*) – The Indian word, gurmar means "sugar destroyer." This stimulates insulin secretion from the pancreas without affecting insulin sensitivity. It may also decrease glucose absorption in the intestine, and stimulate beta cell proliferation and function. In two small studies, Gymnema leaves reduced A1C values in both type-1 and type-2 diabetics from 12.8% to 8.25% and 11.5% to 8.55%, respectively, with type-1 diabetics reducing their insulin doses by a mean of 15 U and type-2 diabetics able to discontinue their sulfonylureas. The recommended dose is 400–600 mg daily.

3. Bitter Melon (*Momordica charantia*) – This medicinal plant contains a substance called polypeptide P which reportedly has an insulin like activity, promoting glycogen synthesis, increasing both hepatic glucose uptake and glucose transporter proteins in muscles, which reduces insulin resistance. The largest study conducted with this botanical agent included 100 type-2 diabetic patients with average fasting glucose levels of 160 mg/dl. Following an ingestion of a 75-g glucose load and an aqueous suspension of bitter melon, glucose levels rose to 222 mg/dl compared to previous day control levels of 257 mg/dl. This is available as a liquid and given in capsule form, with one to two capsules (5–15 cc of liquid) 3 times daily being the suggested dose.

4. Fenugreek (*Trigonella foenum-graecum*) – The seeds of this medicinal plant contain trigonelline, nicotinic acid, and coumarin, which reportedly can lower glucose, cholesterol, triglycerides, and raise HDL. This herb can reduce blood glucose in type-1 or type-2 diabetics by enhancing insulin sensitivity. This should be used with extreme caution in patients with peanut allergies and may interact with other anticoagulants and botanicals (like ginger and *Ginkgo biloba*). Ten to hundred grams daily is the recommended dose.

5. Garlic (*Allium sativum*) – This contains allicin (S-allyl cysteine sulfoxide), which is reported to enhance insulin activity through its effects on receptor sites. One needs to ingest 4 g of fresh garlic daily or 200–400 mg in the encapsulated form.

6. Onion (*Allium cepa*) – S-methyl cysteine sulfoxide is responsible for the glucose lowering effect, by stimulating insulin secretion from the pancreas. The usual dose is 400 mg daily.

7. Nopal – This is also known as "prickly pear." This member of the cactus family is believed to decrease glucose absorption and enhance insulin sensitivity when eaten cooked. It appears to exert its major effect on postprandial glucose. In a study published in *Diabetes Care* in 1990, Nopal combined with a sulfonylurea produced a 41-mg/dl reduction in glucose in 3 h compared to placebo.

8. Cinnamon – The active ingredient, hydroxychalcone, increases glucose uptake and glycogen synthesis by increasing insulin sensitivity. In a randomized trial published in diabetes care in 2003, 60 patients with type-2 diabetes were given cinnamon 4 times daily in 1, 3, and 6 g doses. Statistically significant reductions in fasting blood glucoses were observed at all doses, with reductions from 209 to 157 mg/dl with 1 g, 205–169 mg/dl with 2 g, and 234–166 mg/dl with the 6 g dose. A meta-analysis in 2008 published in the journal, *Diabetes Care* revealed no significant effect of cinnamon on A1C, fasting glucose, or lipid levels. The recommended usage is ½ to one teaspoonful of ground cinnamon daily on food or cereal.

9. Milk Thistle – The active ingredient in this member of the aster family is silymarin, which possesses antioxidant and liver protecting properties. This product was studied in 1997 in a review in the *Journal of Hepatology* in which 60 patients with type-2 diabetes and cirrhosis were randomized to placebo or 600 mg daily of silymarin. Fasting glucose dropped significantly from 190 to 165 mg/dl at 12 months with a reduction in A1C from 7.9 to 7.2% and decreased insulin dosage from 55 to 45 U daily.

10. Aloe – The high fiber content of the gel component may be responsible for its glucose lowering capability in both type-1 and type-2 diabetics. Only limited data support its use with the dose ranging from 50 to 200 mg daily of the gel form, since the juice form is a potent laxative.

Other herbs that have been reported to potentially lower blood glucose include guayusa (*Ilex guayusa*), cultivated mushroom (*Agaricus bisporus*), shiitake mushroom (*Lentinus edodes*), and blueberry leaf (*Vaccinium myrtillus*) for insulin dependent diabetes. While European mistletoe (*Viscum album*), maitake mushroom (*Grifola frondosa*) have been shown to be effective in insulin dependent diabetes.

Green tea contains flavonoids which are catechin related compounds that exert a protective effect on pancreatic beta cells, but do not induce their regeneration. Catechins have also been shown to have an inhibitory effect on intestinal glucose transporters, decreasing glucose absorption, while also upregulating glycogenesis and downregulating glycogenolysis. Caffeine intake from coffee, black tea, green tea, and oolong tea was associated with a lower risk for self reported type-2 diabetes in a clinical trial of 17,413 Japanese adults (10,686 women) published in the *Annals of Internal Medicine* in 2006. Of interest is the presence of catechins or flavonoids in red table wines, dark chocolates, and black grapes [44]. The possibility of cardiovascular benefits in consuming these substances has received considerable attention recently.

Flavonoids are very potent compounds and intake should be restricted to only foods and not supplements. Two reports have linked a high intake of flaveonoids to increased risk of fetal gene damage and risks for leukemia in infants.

Flavonoids in cocoa powder and dark chocolate reduced low density lipoprotein oxidative susceptibility as well as prostaglandin levels in some studies, but the clinical importance or relevance of this effect is not known. Flavonoid rich cocoa as well as black grapes seem to have antiplatelet effects and delay clotting time. Purple grape juice and tea have been shown to significantly increase brachial artery dilatation in patients with cardiovascular disease [26].

Most recently the antioxidant effect of flavonoids and other polyphenols have been of interest, particularly their role in cancer prevention and inhibition of oxidation of low density lipoproteins. Moderate ingestion of tea has been shown in some studies to protect against cancer, cardiovascular disease, and kidney stones. The flavonoid content of herbal teas is much lower that the green teas. The consumption of one to two cups of tea daily has been associated with a decreased mortality from stroke in men by 50% and from cancers of the mouth, pancreas, colon, esophagus, skin, lung prostate, and bladder by 20–40%. These data, however, reflect association rather than direct causation. Hence it is not prudent at the present time to officially recommend the consumption of large amounts of phenolics in foods or supplements without further convincing data. Clinical trials currently in progress may help to clarify some of these intriguing therapeutic possibilities.

Currently none of these herbs have the endorsement of the ADA and need more clinical based evidence before achieving that plateau with published data, even in reputable journals involving small cohorts. The list is supplied here as a guideline and source of information for physician when being asked about these substances, while giving some insight into their potential for drug-herb interactions – particularly hypoglycemia.

The same precautions regarding the use of alcohol that apply to the general population are applicable in the diabetic. Women during pregnancy and patients with advanced neuropathy, severe hypertriglyceridemia, history of alcohol abuse, or pancreatitis should abstain from alcohol ingestion. Alcohol has been shown to have both hyper and hypoglycemic effects in people with diabetes. This depends largely on the amount of alcohol acutely ingested, whether the use is chronic or excessive and binged and whether food is concomitantly consumed. Some clinical trials have suggested that light to moderate alcohol ingestion may be associated with increased insulin sensitivity and decreased risk for coronary disease.

Although a strong association exists between chronic excessive intake of alcohol and blood pressure in men and women when the intake is greater than 30–60 g/day, light to moderate amounts of alcohol (2–4 oz of 100% alcohol or its equivalent daily) do not raise blood pressure. If individuals choose to drink alcohol, daily intake should be limited to one drink for adult women and two adult men with portions limited to 1.5 oz of distilled spirits, 5 oz of wine, and 12 oz of beer. Ideally the alcohol should be ingested with food to avoid the risk of hypoglycemia. The risk of developing type-2 diabetes may be modified by moderate alcohol consumption with reduction in cardiovascular outcomes compared to nondrinkers. This risk reduction may be related to an increase in insulin sensitivity and adiponectin concentrations, and thus reduced adipocyte inflammation. Alcohol ingestion has also been shown to reduce hepatic glucose production and growth hormone release in the early morning hours abolishing the dawn phenomenon in insulin dependent diabetics,

Table 2
Basic nutrition principles

Medical nutrition therapy should be individualized according to the metabolic profile, desired goals, and clinical outcomes in accordance with the usual dietary habits of the patient

Regular monitoring of glucose, A1C, lipids, blood pressure, renal function, body weight, and quality of life are crucial to assess the ongoing needs of the patient and ensure successful outcomes

Family members of individuals with type-2 diabetes should be encouraged to engage in regular physical activity and dietary management to decrease their risk of developing the disease

From American Diabetes Association [46]

while increasing hepatic insulin sensitivity and inhibiting lipolysis by blocking free fatty acid release from adipose tissue.

In summary, nutrition in the treatment of diabetes is intended to stabilize blood sugar levels, prevent secondary disease including micro and macrovascular disease, stabilize body weight, and improve overall health by maintaining sound nutritional status. These nutritional principals include the reduction of fat to prevent cardiovascular disease and control of carbohydrate and protein along with total caloric intakes to regulate weight and glycemia.

These general goals can be achieved by avoiding foods high in sugar such as honey, desserts, candy, soft drinks and pies, as well as avoiding the fatty foods, saturated fats, dairy products, lunch meats, and cheese. Foods should be consumed at regular intervals, avoiding meal skipping and irregular dietary habits with ingestion of fish and lean meats in moderation and consumption of high fiber foods including vegetables, cereals, dried beans, and whole grains.

Diet plays a major role in regulating fat, protein, and carbohydrate homeostasis in patients with diabetes. Unfortunately most physicians do not have the time or the knowledge to develop an individualized diet plan for each patient. Hence the importance of certified diabetic educators and dietitians are critical in formulating plans and cooperating with the physician for achieving goals and utilizing the basic nutrition principles outlined in Table 2. Full utilization and cooperation with these trained professionals has proven to be invaluable in helping patients achieve their dietary goals.

REFERENCES

1. Anderson JW. Nutritional management of diabetes mellitus. Modern nutrition in health and disease, 9th ed. Baltimore: Williams & Wilkins; 1999:1365.
2. Blackburn G, Waltman B. Physician's guide to the new 2005 dietary guidelines: how best to counsel patients. Cleve Clin J Med. 2005; 72(7):609–618.
3. Foster GD, et al. A randomized trial of a low carbohydrate diet for obesity. N Engl J Med. 2003; 348:208202090.
4. Finkelstein EA, Ruhm CJ, Kosa KM. Economic causes and consequences of obesity. Annu Rev Public Health. 2005; 26:239–257.
5. Hodge AM, English DR, O'Dea R, Gilkes GG. Glycemic index and dietary fiber and the risk of type-2 diabetes. Diabetes Care. 2004; 27:2701–2706.
6. Jenkins D, Kendall C, McKeown-Eyssen G, Josse R. Effect of a Low glycemic Index or a High Cereal Fiber Diet on Type-2 Diabetes. JAMA. 2008; 300(23):2742–2753.
7. Tuttle K, Milton J. The Eco Atkins diet. Arch Intern Med. 2009; 169(11):1027.
8. Nathan DM, Buse JB, Davidson MB, Heine RJ, Holman RR. Management of hyperglycemia in type-2 diabetes: A consensus algorithm for the initiation and adjustment of therapy: a consensus statement from the American Diabetes Association and the European Association for the Study of Diabetes. Diabetes Care. 2006; 29:1963–1972.
9. Samaha FF, et al. A low carbohydrate as compared with a low fat diet in severe obesity. N Engl J Med. 2003; 348:2074–2081.
10. Corella D, Peloso G, Arnett D. APOA2, dietary fat and body mass index. Arch Intern Med. 2009; 169(20):1897–1906.
11. Gardner C, Kiazand A, Sofiya A, Kim S. Comparison of the Atkins, Zone, Ornish, and LEARN diets for change in weight and related risk factors among overweight Premenopausal Women. JAMA. 2007; 297(9):969–977.
12. Samaha FF, Iqbal N, Seshadri P, Cicano KL. A low carbohydrate diet as compared to a low fat diet in severe obesity. N Engl J Med. 2003; 348(21):2074–2081.

13. Ludwig DS. The glycemic index: physiological mechanisms relating to obesity, diabetes, and cardiovascular disease. JAMA. 2002; 287:2414–2423.
14. Hooper L, Thompson RL, Harrison RA. Omega 3 fatty acids for prevention and treatment of cardiovascular disease. Cochrane Database Syst Rev. 2004;(4):CD003177.
15. Baraona E, et al. Pathogenesis of alcoholic hypertriglyceridemia and hypercholesterolemia. Trans Assoc Am Physicians. 1983; 96:306–315.
16. Daviglus ML, Stamler J, Orencia AJ. Fish consumption and 30 year risk of fatal myocardial infarction. N Engl J Med. 1997; 336(15):1046–1053.
17. Hu F, Bronner L, Willett W. Fish and omega-3 fatty acid intake and risk of coronary artery disease in women. JAMA. 2002; 87(14):1815–1821.
18. Burr ML, Fehily M, Rogers S, Welsby E. Diet and re-infarction trial (DART). Eur Heart J. 1989; 10(6):558–567.
19. Marchioli R, Valagussa F. GISSI-Prevention trial. Eur Heart J. 2000; 20(12):949–952.
20. Meigs JB, Mittleman MA, et al. Hyperinsulinemia, hyperglycemia, and impaired hemostasis. The Framingham Offspring Study. JAMA. 2000; 238:221–228.
21. Hu F. Fish, omega-3 fatty acid intake and CHD risk in diabetic women. Cardiology Review. 2004; 21(1).
22. Harper CR, et al. The fats of life: the role of omega-3 fatty acids in the prevention of coronary heart disease. Arch Intern Med. 2001; 161:2185–2192.
23. Saydah SH, Loria CM, et al. Subclinical states of glucose intolerance and risk of death in the U.S. Diabetes Care. 2001; 24:447–453.
24. Atkinson RI, et al. Effects of calorie restriction and weight loss on glucose and insulin levels in obese humans. J Am Coll Nutr. 1985;4:411–419.
25. The Heart Outcomes Prevention Evaluation Study Investigators. Vitamin E supplementation and cardiovascular events in high risk patients. N Engl J Med. 2000; 342:154–160.
26. Young IS. Antioxidants in health and disease. Clin Pathol. 2001; 54:176–186.
27. Kushi LH, Folsom AR, Prineas RD, Mink PJ, Wu Y. Dietary antioxidant vitamins and death from coronary artery disease in postmenopausal women. N Engl J Med. 1996; 334:1156–1162.
28. Klipstein-Grobusch K, Geleijnse JM, den Breejen JH. Dietary antioxidants and the risk of myocardial infarction in the elderly: the Rotterdam study. Am J Clin Nutr. 1999; 69:261–266.
29. Losonczy KG, Harris TB, Havlik RJ. Vitamin E and vitamin supplement use and risk of all cause and coronary heart diseases mortality in older persons: the Established Populations for Epidemiologic Studies of the Elderly. Am J Clin Nutr. 1996; 64:190–196.
30. Mantzoros CS, Williams CJ, Manson JE, Meigs JB, Hu FB. Adherence to the Mediterranean dietary pattern is positively associated with plasma adiponectin concentrations in diabetic women. Am J Clin Nutr. 2006; 84:328–335.
31. Tribble DL. AHA Science Advisory. Antioxidant consumption and risk of coronary heart disease: emphasis on vitamin C, vitamin E, and beta-carotene. Circulation. 1999; 99:591–595.
32. Knekt P, Reunanen A, Jarvinen R. Antioxidant vitamin intake and coronary mortality in a longitudinal population study. Am J Epidemiol. 1994; 139:1180–1189.
33. Enstrom JE, Kanim LE, Klein MA. Vitamin C intake and mortality among a sample of the United States population. Epidemiology. 1991; 3:194–202.
34. Shepherd J. Raising HDL and lowering CHD risk: does intervention work? Eur Heart J Suppl. 2005; 7(suppl F):F15–F22.
35. The ATBC Study Group. The alpha-tocopherol beta carotene lung cancer prevention study. Ann Epidemiol. 1994; 4(1):1–10.
36. Stephens NG, et al. Randomized, controlled trial of Vitamin E in patients with coronary artery disease. Cambridge Heart Antioxidant Study. Lancet. 1996; 347:781–786.
37. Anderson RA. Chromium metabolism and its role in disease processes in man. Clin Physiol Biochem. 1986; 4:31–41.
38. Cefalu WT. Improvements in fasting insulin levels and glucose tolerance in chromium treated corpulent rats. J Nutr. 2002; 132:1107–1114.
39. Gulland J. Growing evidence supports role of chromium in prevention treatment of diabetes. Hollistic Primary Care. 2003; 4:8.

40. Vivekananthan DP, et al. Use of antioxidant vitamins for the prevention of cardiovascular disease: meta-analysis of randomized trials. Lancet. 2003; 361:2017–2023.
41. Stranges S, Marshall JR, Natarajan R, Donahue R. Effects of long term selenium supplementation on the incidence of type-2 diabetes. Ann Intern Med. 2007; 147:217–223.
42. Chen J. Salsalate seems effective for type-2 diabetes; the TINSAL-T2D trial. Ann Intern Med. 2010; 152:346–357.
43. Bremness L. HERBS. Mifflin Company, Boston; 1994.
44. Iso H, Date C, Wakal K. The relationship between green tea and total caffeine intake and risk for self reported type-2 diabetes among Japanese adults. Ann Intern Med. 2006; 144:554–562.
45. Franz M. Diabetes: nutrition recommendations for 2002. Pract Diabet. 2002; 19:15–18.
46. American Diabetes Association. Evidence based nutrition principles and recommendations for the treatment and prevention of diabetes and related complications. Diabetes Care. 2002; 25:S50–S55.

SUPPLEMENTARY READINGS

Atkins RC. Dr. Atkins' New Diet Revolution. New York: Avon Books; 1998.
Blumenthal M, et al. Herbal Medicine. Integrative Medicine Communications, Newton; 2000.
Bonow RO. Diet, obesity and cardiovascular risk. N Engl J Med. 2003; 348:2082–2090.
Diabetes Prevention Research Group. Reduction in the evidence of type 2 diabetes with life style intervention or metformin. N Engl J Med. 2002; 346:393–403.
Halliwell B, et al. Free radicals in biology and medicine, 2nd ed. Oxford: Clarendon Press; 1989.
Hasnain B, et al. Recent trials of antioxidant therapy: what should we be telling our patients? Cleve Clin J Med. 2004; 71(4):327–334.
Rotbaltt M, et al. Evidence based herbal medicine. Hanley & Belfus, Philadelphia; 2001.
Tuomilehto J, et al. Prevention of type 2 diabetes mellitus by changes in lifestyle among subjects with impaired glucose tolerance. N Engl J Med. 2001; 344:1343–1350.
Weber P, et al. Vitamin E and human health: rationale for determining recommended intake levels. Nutrition. 1997; 13:450–460.
Yanovski SZ, et al. Obesity. N Engl J Med. 2002;346:591–602.

5   Obesity and the Metabolic Syndrome

Key Words: The Metabolic syndrome, Obesity, Weight reduction, Body measurement, The National Cholesterol Program-Adult Treatment Panel (NCEP)

INTRODUCTION

The clustering of abnormal laboratory test data and body measurements, listed in Table 1, encompassing parameters that should be measured on a regular basis in physician offices, collectively referred to as "The Metabolic Syndrome" represents an important risk stratification determination with its awareness and applicability to primary care increasing worldwide. A recent review found that greater than 66% of physicians consider this syndrome in the diagnosis, treatment, and management of their patients. These physicians felt that greater than 20% of their patients had metabolic syndrome with over 94% of physicians expecting patients diagnosed with metabolic syndrome to increase within the near future [1].

This heightened awareness reflects both the increased amount of medical literature supporting this syndrome as well as the obesity problem not only in the USA, but worldwide. In the past several decades obesity has reached almost epidemic proportions in the USA especially among children, adolescents, and young adults.

The prevalence of obesity is increased among non-Hispanic, African American, and Mexican American women especially. Various environmental, cultural, genetic, and behavioral factors have been identified as causative agents in this regard. Obesity is, of course, a great public health concern because it is directly related to the development of diabetes, hypertension, osteoarthritic changes, and ultimately congestive heart failure.

From: *Current Clinical Practice: Type 2 Diabetes, Pre-Diabetes, and the Metabolic Syndrome*
Edited by: R.A. Codario, DOI 10.1007/978-1-60327-441-8_5
© Springer Science+Business Media, LLC 2011

Table 1
Criteria for diagnosing metabolic syndrome

Waist circumference

>35 in. (88 cm) in women

>40 in. (102 cm) in men

Triglycerides

>150 mg/dl

HDL

<40 mg/dl in men

<50 mg/dl in women

Blood pressure

>130/85 mmHg or treated hypertension

Fasting glucose

>100 mg/dl

From NCEP ATP III [74] and Genuth [75]
Three of five of these conditions is diagnostic

Various types of classification systems have been used to determine weight. However, regardless of the system used, overweight children often become overweight adults and therefore more likely to experience the problems associated with this condition including higher morbidity and mortality.

THE METABOLIC SYNDROME

The National Cholesterol Program-Adult Treatment Panel (NCEP-ATP III) guidelines indicate that the metabolic syndrome may be diagnosed when a patient has three or more of five clinically identifiable risk factors. These five factors include:

1. Abdominal obesity with a waist circumference in men greater than 102 cm (40″) and for women, greater than 88 cm (35″).
2. Triglyceride count equal to or greater than 150 mg/dl.
3. HDL level less than 40 mg/dl in men and 50 mg/dl in women.
4. Blood pressure equal to or greater than 130/85 mmHg.
5. Fasting blood glucose equal to or greater than 100 mg/dl.

The metabolic syndrome and obesity are increasing in epidemic proportions worldwide [2]. The metabolic syndrome has been associated with various names since being originally described by Reaven [3]. These names include:

1. Diabesity
2. Syndrome X
3. Deadly quartet
4. Deadly pentad disease
5. Dysmetabolic syndrome

6. Polymetabolic syndrome
7. Coronary risk syndrome
8. Insulin resistance syndrome
9. Atherothrombogenic syndrome
10. Hormonal metabolic syndrome
11. Hyperinsulinemia/insulin resistance syndrome
12. Dyslipidemic hypertension
13. Obesity/insulin resistance syndrome
14. Vascular multi-risk metabolic syndrome
15. Metabolic cardiovascular risk syndrome
16. Metabolic and hemodynamic disorder syndrome.

At the central core of this syndrome is insulin resistance, which is associated with

1. Obesity
2. Advanced age
3. Sedentary life style
4. Genetic inheritance
5. Hyperglycemia
6. Impaired glucose tolerance
7. Hyperinsulinemia
8. Altered fibrinolysis
9. Hypertension
10. Decreased HDL
11. Increased triglycerides and
12. Increase in small dense LDL

According to data in the *Journal of American Medical Association*, it is estimated that 47 million have metabolic syndrome with the incidence of the syndrome arising progressively as individuals begin to age, reaching a peak between the ages of 60–69 [4], with the prevalence increasing from 10% in the 30–39 year age group to 45% in the 60–69 year age group [5].

There is also a significant degree of association of the individual components of this syndrome with enhanced cardiovascular morbidity and mortality, and type-2 diabetes with reversal of these abnormalities being associated with attenuation in risk.

Univariate analyses of non-diabetic hypercholesterolemic Scottish men who met the ATP III criteria for the metabolic syndrome have demonstrated an increase in coronary heart disease by 76% and tripled the risk of developing type-2 diabetes [6].

In a study of 4,483 patients aged 35–70 years from Finland and Sweden, the prevalence of the metabolic syndrome increased in a stepwise fashion with progressive glucose intolerance, while cardiovascular mortality increased by 80% in those with metabolic syndrome, tripling the risk of coronary heart disease and doubling the risk of myocardial infarction and stroke [7].

Lakka evaluated the impact of metabolic syndrome on 2,682 middle aged Finnish men with no known cardiovascular disease or diabetes and found that death from coronary heart disease was 2.9–4.2 times more likely with the presence of the metabolic syndrome, doubling the risk of all cause mortality [8].

The San Antonio Heart Study evaluated 2,815 men and women over a 13-year period of time and found that deaths from cardiovascular disease were 2.53 times more likely in those with the metabolic syndrome with all cause mortality of 1.47.

Those within the group who did not have diabetes or cardiovascular disease (2,372 in total), death from cardiovascular disease was still doubled in those with the metabolic syndrome [9].

It is of particular interest to note that concomitant presence of the metabolic syndrome and diabetes enhances cardiovascular risk as shown in cross sectional data from the National Health and Nutrition Examination Survey (NHANES) III, which demonstrated that the prevalence of coronary heart disease was 7.55 in individuals greater than 50 years who had neither diabetes or the metabolic syndrome, but 19% in those with both the metabolic syndrome and diabetes [10].

The fact that multiple factors included within the metabolic syndrome cluster together and occur by coincidence pales in its comparison to its value as an important risk stratification strategy for all health care providers and patients alike.

Treatment of the syndrome consists primarily of three therapeutic strategies:

1. Weight loss and increased physical activity designed to reverse the direct causes of the condition.
2. Direct pharmacotherapy of the various risk factors including dyslipidemia, elevated blood pressure, the prothrombotic state, and concomitant insulin resistance.
3. Dietary management focusing not only on macronutrients with high protein and low cholesterol, saturated and trans fats along with caloric, sodium, and simple sugar restriction, but also emphasizing whole grains, fruits, and vegetables.

Significant benefit has been demonstrated in reducing cardiovascular risk with a pharmacologic modification of the risk factors, but clearly reversal of the root causes by weight reduction and physical activity is extremely important and critical to management of the condition.

Obesity represents a major component of the metabolic syndrome and has a significant association with insulin resistance. Clearly most individuals with a metabolic syndrome are overweight or frankly obese and indeed most people with insulin resistance have truncal obesity, and for these patients weight reduction must be the top priority. It is this truncal, central, visceral, or predominately upper body distribution of body fat that has a stronger association for cardiovascular disease than just being overweight or possessing an increased body/mass index [11]. Table 2 classifies obesity and outlines the increased cardiovascular risk associated with progressive weight gain. Clearly, the greater the weight, the greater are the medical risks.

The insulin resistance associated with this syndrome appears to be associated with abnormalities of and increases in fatty acid metabolism. Increased amounts of free fatty acids not only promote insulin resistance, but also elevation of blood pressure, reduction of high density lipoprotein levels and increased triglyceride concentration. The increased visceral obesity in these patients is associated with an increased release of free fatty acids into the portal blood, resulting in hepatic overproduction of triglycerides with subsequent diminished synthesis of high density lipoprotein cholesterol. Not to be overlooked is the fact that insulin resistance and subsequent free fatty acid elevations also contribute to pro-inflammatory, pro-adhesive, and pro-thrombotic states in addition to impaired glucose tolerance initiating, enhancing, and promoting atherogenesis, summarized in Table 3.

Table 2
Classification of overweight and obesity

| | *BMI* | *Class* | *Risk for diabetes, cardiovascular disease, hypertension* | |
| | | | *Waist circumference* | |
			Men <40" *Women <35"*	*Men >40"* *Women >35"*
Underweight	<18.5	–	–	–
Normal	18.5–24.5	–	–	–
Overweight	25.0–29.9	–	Increased	High
Obesity	30.0–34.9	I	High	Very high
	35.0–39.9	II	Very high	Very high
Extreme obesity	>39.9	III	Extremely high	

From Flegal et al. [76]

Table 3
Hypercoagulation/inflammation

Obesity promotes pro-inflammatory factors

Inflammation is a major contributor to atherogenesis

Pro-inflammatory and prothrombotic factors enhance cardiovascular risk

From Vega [28]

Metabolic syndrome has become such a risk for arteriosclerotic vascular disease that a strong support exists for elevating this to the coronary artery disease to an equivalent status indicating that an LDL of 100 mg/dl or less would be ideal to reduce risk in this population. Cardiovascular risk can be increased in the short-term for some patients and in the longer-term for others. The American Heart Association and the National Heart, Lung and Blood Institute scientific statement recommend targeting the specific components of the metabolic syndrome for drug therapy when 10 year absolute risks are high or moderately high with the Framingham risk scoring (FRS) to be used for those patients with no overt coronary artery disease or diabetes [12]. However, even the FRS can underestimate the severity of risk with the metabolic syndrome, especially women and patients under the age of 50 [13]. Hence ATP III concedes that "the presence of the metabolic syndrome provides the option to intensify LDL lowering therapy after LDL-cholesterol goals are set with the major risk factors" [14].

Due to the fact that the FRS may underestimate global cardiovascular risk in women, the Reynolds Risk Score has been developed. The score includes hs-CRP and family history (myocardial infarction before age 60 in either parent) in addition to the other parameters measured in the FRS [15].

Despite the fact that no formula or algorithm currently exists for calculating or measuring the risk for cardiovascular disease in patients with the Metabolic Syndrome, lipoprotein abnormalities, particularly low density lipoprotein particle numbers and other surrogate markers measure the risk of coronary artery disease. Although some have suggested that this syndrome is nothing more than the additive risks of the various components support, its evolution as an independent risk factor for cardiovascular disease is enhanced by published data.

A prospective Finnish trial of 1,209 men 42–60 years of age with no evidence of carcinoma, diabetes, or cardiovascular disease indicated that all cause mortality and cardiovascular disease risk was increased in those with the metabolic syndrome [16]. Individuals who experienced myocardial infarction have been shown to have a higher incidence of this syndrome in retrospective analyses. The Prospective Cardiovascular Munster (PROCAM) study showed that the coexistence of the syndrome with diabetes enhances cardiovascular and cerebrovascular risk [17]. Total LDL particle number can be significantly higher than one would expect by just measuring the LDL cholesterol level in these patients (according to data in the Framingham Offspring Study). The study also revealed that total small LDL particles were increased commensurately with the amount of metabolic syndrome risk factors. A retrospective analysis of the West of Scotland Study patient population showed that individuals with all five factors within the metabolic syndrome were almost 25 times more likely to develop diabetes and 3.6 times more likely to experience a cardiovascular event [18]. This data resemble follow-up studies from the Framingham Offspring Study, which showed that the clustering of risk factors within the metabolic syndrome increased coronary-heart-disease risk over time with men having three or more metabolic risk factors increasing their cardiac risk twofold, while women experience a fivefold increase. Surrogate markers of subclinical coronary artery disease include ankle-brachial indices, calcium scores of the coronary arteries, carotid intima-media thickness, two-dimensional echocardiography, and brachial artery reactivity evaluation.

According to ATP-III there are three categories of risk of arteriosclerotic vascular disease.

These include:

1. Underlying risk factors
    (a)   Obesity
    (b)   Sedentary life style
    (c)   Atherogenic diet
2. Major risk factors
    (a)   High LDL cholesterol
    (b)   Diabetes
    (c)   Smoking
    (d)   Low HDL cholesterol (<40 mg/dl)
    (e)   Hypertension (140/90 mmHg or on BP medication)
    (f)   Male gender
    (g)   Age >45 for men and >55 for women
    (h)   Family history of premature coronary artery disease in first degree relative (male <55 and female <65)
3. Emerging risk factors
    (a)   Metabolic syndrome
    (b)   Elevated triglycerides (>150 mg/dl)
    (c)   Elevated lipoprotein (a)

(d)   Elevated lipoprotein-associated phospholipase A2 (Lp-PLA2)
(e)   Elevated small, dense LDL
(f)   Elevated fibrinogen
(g)   Elevated homocysteine
(h)   Increased remnant lipoproteins
(i)   Increased high sensitivity CRP
(j)   Impaired fasting glucose (>100 and <125 mg/dl)
(k)   Elevated urine microalbumin/creatinine ratio
(l)   Increase carotid intimal thickening
(m)   Arteriosclerotic peripheral vascular disease
(n)   Increased coronary arterial calcification (CAC) measured by electron beam computerized tomography [19]

Rader and Szapary recommend the following guidelines for risk factor consideration [2].

1. The traditional factors are most important – Compelling clinical evidence now makes it clear that these traditional risk factors contribute to arteriosclerotic vascular disease and that correcting the abnormalities in these risk factors will reduce the risk of cardiovascular events. These factors must be corrected before giving great consideration to the other emerging factors, otherwise little benefit will accrue.
2. Emerging risk factors should never be used as a reason for diminishing or ignoring the risk conferred with abnormalities in the traditional risk factors. Therefore, physicians should not be less aggressive in their management of patients because the hs-CRP level or the CAC score is normal.
3. Emerging risk factors can increase risk – Recent data suggest that the presence of an elevated hs-CRP should lower LDL goals by as much as 30 mg/dl. In patients with moderate risk according to FRS, the presence of an elevated emerging risk factor may necessitate moving that patient into the high risk category.
4. These emerging risk factors should not be used to assess risk on a routine basis – The emphasis placed on these various factors may change depending upon new clinical data. At this time the ATP III views the use of emerging risk factors as an option only for selected individuals based on clinical judgment. These factors, however, should not be given stronger emphasis than the major risk factors.
5. These emerging risk factors should not generally be used as therapeutic targets, but aids to gauge prognosis. More clinical evidence is needed to endorse serial measurements of these factors. Even the Framingham score lacks scientific relevance with repeated calculations as does the hs-CRP [20]. Until outcomes data support a direct relationship in this regard, the relevance of repeatedly evaluating factors in this class remains to be elucidated.

It behooves the physician to heighten awareness to the presence of metabolic syndrome and aggressively reduce risk factors in this patient population. Even though FRS may underestimate risk in this patient population, it still remains an indispensable modality, with intensive LDL lowering therapy critical even after lipid goals are achieved.

Some of the emerging or what Szapary and Rader refer to as "advanced" laboratory tests are the hs-CRP, homocysteine, lipoprotein (a), lipoprotein associated phospholipase A2, vertical analysis profile or VAP testing including quantifying small, dense, and large buoyant LDL and fibrinogen.

Elevations of one or more of these factors might warrant more aggressive treatment in selected patients at risk. For example, clinical trials for 27,393 women published in the *New England Journal of Medicine* have shown that, when followed for an 8 year period, patients with a high hs-CRP and a low LDL were at greater risk for vascular disease than those with a high LDL and a low hs-CRP. Greatest risk existed for those with a low hs-CRP and low LDL [21].

The American Heart Association and the Centers for Disease Control have issued a statement on the use of hs-CRP and other inflammatory markers. Their recommendation for evaluations and treatment in the primary prevention setting is that the current weight of evidence supports consideration for the measurement of hs-CRP in patients at moderate risk according to the Framingham score (10–20%). Although acknowledging that hs-CRP is an independent risk factor, they did not recommend using other inflammatory markers [22].

The current recommendation is that an elevated hs-CRP places a patient at risk for a vascular event and not to be used in a serial way to gauge progress or prognosis. Those individuals with hs-CRP levels greater than 10 mg/l should merit a search for other inflammatory causes like inflammatory bowel disease, arthritis, collagen vascular disease, vasculitis, etc.

Non invasive methods of evaluating arteriosclerosis are useful in detecting subclinical evidence of disease which may warrant changing a patient's status from primary prevention to secondary prevention, which can affect the aggressiveness of therapy.

The primary noninvasive test available is the ultrasound and Doppler examination along with the ankle brachial index (ABI). This test can be used to evaluate peripheral arterial disease. The ABI measures the ratio between blood pressure in the ankles and the arm. ABIs less than 0.90 are diagnostic of peripheral arterial disease, which is a known coronary artery risk equivalent, while ABIs greater than 1.5 are indicative of an increased risk for cardiovascular disease. Reduced ABI readings (<0.90), even in asymptomatic patients, would justify starting statin therapy and targeting an LDL of <100 mg/dl.

Increases in carotid intimal thickening have been associated with coronary arteriosclerotic disease. The NCEP currently recognizes carotid artery disease as a coronary artery risk equivalent [23].

EBT scores >100 have reasonable test characteristics for angiographically proven coronary artery disease with a specificity of 77% and sensitivity of 89%. This also correlates with CAD mortality as well. The AHA position statement conceded that elevated CAC scores in intermediate risk patients could help guide medical therapy. Addition of CAC scores to prediction models based on traditional risk factors can improve risk classification. A recent prospective study in Circulation showed that CAC scoring combined with FRS added substantially to global risk prediction when CAC scores are greater than 100 in subjects with an FRS >10% [24].

Lipid abnormalities associated with metabolic syndrome include low HDL cholesterol, elevated triglycerides, and a predominance of small dense low density lipoprotein or LDL particles. The predominance of small, dense LDL instead of large buoyant LDL also confers increased risk. This is not to say that large, buoyant LDL is not atherogenic, but that the smaller, dense LDL molecule is more atherogenic [25].

Elevated serum triglyceride levels represent an independent risk factor for coronary heart disease especially in women. Triglyceride levels greater than 500 mg/dl are associated with an increased risk of pancreatitis. Excessive alcohol intake, high carbohydrate diets greater than 60% of the total calories, diabetes, genetic disorders, physical inactivity, obesity, overweight status, and certain medications like estrogens, beta blockers, thiazide diuretics, anti-retroviral agents, and steroids may also raise triglyceride levels.

Interestingly, recent reports indicate that patients taking olanzapine for schizophrenia may be at increased risk for developing metabolic syndrome. This study found that the risk for metabolic syndrome was increased by almost 20% for schizophrenic patients taking this drug [26].

Drug therapy in addition to life style changes is often necessary in patients with triglycerides greater than 200 mg/dl and should be strongly considered even with triglycerides greater than 150 mg/dl particularly if the HDL is lower than normal or if the triglyceride/HDL ratio is greater than 4:1. Insulin resistance begins to increase significantly when this ratio is exceeded as does the likelihood of producing more atherogenic small, dense LDL cholesterol. The fibrates as a class including gemfibrozil and fenofibrate have been extremely effective in reducing triglyceride levels [27]. Omega-3 fatty acids have also shown to be efficacious in this regard as well as the thiazolidinediones (pioglitazone) [13].

Individuals with hypertriglyceridemia often have elevations in their non HDL cholesterol levels as well. The non HDL cholesterol is equal to the sum of the low density lipoprotein (LDL) plus the very low density lipoprotein (VLDL) and is also equal to the total cholesterol level minus the level of the HDL.

Many feel that the non HDL cholesterol is just as important a parameter (maybe even more important) than the LDL, representing the atherogenic particles circulating in the blood stream and correlating well with apolipoprotein B levels. Normal levels of the non HDL cholesterol are 30 mg/dl greater than the LDL.

Niacin has also been shown to be efficacious in reducing triglyceride levels, with the extended release preparation associated with less side effects, smoother continuous drug delivery, and less hyperglycemic effects than its shorter acting (crystalline) or sustained release preparation which has been reported to cause irreversible hepatocellular injury.

Low HDL cholesterol levels now represent a strong and independent predictor of coronary heart disease. Low HDL cholesterol can be decreased by several factors associated with insulin resistance including type-2 diabetes, increased weight, cigarette smoking, physical inactivity, high carbohydrate consumption, elevated triglycerides, certain drugs such as anabolic steroids (particularly testosterone preparations), progesterone, and beta blockers [28].

In individuals with low HDL cholesterol levels, the first objective is to normalize the LDL cholesterol. Once the LDL cholesterol is at goal, which is less than 100 mg/dl for individuals with known coronary disease or any coronary artery disease equivalent (diabetes, abdominal aortic aneurysm, carotid atherosclerotic disease, peripheral vascular disease and soon the metabolic syndrome) and less than 130 in other individuals, the next step is to raise the HDL to desired levels (45 mg/dl in diabetic men and 44 mg/dl in diabetic women). If the triglycerides are elevated greater than 500 mg/dl then attention should be given to its reduction to minimize the risk of pancreatitis.

Ongoing Framingham data indicate that careful consideration must also be given to the ratio of the LDL cholesterol to the HDL cholesterol with levels greater than 2.0 being associated with increased risk, along with the ratio of the total cholesterol to the HDL – with ratios less than 4 being desirable.

Plasma triglyceride concentration (>130 mg/dl), the ratio of triglyceride to high density lipoprotein cholesterol (>3.0) and serum insulin levels (>109 pmol/l) may also be useful metabolic parameters in identifying insulin resistant individuals [29].

Clearly, type-2 diabetes is associated with a marked increase in the risk for coronary artery disease. Although the correlation between hyperglycemia and macrovascular disease is well established, the groundwork for this atherogenic disaster may be laid in the pre-diabetic state during which time macrovascular disease likely originates.

In the San Antonio Heart Study those individuals who started with normal glucose tolerance and later developed type-2 diabetes were noted to have increased triglycerides, systolic blood pressure, and decreased HDL before they developed diabetes [30]. Recently interest has focused on the role of impaired fibrinolysis and accelerated thrombogenesis to explain the subclinical inflammatory state associated with insulin resistance and the metabolic syndrome or the pre-diabetic state [31].

The Insulin Resistance Atherosclerosis Study (IRAS) found that insulin resistance is significantly associated with higher hs-CRP levels, higher fibrinogen, and higher plasminogen activator inhibitor-1 (PAI-1) levels. These elevated PAI-1 and CRP levels predict the development of type-2 diabetes. Pharmacologic therapeutic modalities designed to improve insulin sensitivity, like thiazolidinediones and metformin, have been shown to reduce elevations in these nontraditional risk factors [32].

Biguanides (metformin) improve insulin sensitivity at the hepatic level, whereas thiazolidinediones are more efficacious in improving insulin sensitivity in the peripheral adipose tissue. It has not yet been demonstrated that these drugs can decrease cardiovascular mortality and morbidity in patients with the metabolic syndrome. However, clinical trials are currently being conducted with the early results, particularly in the area of inflammatory markers, being very encouraging.

The thiazolidinediones directly target insulin resistance by stimulating peroxizome proliferator activated receptor (PPAR) alpha and gamma. Thiazolidinedione therapy has been shown to reduce the development of diabetes in patients in the TRIPOD trial of Hispanic gestational diabetics and to preserve beta cell function in certain animal models [33].

The Diabetes Prevention Trial showed that the therapeutic life style modification of diet along with exercise was more effective than metformin (61 vs. 38%) in delaying or preventing the development of diabetes [34]. Clinical trials such as RECORD (the Rosiglitazone Evaluation for Cardiac Outcomes and Regulation of Glycemia and Diabetes) and BARI-2D (Bypass Angioplasty Revascularization Intervention Type-2 Diabetes) study as well as the DREAM (Diabetes Reduction assessment with rosiglitazone and ramipril medication) and ADOPT (Avandia Diabetes Outcomes and Progression) trials have shed more light on the efficacies of these agents in terms of risk reduction which will be discussed in Chap. 14.

Recently adiponectin and TNF-alpha (tumor necrosis factor alpha) have been shown to play an important role in adipose tissue expression of cytokines like interleukin-6 and may be linked to development of tissue lipid accumulation and subsequent insulin resistance syndrome. It is known that adipose tissue secrets several cytokines including interleukin-6, leptin resistant adiponectin, and tumor necrosis factor. Previous studies have indicated that TNF-alpha secretion from the adipose tissue has been associated significantly with obesity-related reduction in insulin sensitivity [35]. Recent advances in clinical obesity research have demonstrated that adipose tissue functions as an endocrine organ producing a variety of secretins that subsequently affect vascular function, energy storage, insulin sensitivity, and appetite. A significantly greater proportion of free fatty acids are secreted with increasing intra-abdominal, pancreatic, and hepatic fat deposition along with pro-inflammatory adipokines including angiotensin-II [36].

Indeed, the development of the metabolic syndrome is associated with an unbalanced production of these pro-inflammatory molecules that play a significant role in insulin resistance, hypertension, and atherosclerosis. Adiponectin is the most prolific protein secreted by the adipocytes, improving endothelial function, inhibiting inflammation, decreasing hepatic glucose production, enhancing skeletal muscle glucose uptake, and inhibiting arterioosclerosis. This protein consists of 244 amino acids, similar in structure to complement C1Q and the TNS family as well as collagens 8 and 10. It is significantly expressed in the plasma and activates two receptors primarily located in the liver. Once activated, these receptors mediate endothelial function, glucose metabolism, and transport.

Hypoadiponectinemia is directly related to insulin resistance. Intraperitoneal adiponectin injections into rodents with type-1 and type-2 diabetes demonstrated significant reduction in plasma glucose levels while enhancing insulin secretion [37]. Its effects on plasma glucose appear to be mediated through an inhibition of hepatic glucose production by inhibiting gluconeogenesis, while suppressing glucose-6 phosphate and phosphoenol pyruvate carboxykinase expression. Its effects on insulin activity can also be seen by its suppressive effect on free fatty acid influx in the liver thereby playing a role inhibiting hepatocyte fatty degeneration and subsequent steatohepatitis.

A negative correlation exists between visceral fat and insulin resistance with adiponectin with its expression being reduced in diabetes, cardiovascular disease, and metabolic syndrome. Adiponectin levels tend to be higher in men than woman and increase with weight loss [38]. Inhibition of the renin-angiotensin-aldosterone system (RAAS) or the endocannabinoid receptor-1 system in humans increases circulating levels. Thiazolidinediones, by virtue of their PPAR-gamma agonist activity enhance adiponectin expression by two- to threefold not only in type-2 diabetics, but in non diabetics as well [39].

In addition to improving endothelial function, adiponectin has been shown to inhibit vascular smooth muscle cell proliferation, endothelial inflammation, and neointimal thickening, while reducing macrophage cholesterol ester formation. In the presence of vascular inflammation, plaque progression is enhanced causing plaque instability generating metabolic sequence of events leading to enhanced thrombosis and ultimately cardiovascular events.

Macrophages incubated with adiponectin demonstrated a dose dependent increase in interleukin-10 which is an anti-inflammatory cytokine, enhancing the production of the tissue inhibitor for metalloproteases.

By enhancing endothelial nitric oxide production, adiponectin may also play a role in blood pressure reduction. Hypoadiponectinemia is identified as a risk factor for the development of hypertension.

Interestingly in humans, adiponectin levels are decreased in obese patients, as well as those individuals with insulin resistance, and type-2 diabetes. More obese individuals show lower adiponectin levels than normal weight individuals. The expression of adiponectin from adipose tissue appears to be significantly higher in lean subjects and women and further levels of adiponectin are associated with higher degrees of insulin sensitivity and lower TNF-alpha expression. The prothrombotic state associated with increased thrombotic activity and decreased fibrinolytic activity reflected by increased concentration and activity of coagulation factors along with an overexpression of plasminogen activator inhibitor are all hallmarks of the metabolic syndrome [40].

Leptin is a 167 amino acid human leptogene product [41]. Human obesity is characterized by elevated levels of leptin consistent with leptin resistance. This protein is a metabolic symbol for energy deficiency, with weight loss and caloric restriction resulting in a rapid decline in leptin levels. This subsequently stimulates the hypothalamus to increase appetite. Leptin has also been shown to accelerate wound healing, cell growth and angiogenesis, enhancing sympathetic activity via several hypothalamic neuropeptides, resulting in increases in blood pressure and energy expenditure.

Regulation of body-fat stores is critical to prevent excessive body-weight changes, while adipocyte production of leptin is proportional to the adipose tissue mass, with sympathetic blockade enhancing leptin expression as well as food intake, insulin, and steroids.

Leptin has also been demonstrated to have several non-sympathetic actions in the cardiovascular system with high doses increasing endothelial generation of nitric oxide and promoting angiogenesis [42]. At the kidney level, high doses enhance diuresis and natriuresis while leptin receptors have been demonstrated on the platelets promoting platelet aggregation and enhancing insulin mediated glucose uptake via peripheral receptors, with mitogenic effects on vascular smooth muscle increasing the risk of myocardial hypertrophy and vascular atherosclerosis and hypertrophy. Despite these non-sympathetic depressor actions of leptin, its overall effect is that of a pressor.

The circulating levels of this hormone represent a barometer of energy stores, particularly in adipose tissue, playing an important role in directing neuroendocrine function and metabolic regulation in conserving energy and even preventing fertilization by inducing hypothalamic hypogonadism via central nervous system receptors. Leptin deficiency states have been reported in lipoatrophy and those individuals with exercise or diet induced amenorrhea. Leptin replenishment in these individuals results in improved metabolic function and restoration of ovulation.

Clot formation and subsequent dissolution depend on a balance between two processes, fibrinolysis/thrombolysis and coagulation. Hyperfibrinogenemia has been associated with an increased risk for cardiovascular disease and acts synergistically with dyslipidemia and hypertension to promote this type of disease. Visceral obesity and insulin resistance have been associated with increased levels of PAI-1, predisposing these individuals to cardiovascular disease, hyperglycemia, and hyperinsulinemia.

This is why low dose aspirin, 81–160 mg/day, is routinely recommended for prevention of cardiovascular complications in these individuals. Clopidogrel (Plavix) may be of benefit in aspirin intolerant patients to prevent stroke, having already demonstrated its efficacy in peripheral arterial diseases and coronary artery disease, particularly in the post myocardial infarction (acute coronary syndrome) and stenting period. Prasugrel (Effient), a P2Y12 platelet inhibitor, a thienopyridine, has also been approved to reduce the risk of thrombotic cardiovascular events in patients with acute coronary syndrome who are to be managed with percutaneous coronary intervention.

The predominance of small, dense LDL instead of large buoyant LDL also confers increased risk especially in patients with metabolic syndrome. This is not to say that large, buoyant LDL is not atherogenic, but that the smaller, dense LDL molecule is more atherogenic [14].

Reduction of non HDL cholesterol is a secondary target if the triglyceride levels are elevated. Drug therapy for individuals with lone HDL reductions and normal triglycerides and LDLs is generally reserved for those individuals who are at high risk such as existing coronary disease or coronary heart disease equivalents [25]. On occasions, combination therapy with statins and niacin can be considered along with a combination of statin and fenofibrate in well selected individuals. This topic will be dealt with in greater detail in the section on lipids.

Blood pressures greater than 130/85 – a criteria for metabolic syndrome – have been associated with an important risk factor for stroke and myocardial infarction. Beginning at 115/75, cardiovascular disease risk doubles with each incremental increase of 20/10 mmHg. JNC-7 guidelines classify patients with a systolic blood pressures of 120–139 mmHg or diastolic blood pressures of 80–89 mmHg as being pre-hypertensive.

Patients with hypertension are twice as likely to develop diabetes over a 4–5 year period of time with hypertension being twice as prevalent in individuals with type-2 diabetes compared to non-diabetics. Although diet and other therapeutic life style changes are important steps to treating blood pressure and hypercholesterolemia, most patients will require pharmacologic intervention in order to attain treatment goals.

Various classes of antihypertensive agents can be used with success in patients with diabetes and those with metabolic syndrome [43]. These include the thiazide diuretics, angiotensin converting enzyme (ACE) inhibitors, angiotensin receptor blockers (ARBs), direct renin inhibitors, calcium-channel blockers, and beta blockers. Concerns of effects on lipid parameters and glucose should be taken into account when prescribing diuretics and non selective beta blockers, particularly as solo therapy.

A more detailed discussion of their use in diabetics will follow in a later chapter.

Nonetheless, various clinical trials have demonstrated improved outcome improvement in cardiovascular disease including stroke in diabetic patients with blood pressure lowering therapy.

OBESITY

The overwhelming majority of type-2 diabetics are overweight or frankly obese and obesity is not only associated with insulin resistance, but also increased mortality, hypertension, congestive heart failure, and increased cardiovascular risks. Although genetic predisposition is certainly a significant contributing factor, atherogenic diets, physical activity, and high caloric intake (particularly carbohydrates) contribute to obesity, which enhances the genesis of the metabolic syndrome, which enhances the risk for insulin resistance, promoting accelerated arteriosclerotic vascular disease, and the prothrombotic and proinflammatory state.

Obesity in the United States population has increased steadily over the past 40 years and crosses all educational ethnic age and gender groups. More than two-thirds of the United States adult population is obese or overweight. Alarming is the fourfold increase in obesity from 1996 to 2004. Larger proportions of minorities and women compared to nonminority and men are overweight and obese. The age adjusted prevalence of obesity doubled from 15 to 35% during the interval from NHANES 2 which was 1976–1980 and NHANES 3 from 1999 to 2000 [4]. The National Center for Health Statistics released data in 2007, which indicated that 25.6% of US adults had a BMI (body mass index) greater than 30 kg/m^2, while 69% of all adults did not meet the national standards for physical activity! Elevated BMI increases the risk for diabetes, but this risk can be modestly attenuated by physical activity.

Diabetes and obesity are closely related with a 4.5% increase in the risk for diabetes with every 5 kg weight gain, with women possessing a 25% increased relative risk for diabetes with each unit of BMI greater than 22. Not only does obesity increase cardiovascular and diabetes risk, but also enhances risk for colon, prostate, gall bladder, breast, and pancreatic cancers [44].

An often overlooked association is that between depression and obesity. Dysthymia or major depression can be seen in up to 12% of patients with diabetes as well.

The concomitant presence of depression and diabetes can not only influence the capacity to adhere to therapeutic lifestyle changes, but can also be associated with the development of microvascular and macrovascular disease with depression in diabetes associated with double the likelihood of having three or more cardiovascular risk factors compared to diabetics without depression. Various metabolic, biochemical, genetic, emotional, cultural, and psychosocial factors can be interrelated in causing of obesity, which contributes to the cascade of associated complications indentified with insulin resistance and hyperinsulinemia.

Various metabolic markers can identify those individuals who are overweight and insulin resistant. In non-diabetic normotensive overweight volunteers, insulin concentration, the ratio of triglyceride to high density lipoprotein cholesterol concentration, and levels of plasma triglyceride can help identify overweight individuals who are significantly insulin resistant and at increased risk for various adverse outcomes.

The entity of prediabetes is intimately associated with the metabolic syndrome. It is well known that individuals that will ultimately develop type-2 diabetes experience a progressive development of glucose intolerance over a period of time, beginning with normal glycemia to impaired glucose tolerance and overt diabetes. Increased risk factors for this condition would include not only obese individuals but those individuals with impaired glucose tolerance, hypertension, women with a history of gestational diabetes, specific ethnic groups such as Asians, Pacific Islanders, Hispanics, African Americans, Native Americans, and especially those individuals with first degree relatives having type-2 diabetes [45].

There is a 40% life time risk of developing type-2 diabetes in individuals whose first degree relatives have the condition. The probability of developing diabetes is also increased when siblings have been affected with diabetes. These all indicate an important contribution of inherited factors in the pathogenesis of the disease.

The Physician's Health Study, a prospective cohort evaluation of 20,757 men who did not have diabetes at baseline reported 1,836 incident diabetes cases over a 23.1 year follow up with the incidence increased in overweight inactive men compared to those active men with normal BMIs (hazard ratios of 6.57 and 2.39, respectively) [46].

Relatively less well known is obesity related cardiorenal syndrome. This condition has been described in obese patients with normal ejection fraction, diastolic dysfunction, and eccentric left ventricular hypertrophy. These patients can go on to develop pulmonary hypertension and right heart failure with or without obstructive sleep apnea. Increases in total blood volume, epicardial fat, and accelerated tissue demands often accompany the obese state leading to increased left ventricular stroke work, high output cardiac states, and ultimately increased intraventricular wall stress with left ventricular enlargement.

The waist to hip ratio has been a common way of measuring body fat distribution with a direct relationship being demonstrated between an increase in this ratio and the risk for type-2 diabetes.

Gestational diabetes is now a well known accepted risk factor for subsequent developmental of type-2 diabetes. After 28 years of follow-up, women with a history of gestational diabetes demonstrated a 50% incidence of development of type-2 diabetes. Various risk factors predicted a future development in these women, including hyperglycemia during pregnancy and immediate post delivery period, family history of diabetes, increased prepregnancy weight, age, and number of deliveries.

Prevention strategies in these individuals should emphasize weight reduction, physical activity, avoidance of overweight, and cigarette smoking. These individuals are clearly more insulin resistant than the general population and all attempts to reduce insulin resistance are of benefit in these individuals.

It has indeed been suggested by many authors that the metabolic syndrome should be equated with diabetes as a coronary risk equivalent. Individuals with impaired glucose tolerance have an increase risk of overall coronary heart disease and angina as well as intimal wall thickness of the carotids. Hence it should be clearly understood that the pre-diabetic patient is not only prone to developing diabetes, but is also at increased cardiovascular risk.

Several epidemiologic trials since 1999 including the Chicago Policemen Trial [47], The Diabetes Intervention Study [48], Honolulu Heart Study [49], and the Islington Diabetes Survey [50] have all indicated that as postprandial glucose rises from 150 to 200 there is a correspondingly progressive increased risk of fatal and non-fatal myocardial infarction.

Clearly, macrovascular disease begins with insulin resistance and then although the diabetic patient may suffer from their microvascular disease, they will ultimately die from their macrovascular disease. Small wonder then that many authors feel that diabetes, prediabetes, the metabolic syndrome, and cardiovascular disease have multiple etiologies in common.

The presence of insulin resistance doubles the annual risk of a coronary heart disease event independent of the presence of type-2 diabetes. Further evidence of the importance of insulin resistance comes from the Bruneck study, which looked at 4,800 patients between the ages of 40–79, using the HOMA (The Homeostasis Model Assessment) method, a technique that allows beta cell function and insulin resistance to be estimated by measuring glucose and fasting of plasma insulin [51].

In this study the number of metabolic abnormalities correlated with a degree of insulin resistance and the more abnormalities that were demonstrated, the greater the likelihood of insulin resistance.

The San Antonio Heart study looked at two subgroups of patients based on insulin resistance during a 7-year follow-up study [31]. Curiously, only the more insulin resistant converters showed proatherogenic profiles such as hypertension and dyslipidemia, while those individuals who were less insulin resistant had blood pressure and lipid profiles comparable to subjects who do not develop diabetes.

The Botnia study in Western Finland found that insulin resistance syndrome was significantly predictive of cardiovascular mortality and morbidity across a broad spectrum of glucose levels indicating that it is insulin resistance which increases cardiovascular risk in both impaired glucose tolerance and type-2 diabetes [52].

Hence although significant clinical benefits can be demonstrated by improvement in the hyperglycemic state, therapeutic modalities targeting insulin resistance will demonstrate additional benefits allowing for a greater impact on the incidence of cardiovascular events. This can be appreciated when one realizes that the UKPS trial demonstrated the – efficacy of sulfonylureas, metformin, and even insulin in statistically and significantly reducing the risk of microvascular complications which are responsible for 80% of diabetes related morbidity [53].

In recent years a great deal of attention has been devoted to the endothelium in understanding the pathophysiology of vascular health and cardiovascular disease. It is well known that the endothelium plays an important role in regulating vascular tone, vascular smooth muscle migration, thrombosis, thrombolysis, and coordinating responses to various chemical and mechanical stimuli. It is the endothelial cells that are responsible for synthesizing and releasing various growth modulators and vasoactive substances and allow the endothelium to respond to these stimuli. Partial or complete loss of a proper balance between vasodilators and vasoconstrictors, inhibitor and growth promoting factors, anticoagulant and procoagulant factors, and atherogenic and proatherogenic factors result in endothelial dysfunction [54].

Endothelial dysfunction is not only a critical event in the subsequent development of the microvascular complications of diabetes, but actually precedes the clinically detectable plaque in the coronary disease and serves as a pivotal event in the atherogenic process.

Abnormalities in vascular endothelial reaction have been demonstrated in both type-2 diabetes and in the prediabetic state. These abnormal responses suggest that multiple abnormalities in the nitric oxide pathway are likely to be present. These would include an abnormality in signal transduction in the vascular smooth muscle, increased deactivation of nitric oxide by various reactive oxygen substrates, and direct reduction in nitric oxide production.

Reductions in the quantity and the action of nitric oxide in the insulin resistance syndrome can be affected by the host of metabolic abnormalities associated with the condition. Insulin is known to enhance vasodilatation in a nitric oxide dependent fashion; however, this mechanism is attenuated in patients with type-2 diabetes, and in overweight and obese, or euglycemic insulin resistant individuals.

It is likely that those individuals with insulin resistance may also be resistant to the vasodilatory and subsequent vasoprotective effect of insulin induced nitric oxide production. As the result of the close association between insulin resistance and cardiovascular disease, therapeutic approaches targeting insulin resistance play an important role for physicians in primary care.

Clearly understanding the interrelationships between genetic factors and metabolic abnormalities in determining risk for cardiovascular disease in those individuals in the prediabetic and/or metabolic syndrome state can play a significant role in reducing mortality and morbidity.

The United States has the greatest percentage of people over the age of 15 with a BMI greater that 30 kg/m^2 [55]. Obesity is among the top four risk factors for cardiovascular disease; the others are smoking, diabetes, and hypertension while obesity itself increases the risk for many other diseases including carcinoma, heart failure, steatohepatitis, pulmonary fibrosis, and diabetes. Combining all four factors increase cardiovascular risk 21 fold.

Most of the detrimental effects of obesity are related to inflammatory processes, enhanced oxidative stress, and ectopic fat deposition. Central to this entire process is the adipocyte, which increases in size with excessive caloric intake, overwhelming the storage capacity of these cells. These cells can then undergo apoptosis or cell death. This causes monocytes and macrophages to be recruited into the visceral fat to phagocytize these deceased adipocytes increasing the production of chemo-attractant protein-1. This causes more monocytes and macrophages to migrate into adipose tissue so that obese individuals can possess up to 50% of the visceral adipocyte population as macrophages compared to only 5–10% in non-obese individuals.

Fat cells release many inflammatory substances like leptin, interleukin-6, PAI-1, and angiotensinogen. Increased levels of angiotensinogen cause the adipocyte to become a pressor organ, activating the RAAS, leading to hypertension and increased vascular oxidative stress, accelerated atherogenesis, and enhanced cardiovascular risk.

These altered adipocytes may also contribute directly or indirectly to reduced production of beneficial adiponectin, which possesses anti-inflammatory properties and increases insulin sensitivity by downgrading hepatic glucose production and improving skeletal muscle glucose uptake. We can therefore see an entire legion of inflammatory cytokines from these altered or angry adipocytes producing a variety of systemic problems due to the accumulation of increase amounts of free fatty acids. These include: enhanced cardiac insulin resistance resulting in left ventricular dysfunction, fibrosis and ventricular hypertrophy, hepatocyte injury producing steatohepatitis (non-alcoholic steatohepatitis), impaired endothelial function, pancreatic beta cell apoptosis, and even Alzheimer's disease.

Benefits for treating the obese individual with agents that decrease RAAS activity were shown in the MADE-ITT (Metabolic Assessment of Diovan's Efficacy in comparison to Thiazide Therapy) trial [56]. In this study, individuals with an average BMI of 36 kg/m^2 were given valsartan (Diovan) a diuretic once daily, or a combination of both. In this study, the greatest reduction in blood pressure was with combination therapy. However, C-reactive protein levels decreased with the ARB and increased with the diuretic.

Recent attention has been devoted to the endocannabinoid system, consisting of CB1 and CB2 receptors, and signaling molecules and their subsequent impact on metabolic functions. CB1 receptors are located peripherally in adipose, muscle, gastrointestinal tract, liver tissue, and centrally in the nucleus accumbens in the hypothalamus, playing an important role in regulating energy homeostasis as well as glucose and lipid metabolism.

CB2 receptors are allocated on cells in the immune and hematopoietic system and not believed to be involved in energy regulation. Overactivity of the endocannabinoid system in adipose tissue decreases adiponectin promoting insulin resistance, increased intra-abdominal adiposity, and dyslipidemia.

The Diabetes Prevention Program Study involved 4,000 subjects at 25 different centers with a 3-year enrollment phase [57]. Subjects were followed for 3–6 years. The trial had a 90% power to detect a 33% reduction in progression to diabetes. The intensive life style intervention group received training in diet, exercise, and behavior modification and was placed on a low fat hypercaloric diet. The significant reduction in development of Type II diabetes with weight loss and life style changes even with a modest weight loss of 5% showed the value of these modifications [34].

Weight control enhances LDL lowering and reduces all risk factors while physical activity reduces the LDL, increases the HDL and can lower the LDL. The complicated interrelationships of the metabolic syndrome in both android (males) and gynoid (females) centers around insulin resistance, and the development of hyperinsulinemia with subsequent impaired glucose tolerance, hypertension, dyslipidemia, and arteriosclerotic vascular disease [58].

Weight reduction in obesity remains an important yet very elusive goal in therapy. Various diets have been promulgated through the years. The goals are to achieve a 1–2 weight pound reduction per week reducing weight circumference and preventing weight gain. National Guidelines provide for three types of diet, the moderate calorie deficient diet which allows for a deficit of 500–1,000 kcal/day, the low calorie diet which balances five food groups with 1,000–1,200 kcal/day in women, and 1,200–1,600 kcal/day in men and a very low calorie diet which involves 800 kcal in 1 g/kg of protein. This latter diet requires special monitoring in vitamin supplementation along with medical supervision.

These diets can be divided into the following:

Balanced diets (Weight Watchers, Jenny Craig, LA Weight Loss, Medifast)
Low fat diets (Pritikin, Dean Ornish)
Low carbohydrate diets (Atkin's and the South Beach) [27].

Obesity is based on the body/mass index (BMI). The BMI is calculated by dividing the weight in kilograms by the square of the height in meters (kg/m^2). More than half of adults in the USA are considered overweight with a BMI of >25 with one-third being obese with a BMI >30.

Basically any diet can be effective if there is a deficit of caloric intake relative to caloric expenditure. In patients on diet alone there is in general a 5–6% reduction in body weight over the first 6 months of treatment, with the weight slowly returning over a 12–24 month period. Compensatory changes in energy expenditure oppose maintenance of lower body weight.

The Atkins diet recommends induction of weight loss with only 20 g of carbohydrate daily with consumption of green salads and other vegetables, plus liberal amounts of fat and protein. Carbohydrate intake gradually increases with the maintenance program. However, the adverse effects of this diet make it an unwise option – particularly for diabetics. Endothelial function can be reduced by 50% compared to patients on a low fat diet in a study of 70 men and women 16–60 years of age with body mass indices between 27 and 40 kg/m^2 and metabolic syndrome [59].

Carbohydrate restriction leads to ketosis with fat from adipose tissue being the major source of energy. Ketosis can suppress appetite and have a diuretic effect. The low carbohydrate diets are usually associated with quick weight loss in the first 1–2 weeks.

A study comparing low carbohydrate diets (<30 g daily) with a low fat calorie restricted diet in 132 severely obese patients with a mean BMI of 43 with a high prevalence of diabetes and the metabolic syndrome showed that after 6 months, the 43 patients still on the low carb diet lost a mean of 5.8 kg, compared to 1.9 kg lost by the 36 patients still on the low fat, low calorie diet.

At least for the first 6 months of a high fat, low carbohydrate diet, there appear to be no adverse effects on risk factors for atherosclerosis, although carotid intimal thickening can occur while choosing high saturated fat alternatives to carbohydrates. Ketosis can cause bad breath and prolonged ketosis may increase the risk of osteoporosis due to calcium loss from bone. The safety of this diet long term remains to be demonstrated.

The South Beach Diet adds more grain and fiber to the regimen and appears to offer a more practical alternative for many individuals who have difficulty in restricting carbohydrate intake.

Nonetheless it is important to understand that with both of these diets significant attention has to be devoted in reduction of trans fatty acid and saturated fat content particularly in those individuals who have existing arteriosclerotic vascular disease or are prone toward arteriosclerotic deposition. This seems to be a more prudent approach until further study has been completed.

Medications currently available by prescription to aid in weight reduction are:

1. Sympathomimetic Amines – Methamphetamine (Desoxyn) and phentermine (Ionamin) are controlled substances. Phentermine was used with fenfluramine as "Phen-Fen" until the combination was associated with heart valve abnormalities. These drugs are approved for short term use only and are moderately effective when used in conjunction with diet. Adverse effects include dry mouth, hypertension, nervousness, insomnia, and sexual dysfunction.

2. Orlistat (Xenical) – This lipase inhibitor decreases absorption of fat from the gastrointestinal tract. Adverse effects include flatulence and oily spotting with discharge and fecal urgency. Although weight loss of up to 8.5 kg is possible with this agent, its tolerability makes it challenging to take [60].

3. Sibutramine (Meridia) – This drug is a serotonin, norepinephrine, and dopamine reuptake inhibitor. This medication has been used to promote weight loss over a prolonged period of time safely. Side effects include hypertension, dry mouth, and insomnia and should not be used with SSRIs (selective serotonin reuptake inhibitors). Weight loss of up to 4.5 kg after 1 year of therapy has been reported.

4. SSRIs – Although some reports can indicate that these drugs may cause weight gain, other studies show weight loss with these products. This can be seen especially with those patients who tend to eat when depressed. Sexual dysfunction and decreased libido remain the major problem with this class.

5. Bupropion – (Wellbutrin SR) – This non SSRI has been modestly effective in promoting weight loss in doses of 300–400 mg daily. This drug is generally well tolerated, but can increase the risk of seizures. This is less likely with the sustained release preparation.

6. Zonisamide (Zonegran) – This antiepileptic drug causes weight loss as a side effect. In a 16-week trial of 60 patients, and a mean BMI of 36.3, average weight loss was 5.9 kg compared to 0.9 kg with the placebo group. A 16-week extension study showed a further 3.3 kg weight loss compared to 1.5 kg with placebo. Cognitive problems, difficulty in concentrating, and rare reports of Stevens–Johnson syndrome have been reported [61].

7. Topiramate (Topamax) – This antiepileptic drug was evaluated in a double blind trial in 385 patients on a reduced calorie diet. Here, 64–384 mg daily of topiramate for 6 months led to a 4.8–6.3% weight loss compared to 2.6% for placebo. Paresthesias, somnolence, and difficulties with concentration and attention were reported side effects [62].

8. Metformin – (Glucophage) – In the Diabetes Prevention Program, patients with impaired glucose tolerance lost 2.1 kg compared to 0.1 kg weight loss with placebo. The (Biguanides and the Prevention of the Risk of Obesity) BIGPRO trial in 1994 evaluated this drug in non diabetics and found similar weight loss with this product in that population. This drug has not been formally approved for use in impaired glucose tolerance or for weight loss in non-diabetics [63].

9. GLP-1 receptor agonists. Agents like exenatide and liraglutide can cause significant weight reductions in diabetic patients. In clinical trials baseline body weight after 30 weeks of therapy with exenatide (Byetta) 10 μg twice daily decreased by 2.8 kg in combination with metformin (0.3 kg with placebo), 1.6 kg in combination with a sulfonylurea (0.6 kg with placebo), and 1.6 kg with metformin and sulfonylurea (0.9 with placebo) [64]. Weight loss was even higher when therapy was continued for 52 weeks (up to 3.6 kg) with 2 and 3 year extension data showing weight reductions of 5 kg. Liraglutide (Victoza) therapy has been reported to reduce weight whether used alone or in combination with metformin. In a double blinded 26-week study, liraglutide in combination with metformin reduce weight by 2.8 kg at the 0.6 mg dose and 4.4 kg with the 1.8 mg dose given once daily. Monotherapy for 52 weeks with liraglutide demonstrated weight reduction of 2.05 kg with the 1.2 mg dose and up to 2.45 kg with the 1.8 mg dose compared to sulfonylurea therapy [65]. In the LEAD-6 trial, liraglutide once daily resulted in similar weight reductions to twice daily exenatide (2.8–4.1 kg) [66].

10. Pramlintide (Symlin) – Adjunctive treatment of type-2 diabetics with both glargine (Lantus) and basal insulin (neutral protamine hagedorn, lente, or ultralente) has resulted in significant weight reductions compared to placebo of 2.3 kg with basal insulin and 2.8 kg with glargine. This agent can be effective in preventing or diminishing weight gain often associated with tighter glycemic control in type-2 diabetics.

11. Rimonabant – This selective cannabinoid-1 receptor blocker has been shown to reduce body weight and improve cardiometabolic risk factors in obese patients, but has had significant depression associated with its use – particularly with higher doses of 20 mg daily. The impressive data in the Rimonabant in Obesity (RIO)-LIPIDS Study and the RIO-North America Study were tempered by the high discontinuation rates and mental health side effects causing the drug to fail its first audition for approval with the FDA [67].

12. Phentermine/topiramate controlled release (Qnexa) – Once daily; low dose phentermine and topiramate CR have been shown to have favorable effects on weight, glycemic control, and blood pressure after 28 weeks. Both products were associated with adverse effects at their recommended doses. However, when combined at lower doses in a once daily preparation, significant reductions in blood pressure and weight resulted in phase three trials. This drug has not been FDA approved.

Surgery for weight reduction, especially bariatric procedures, involves less complications, and better outcomes in experienced hands. Surgical procedures for severe obesity increased from 16,000 cases yearly in the decade of the 1990s to 103,000 in 2003, 107,000 in 2005, and over 200,000 in 2008, due to the failure of diet and exercise, and improved, safer surgical methods.

The surgical treatment of obesity has resulted in some impressive improvements in surrogate outcomes. Data from two meta-analyses revealed that 70% of patients have improved lipid parameters, resolution of obstructive sleep apnea occurred in 85.7%, glycemic control improved in 86% of diabetics and 77% had complete resolution, while hypertension improved in 86% and was completely eliminated in 61.7% [68].

Indications for surgery are those patients with a BMI greater than 40 kg/m² or greater than 35 kg/m² with other serious comorbidities like sleep apnea and uncontrolled diabetes in whom previous nonsurgical weight loss measures have failed. These procedures should not be performed in individuals with severe cardiac disease, drug or alcohol abuse, high anesthesia risk, binge eating disorders, or major psychiatric diseases.

In general, there are three types of bariatric procedures: restrictive, malabsorptive, and combined malabsorptive/restrictive [69].

The restrictive procedures maintain absorptive function of the small intestine while limiting caloric intake. These procedures can be reversed if necessary and are generally easier and safer to perform compared to the malabsorptive ones. However, patients generally lose less weight and are more likely to gain weight long term. Included in these procedures are: gastric banding, sleeve gastrectomy, vertical banded gastroplasty, and laparoscopic adjustable gastric banding.

In vertical banded gastroplasty, staples are used to create a 15–20 ml gastric pouch in the upper stomach, with a small calibrated opening in the rest of the stomach. Mean weight loss is as high as 60% in the initial postoperative period, although many patients can regain lost weight over 5–10 years. Complications include reflux, stenosis, and staple line breakdown with 15–20% of patients requiring a second procedure to correct outlet stenosis or sever reflux. There is no malabsorption with this technique with perioperative mortality less than 1%. This procedure is the least efficacious with weight loss of 35–50%, short-term only. Reoperation rates are high due to reservoir breakdown or component deterioration [70].

Malabsorptive procedures such as biliopancreatic diversion and jejunoileal bypass shorten the length of the small intestine thereby reducing nutrient absorption. Although greater weight reductions are achieved with this technique, side effects such as diarrhea, nutritional deficiencies, problems with the stoma and intestinal dumping have limited their use to such an extent that they are rarely used in this country.

In the biliopancreatic bypass with duodenal switch, the greater curvature of the stomach is resected, leaving a small gastric pouch (100–250 ml) and the proximal duodenum is anastomosed to the distal 250 cm of ileum, bypassing the duodenum, the entire jejunum, and the rest of the ileum. Perioperative mortality is 1% higher than the other procedures along with metabolic malabsorptive anemia, along with fat soluble deficiencies and protein calorie malnutrition [43].

Malabsorptive/restrictive surgeries such as the Roux-en-Y bypass restrict oral intake by creating a small pouch, which results in mild degrees of malabsorption with enhanced gastrointestinal transport. Patients can lose up to 70% of their excess weight over a 10 year period although intestinal obstruction, dumping syndrome, and stomal problems can complicate this procedure.

Roux-En-Y-gastric bypass is the treatment of choice for patients >100 lb over desired weight or BMI > 40. The first portion (20–30 ml) of the stomach is clipped with staples and anastamosed to the jejunum, bypassing most of the stomach, the entire duodenum and the first 15–20 cm of the jejunum. Mean weight loss is 65–75% or 35% of initial weight. This procedure can reverse the glycemia of type-2 diabetes if done early. Perioperative mortality is less than 1% with deficiencies of calcium, iron, vitamin D, folate, and vitamin B12 commonly occurring due to malabsorption along with zinc, copper, vitamin A, and vitamin K deficiencies. Dumping syndrome and wound infections have been reported with lifelong follow-up necessary to prevent and treat deficiencies and the complications of ulcerations at the gastroenterostomy stoma and the duodenum [71].

Pulmonary embolism and anastomotic leaks are the main causes of postoperative mortality which is 1.1% for diversions or switches, 0.5% for gastric bypass, and 0.1% for banded procedures. Intestinal obstructions, leaks, deep vein thrombosis, wound infections, and hernias cause most nonfatal complications.

The exact mechanism for the resolution of various obesity comorbidities remain to be elucidated. Many result from weight reduction alone, but glucose regulation is improved in some patients well before significant weight reduction. Nonetheless, bariatric surgery can clearly improve lipids, nonalcoholic steatohepatitis, hypertension, insulin sensitivity, and attenuate inflammatory mediators (particularly tumor necrosis alpha and interleukin-6) in addition to causing profound weight reductions. In addition, appetite reduction and early satiety can follow bariatric surgery.

Ghrelin, an appetite stimulating hormone secreted from the fundus of the stomach, falls to extremely low levels following gastric bypass. Also increased following gastric bypass surgery are gastric inhibitory polypeptide or glucose dependent insulinotropic peptide (GIP), as well as plasma protein YY, insulin like growth factor-1, glucagon like protein-1, and adiponectin. All of which play a role in reducing insulin resistance or enhancing insulin sensitivity. Leptin resistance can be corrected with foregut bypass, enhancing glucose uptake, and fatty acid oxidation [72].

In treating the obese patient, recognition and determination of goals is critical. Commitment of the patient to a practically designed program is critical to success. Realistic goals need to be set to avoid patient frustration. Positive reinforcement behavior modification, increased physical activity, and judicious use of pharmacotherapy all play an important role.

Modification of eating and activity habits following a set of principals and techniques can be used in an efficacious way in helping patients battle with obesity. Patients should constantly be reminded of the consequences of overweight and dietary indiscretion, while avoiding being dictatorial or dogmatic.

VanWarmer and Boucher in their review and practical dieting outline the five A's for weight management counseling [73]. These include:

1. Assessing the patient: identifying any biologic, genetic or behavioral risk factors including accurate measurements of height, weight, waist circumference and BMI, and identifying the presence of any other behavioral mediators like barriers to weight loss, social support, or change of status or occupation.
2. Advising the patient including recommending a weight management program and reviewing these recommendations particularly for the diabetic patient and those with specific dietary habits, while recommending helpful stress management techniques. It is important for the physician to give clear respectful advice and to link these recommendations with outcomes data.
3. Set up an agreement with the patient for both short term goals including calorie restriction, glucose monitoring and exercise, and long-term goals – hemoglobin A1C's, lipid profiles and weight reduction, while collaborating on acceptable approaches to changing the patient's life style and stressing achievable goals.
4. Assist the patient with motivation and any problems they may be having, while discussing all available resources to aid the patient in his struggle, sometimes presenting treatment options that have worked for other patients including group sessions.

5. Arranging follow-up to insure proper adherence to techniques and feedback from the patients on their success or lack of success with this program [43].

The authors go on to recommend key messages in any type of counseling program. The first is to emphasize that tight glycemic control is the top priority, not necessarily weight management. Although weight loss may improve glycemic control, better control in some patients may lead to weight gain.

Explaining the pathophysiology of the disease is important to maintain patient compliance as well as self monitoring of the patient's blood glucose, which can give individuals important insight as to how the foods they are ingesting will affect their state of glycemia. Physical activity is always to be encouraged assuming that the individual is capable of such activity. Moderate levels of physical activity for 30–45 min, 3–5 days a week have been shown to be optimum in many exercise protocols.

We must realize that it is the duration of physical activity not the intensity that correlates with benefit. Physical activity will reduce abdominal fat, improve insulin sensitivity and overall cardiovascular health. The initial goal of weight management should be to reduce body weight by at least 10% from baseline.

Key dietary principals in attaining weight reduction must involve a deficit in caloric intake relative to caloric expenditure. Those diets that result in less insulin release particularly in insulin resistant individuals have also been shown to produce more weight loss short-term. The short-term results of many of these diets, particularly the low carb diets appear to be very encouraging, but it is long-term results that tend to be somewhat disheartening.

SUMMARY

The clustering of clinical markers and signs characterized as "The Metabolic Syndrome," easily measurable by providers, serve as an important guideline is assessing risk and in monitoring response to treatment in the prediabetic and diabetic individuals.

REFERENCES

1. Liu S, et al. Dietary carbohydrates, physical inactivity, obesity and the metabolic syndrome as predictors of coronary heart disease. Curr Opin Lipidol 2001;12:395–404.
2. Grundy SM. Coronary plaque as a replacement for age as a risk factor in global risk assessment. Am J Cardiol 2001;88(2A):8E–11E.
3. Reaven GM. Role of insulin resistance in human disease. Diabetes 1988;37:1595–1607.
4. Ford ES, Giles WH, Dietz WH. Prevalence of the metabolic syndrome among US adults: findings from the third National Health and Nutrition Examination Survey. JAMA 2002;287:356–359.
5. Ford ES, Giles WH. Prevalence of the metabolic syndrome among U.S. adults: findings from the third National Health and Nutrition Examination Survey. JAMA 2002;287:356–359.
6. Wilson PW, Kannel WB. Obesity, diabetes and risk of cardiovascular disease in the elderly. Am J Geriatr Cardiol 2002;11:119–123.
7. Ilanne-Parikka P, Laaksonen DE, Eriksson JG. Leisure time activity and the metabolic syndrome in the Finnish Diabetes Prevention Study. Diabetes Care 2010;33:1610–1617.
8. Lakka HM, Laaksonnen D, Lakka T, Niskanen L. The metabolic syndrome and total and cardiovascular mortality in middle aged men. JAMA 2002;288:2709–2716.
9. Burke J, William K, Gaskill S. Rapid rise in the incidence of Type-2 diabetes: the San Antonio Heart Study. Arch Intern Med 1999;159:1450–1456.

10. Lopez-Candales A. Metabolic syndrome X: a comprehensive review of the pathophysiology and recommended therapy. J Med 2001;32:283–300.
11. Nash D. The metabolic syndrome: early clues, effective management. Consultant 2004;May:859–864.
12. Grundy SM, The American Heart Association National Heart, Lung and Blood Institute. Definition of metabolic syndrome. Report of the National Heart, Lung and Blood Institute/American Heart Association conference on scientific issue related to definition. Circulation 2004;109:433–438.
13. Isomaa B, et al. Cardiovascular morbidity and mortality associated with the metabolic syndrome. Diabetes Care 2001;24:683–689.
14. Deen D. Metabolic syndrome: time for action. Am Fam Physician 2004;69(12):2875–2882.
15. Ridker PM, Buring JE, Rifai N, Cook NR. Development and validation of improved algorithms for the assessment of global cardiovascular risk in women. JAMA 2007;297:611–619.
16. Wang J, Ruotsalainen S, Moilanen L. The metabolic syndrome predicts incident stroke. Stroke 2008;39:1078–1083.
17. Cullen P, Shulte H. The Munster (PROCAM) Study. Circulation 1997;96:2128–2136.
18. Sattar N. Metabolic syndrome as a predictor of CHD and diabetes in WOSCOPS. Circulation 2003;108(4):414–419.
19. Polonsky T, McClelland R, Jorgenson N. Coronary artery calcium score and risk classification for coronary heart disease prediction. JAMA 2010;303(16):1610–1616.
20. Ridker PM, Danielson E. Rosuvastatin to prevent vascular events in men and women with elevated hs-CRP. New Engl J Med 2008;359(21):2195–2207.
21. Danesh J, Wheeler JG, Hirschfield GM, Eda S. Reactive protein and other circulating markers of inflammation in predicting coronary heart disease. New Engl J Med 2004;350(14):387–397.
22. Lakka HM, Laaksonen DE, Lakka TA. The metabolic syndrome and total and cardiovascular mortality in middle aged men. JAMA 2002;288:2700–2716.
23. National Heart Lung and Blood Institute. Third report of the National Cholesterol Education Expert Panel on detection, evaluation and treatment of high blood cholesterol in adults. Circulation 2002;106:3143.
24. Raggi P, Gongora MC, Gopal A, Callister TQ. Coronary artery calcium to predict all cause mortality in elderly men and women. J Am Coll Cardiol 2008;52(1):17–23.
25. Linton MF, et al. A practical approach to risk assessment to prevent coronary artery disease and its complications. Am J Cardiol 2003;92(1A):19i–26i.
26. Carulli L, Mazzi F, Rondinella S. Olanzapine metabolic side effects: a weight gain issue? Intern Emerg Med 2008;3(3):237–240.
27. Corella D, et al. The metabolic syndrome: a crossroad for genotype-phenotype associations in atherosclerosis. Curr Atheroscler Rep 2004;6:186–196.
28. Vega Gl. Obesity, the metabolic syndrome and cardiovascular disease. Am Heart J 2001;142:1108–1116.
29. Despres JP. The insulin resistance-dyslipidemic syndrome of visceral obesity: effect on patient's risk. Obes Res 1998;6:8S–17S.
30. Haffner SM, Stern MP, Hazuda HP, Pugh J. Obesity and the metabolic syndrome. The San Antonio Heart Study. Am J Epidemiol 1984;120(5):831–834.
31. Wei M, Gaskill SP, haffner SM, Stern MP. Effects of diabetes and level of glycemia on all cause and cardiovascular mortality. The San Antonio Heart Study. Diabetes Care 1998;21:1167–1172.
32. Festa A, D'Agastino R, Mykkanen L. LDL particle size in relation to insulin, proinsulin, and insulin sensitivity. The Insulin Resistance Atherosclerosis Study. Diabetes Care 1999;22:1688–1693.
33. Ovalle F, Bell DS. Clinical evidence of thiazolidinedione induced improvement of pancreatic beta cell function in patients with type-2 diabetes mellitus. Diabetes Obes Metab 2002;4:56–59.
34. Knowler WC, Barrett-Conner E, Fowler SE, Diabetes Prevention Program Research Group. Reduction in the incidence of type-2 diabetes with lifestyle intervention or metformin. N Engl J Med 2002;346:393–403.
35. Bjorntorp P. Heart and soul: stress and the metabolic syndrome. Scand Cardiovasc J 2001;35:172–177.
36. Hackam DG, et al. Emerging risk factors for atherosclerotic vascular disease: a critical review of the evidence. JAMA 2003;290:932–940.
37. Ginsberg HS. Treatment for patients with the metabolic syndrome. Am J Cardiol 2003;91:29E–39E.
38. Hooper L. Reduced or modified dietary fat for preventing cardiovascular disease. Cochrane Database Syst Rev 2004;2:CD002137.

39. Egan JW, Lebrizzi R. Geerlof JS. The long term effect of pioglitazone as monotherapy or combination therapy on glucose control in patients with type-2 diabetes. Diabetes 2000;49(Suppl 1):A357.

40. Hackman DG, Anand SS. Merging risk factors for atherosclerotic vascular disease: a critical review of the evidence. JAMA 2003;290:932–940.

41. Aizawa-Abe M, Ogawa Y, Mazuzaki H. Pathophysiological role of leptin in obesity related hypertension. J Clin Invest 2000;105(9):1243–1252.

42. Farooqi A, Matarese G, Lord G. Beneficial effects of leptin on obesity. J Clin Invest 2002;110(8): 1093–1103.

43. Wilson PW, Grundy SM. The metabolic syndrome: practical guide to origins and treatment. Circulation 2003;108:1422–1424.

44. Wilson PW, Grundy SM. The metabolic syndrome; a practical guide to origins and treatment. Circulation 2003;108:1537–1540.

45. Snow V, Barry P, Fitterman N. Pharmacological and surgical management of obesity in primary care. Ann Intern Med 2005;142(7):525–531.

46. Physicians' Health Study Research Group. The Physicians' Health Study. New Engl J Med 1989;321(3): 183–185.

47. Stamler R, Stamler, Lindberg HA. Asymptomatic hyperglycemia and coronary heart disease in middle aged men in two employed populations in Chicago. J Chronic Dis 1979;32:805–815.

48. Hanefield M, Fischer S, Julius U. Risk factors for myocardial infarction and death in newly detected NIDDM; the Diabetes Intervention Study. 11 year follow up. Diabetologia 1996;39:1577–1583.

49. Donahue RP, Abbott RD, Reed DM, Yano K. Postchallenge glucose concentration and coronary heart disease in men of Japanese ancestry. Honolulu Heart Program. Diabetes 1987;36:689–692.

50. Jackson CA, Yudkin JS, Forrest RD. A comparison of the relationships of the glucose tolerance test and the glycated hemoglobin assay with diabetic vascular disease in the community. The Islington Diabetes Survey. Diabetes Res Clin Pract 1992;17:111–123.

51. Hsueh WA, Law RE. Cardiovascular risk continuum: implications of insulin resistance and diabetes. Am J Med 1998;105(1A):4S–14S.

52. Groop L, Forsblom C, Lehtovirta M. The Botnia study-metabolic consequences of a family history of NIDDM. Diabetes 1996;95(11):1585–1593.

53. United kingdom Prospective Diabetes Study (UKPDS) Group. Intensive blood glucose control with sulfonylureas or insulin compared with conventional treatment and risk of complications in patients with type-2 diabetes (UKPDS 33). Lancet 1998;352:837–853.

54. Arcaro G, Cretti A, Balzano S. Insulin causes endothelial dysfunction in humans; sites and mechanisms. Circulation 2002;105:576–582.

55. Blackburn GI. The obesity epidemic: prevention and treatment of the metabolic syndrome. Etiology of the metabolic syndrome: potential role of insulin resistance, leptin resistance, and other players. Ann NY Acad Sci 1999;84:11–14.

56. Cooper-DeHoff R, Pepine C. Metabolic syndrome and cardiovascular disease. Clin Cardiol 2007;30(12): 593–597.

57. Lindstrom J, Louheranta J, Mannelin M. The Finnish Diabetes Prevention Study. Diabetes Care 2003;26:12.

58. Malhotra S, Mcelroy S. Associations between metabolic syndrome and psychiatric disorders. Prim Psychiatry 2003;10:37–44.

59. Grundy SM. Atherogenic dyslipidemia and the metabolic syndrome. Circulation 1997;95:1–4.

60. Rao G. Office based stateges for the management of obesity. Am Fam Physician 2010;81(12): 1444–1455.

61. Klein KM. Zonisamide and epilepsy. JAMA 2003;289:1820.

62. Bray GA, Hollander P, Klein S. A 6 month randomized, placebo controlled dose ranging trial of topiramate for weight loss in obesity. Obes Res 2003;11:722–733.

63. Luna B, Feinglos MN. Oral agents in the management of type-2 diabetes mellitus. Am Fam Physician 2001;63:1747–1756.

64. Heine RJ, Van Gaal LF. Exenatide vs. insulin glargine in suboptimally controlled type-2 diabetics. Ann Intern Med 2005;143:559–569.

65. Astrop A, Rosner S. Effects of liraglutide in the treatment of obesity. Lancet 2009;374(9701):1606–1616.

66. Buse J, Rosenstock J, Sistei G, Blonde L. Liraglutide once daily vs. exenatide twice daily for type 2 diabetes. Lancet 2009;374(9683):39–47.
67. Despres JP, Golay A, Sjostrom L. Effects of rimonabant on metabolic risk factors in overweight patients with dyslipidemia. N Engl J Med 2005;353:2121–2134.
68. Brody F. Minimally invasive surgery for morbid obesity. Cleve Clin J Med 2004;71(4):289–298.
69. Nguyen NT, Goldman C, Rosenquist CJ. Laparoscopic versus open gastric bypass: a randomized study of outcomes, quality of life, and costs. Ann Surg 2001;234:279–291.
70. Higa KD, Tienchen H, Boone KB. Laparoscopic Roux-en-Y gastric bypass: technique and 3 year follow up. J Laparoendosc Adv Surg Tech 2001;11:377–382.
71. Crookes PF. Surgical treatment of morbid obesity. Annu Rev Med 2006;57:243–264.
72. Buchwald H, Avidor Y, Braunwald E. Bariatric surgery: a systematic review and meta-analysis. JAMA 2004;292:1724.
73. Boucher JL, Shafer KJ, Chaffin JA. Weight loss, diets, and supplements; Does anything work? Diabetes Spectr 2001;14:169–175.
74. Expert Panel on Detection, Evaluation and Treatment of High Blood Cholesterol in Adults (Adult treatment Panel III). Executive summary of the third report of the National Cholesterol Education Program (NCEP). JAMA 2001;285:2486–2497.
75. Genuth S, Alberti KG, Bennett P. Follow up report on the diagnosis of diabetes mellitus. Diabetes Care 2003;26:3160–3167.
76. Flegal KM, Carroll MD, Kuczmarski RJ, Johnson CL. Overweight and obesity in the United States. Int J Obes Relat Metab Disord 1998;22(1):39–47.

SUPPLEMENTARY READINGS

Bray GA, Hollander P, Klein S. A 6 month randomized, placebo controlled, dose ranging trial of topiramate for weight loss in obesity. Obes Res 2003;11:722–733.

Fenlieb M, Kannel WB, Garrison RJ, McNamara FP. The Framingham Offspring Study. Prev Med 1975;4(4):518–525.

Gadde KM, Franciscy DM, Wagner HR, Krishman KR. Zonisamide for weight loss in obese adults; a randomized controlled trial. JAMA 2003;289:1820–1825.

Greenland P, LaBree L, Azen SP, Doherty TM, Detrano RC. Coronary artery calcium score combined with Framingham score for risk prediction in asymptomatic individuals. JAMA 2004;291:210–215.

Meigs JB, Nathan DM, Wilson PW. Metabolic risk factors worsen continuously across the spectrum of nondiabetic glucose tolerance. The Framingham Offspring Study. Ann Intern Med 1998;128:524–533.

Oparil S. Controlled release phentermine/topiramate (Qnexa) improves blood pressure, weight, and glycemic control. P T 2010;35(6):336, 343.

Ridker PM, Hennekens CH, Buring JE. C-reactive protein and other markers of inflammation in the prediction of cardiovascular disease in women. N Engl J Med 2000;342:836–843.

Serdula MK, Mokdad AH, Williamson DF, Galuska DA, Mendlein JM, Heath GW. Prevalence of attempting weight loss and strategies for controlling weight. JAMA 1999;282:1353–1358.

The Diabetes Prevention Program Research Group. The diabetes Prevention Program: baseline characteristics of the randomized cohort. Diabetes Care 2000;23:1619–1629.

Vague P, Rudnichi A, Fontbonne A. The effect of metformin on the metabolic abnormalities associated with android type body fat distribution. Results of the BIGPRO trial. Diabetologia 1994;37(Suppl 1):236.

Wallace TM, Matthews DR. The assessment of insulin resistance in man. Diabet Med 2002;19:527–534.

6 Oral Agents for Type-2 Diabetes

CONTENTS

Key Words: Oral agent classes, Oral agent combinations, Multiple oral agent therapy, Hyperglycemia, Glycogenolysis, Gluconeogenesis

INTRODUCTION

Clearly oral agents are more popular with patients in the battle for glycemic control. Significant recent advances in oral agents have provided several interesting and synergistic medications to make glycemic control more attainable. These newer agents, by addressing the various causes of hyperglycemia in the type-2 diabetic state can be used synergistically with enhanced glycemic control.

Several landmark clinical trials over a period of many years have emphasized the importance of intensive glycemic control in reducing the microvascular complications of type-2 diabetes. The classical disturbances in this condition are characterized by a combination of insulin resistance and progressive beta-cell deterioration resulting in impaired insulin secretion and release, with the disease demonstrating a wide variance from predominantly insulin resistant to predominantly insulin deficient. Increased hepatic glucose production as the result of enhanced glycogenolysis and gluconeogenesis are also phenotypic hallmarks of this disorder.

Desirable glycemic control requires effective and efficient use of various oral combinations with injectable agents and insulin to achieve this goal. Type-2 diabetes is clearly a heterogeneous, complex, interrelated disease involving multigenic etiologies. The classical disturbances in this condition are characterized by a combination of insulin resistance and progressive beta-cell deterioration resulting in impaired insulin secretion and release,

From: *Current Clinical Practice: Type 2 Diabetes, Pre-Diabetes, and the Metabolic Syndrome*
Edited by: R.A. Codario, DOI 10.1007/978-1-60327-441-8_6
© Springer Science+Business Media, LLC 2011

and increased hepatic glucose production as the result of enhanced glycogenolysis and gluconeogenesis, with the disease demonstrating a wide variance from the predominantly insulin resistant to the predominantly insulin deficient. By addressing all these abnormalities in a synergistic way the agents can be used with optimal efficiency in not only improving the abnormalities associated with this disorder, but even in preserving beta-cell function. Hence early diagnosis is critical to preventing complications, since macrovascular disease begins with postprandial hyperglycemia even in the non-diabetic range, and at the time of development of fasting hyperglycemia, the patient has already lost at least 50% of beta-cell function.

Primary care providers should be especially alerted to those patients who present with fasting glucoses in the impaired range of 100–124 mg/dl with hemoglobin AIC's greater than 6.0%. Thirty percent of these individuals will have an abnormal glucose tolerance test in the diabetic range (>200 mg/dl) when given a 2 hour glucose tolerance test with 75 g of anhydrous glucose. Even if not overtly diabetic, individuals in this category with impaired glucose tolerance (pre-diabetics) have been shown in several clinical trials to have an increased risk of fatal and non fatal myocardial infarction with 10% of these individuals developing microvascular complications of nephropathy, neuropathy, and retinopathy even before developing overt diabetes [1].

The earliest manifestation of type-2 diabetes is elevation of postprandial glucose in association with progressive insulin resistance. In many instances, a loss or delay of early-phase insulin release in response to a mealtime glucose load will aggravate beta-cell deficiency and contribute to the progressive nature of the disorder.

Recently, significant attention has been devoted to the incretin effect mediated by several gastrointestinal peptides. In humans, the major incretins are glucagon-like peptide-1 (GLP-1) and glucose-dependent insulinotropic polypeptide (GIP). Both GLP-1 and GIP increase glucose-dependent and first-phase insulin secretion and are rapidly deactivated by dipeptidyl peptidase-4 (DPP-4), but only GLP-1 suppresses glucagon secretion.

The incretins also have a variety of other systemic effects including appetite suppression by a direct effect on the satiety center, delayed gastric emptying, and an increase in beta-cell neogenesis with apoptosis inhibition (animal and in vitro). Both GLP-1 and GIP are released from the intestinal cells in response to nutrient intake with GLP-1 being synthesized from proglucagon in the L cells of the small intestine and GIP in the K cells of the proximal intestinal mucosa. Close to 95% of individuals with type-2 diabetes in the USA are managed by primary care providers with this disease afflicting approximately 20% of all patients seen in the office setting [2].

The progressive nature of type-2 diabetes is not only confined to the deterioration of beta-cell function, but also the progressive development of severe arteriosclerotic vascular disease. These patients will suffer from their microvascular disease (retinopathy, neuropathy, and nephropathy), but will die from their macrovascular disease including coronary artery disease, complications from peripheral vascular disease, and stroke with many having established micro and macrovascular complications of diabetes at the time of first presentation to their provider.

Elevation of postprandial glucose early in the developing stages of type-2 diabetes, in association with progressive insulin resistance, results in compensatory islet-cell hypertrophy, but eventually insulin production is insufficient to maintain euglycemia. In many instances a loss or delay of early phase insulin release in response to a mealtime glucose load will aggravate beta-cell deficiency and contribute to the progressive nature of the disorder.

For many years oral agents clearly have been popular with patients and physicians in the battle for enhanced glycemic control. As a result of the progressive development of newer and novel oral agents, physicians have at their disposal a wide variety of medications to address the various abnormalities associated with patients with type-2 diabetes. By addressing all these abnormalities in a synergistic way, the agents can be used with optimal efficiency in not only improving the abnormalities associated with this disorder, but even in preserving beta-cell function. Table 1 lists the mechanisms of action of the various agents.

The biguanides and thiazolidinediones (TZD's) enhance insulin sensitivity, with the biguanides being more effective at the liver level and the TZD's more effective at the tissue, particularly the adipocyte level. By addressing insulin sensitivity these agents provide patients with the opportunity to use both endogenous and exogenous insulin more efficiently.

Table 1   Mechanism of action of oral agents

Class	Mechanism of action	Agents
Secretagogues		
Sulfonylureas		Glipizide, glyburide, glimepiride
	Increase insulin secretion Stimulate pancreatic beta cell	
Meglitinides		Repaglinide
Phenylalanines		Nateglinide
Biguanides	Decrease hepatic glucose production	
	Decrease intestinal glucose absorption	Metformin
	Increase peripheral glucose uptake	
	Increase insulin sensitivity	
Alpha-glucosidase inhibitors	Delay in carbohydrate digestion	Acarbose, miglitol
Thiazolidinediones (TZD)	Increase insulin sensitivity Preserve beta-cell function May regenerate beta cells	Pioglitazone Rosiglitazone
DPP-IV inhibitors	Increase insulin release from pancreas Suppresses glucagon Slows Inactivation of glucagon-like peptide-1 (GLP-1) and glucose-dependent insulinotropic polypeptide (GIP)	Sitagliptin Vildagliptin Saxagliptin Linagliptin

From Dailey [*18*]

The sulfonylureas increase insulin secretion from the pancreas, increasing predominately the basal insulin production. These agents are effective in controlling HbA_1C levels primarily by decreasing fasting blood sugar.

The glinides (nateglinide and repaglinide) act by improving bolus insulin secretion when taken before meals. These agents, however, are not effective and are to be taken concomitantly with sulfonylureas. By primarily decreasing postprandial hyperglycemia, these agents are particularly effective early on in the diabetic state when postprandial hyperglycemia is the earliest manifestation of the disease.

The alpha-glucosidase inhibitors (glyset and miglitol) delay carbohydrate uptake and are effective in attenuating postprandial hyperglycemia. Although these agents are not extremely potent, they can be used in a synergistic fashion with other medications and recent data have indicated that acarbose reduced the risk of macrovascular events when compared to placebo.

Several oral agents can address the issue of decreasing hepatic glucose output. Here the biguanides, TZD's, nateglinide, and the sulfonylureas can be effective. Thus, with the oral agents one can see that the diabetic paradigm can be attacked from the four important areas of glucose production, carbohydrate intake, insulin secretion, and peripheral uptake by the tissues.

It is important to understand, however, that there are certain patients who are not candidates for oral agents, since most of the products are metabolized by the liver and excreted by the kidney. They may not be suitable for every patient and the clinician must exert caution when prescribing oral agents in patients with these problems.

The biguanides are contraindicated with creatinine clearances less than 60 (serum creatinine less than 1.4 in women and 1.5 in men) and should not be used in any patient who has a predisposition to developing an acidosis whether it is respiratory or metabolic, especially patients with congestive heart failure, alcoholism, and chronic obstructive pulmonary disease with CO_2 retention.

The TZD's should not be used in New York Heart Association Class III and Class IV patients. These individuals should be warned about the potential for significant edema when insulin is co-administered with these products. Although the original thiazolidinedione (troglitazone) was withdrawn from the market because of severe liver injury requiring transplantation and in some cases death, the newer TZD's (pioglitazone and rosiglitazone) have had rare incidences of hepatotoxicity. These were recently reported in patients with other concomitant, potentially hepatotoxic agents in their system (alcohol and acetaminophen) [3].

The dosage of all the sulfonylureas, except for glipizide, must be reduced in patients with renal insufficiency since these products are metabolically active after being metabolized in the liver. Glipizide metabolites are not metabolically active. Oral agents should not be used in pregnancy because safety data has not established their use.

Children and adolescent diabetics with type-2 diabetes are usually given sulfonylureas and/or metformin because of the clinical experience with these drugs in this age group [4]. Patients in acute hospital settings, especially those in the intensive care unit, should be given insulin for tighter glycemic control which has been shown to significantly improve benefits as we will see in a later chapter. This insulin can be administered with or without appropriately indicated oral agents.

Lets now discuss each group individually.

ORAL AGENT CLASSES

Sulfonylureas

These agents are indicated when hyperglycemia cannot be controlled with exercise, diet, and therapeutic life style changes. They bind to a specific receptor on the pancreatic beta cells which enhances the effect on glucose lowering due to a closure of the potassium dependent adenosine triphosphate channel (K-ATP). Glimepiride (Amaryl) binds to a different protein than the other sulfonylureas, but on the same site as the potassium channel. The subsequent reduction in plasma glucose results in secondary improvement in insulin action. Some concern has been raised recently with regard to the closure of the potassium channel since this channel may play a role in cardiac tissue in coronary artery vasodilatation.

The closing of the potassium pump enhances calcium influx into the myocardial cell enhancing coronary artery vasodilatation. It is argued by some that this impairment of the potassium pump also impairs coronary artery vasodilatation during acute ischemic events. Hence recent studies have raised the question about the prognosis of patients who present with acute myocardial ischemia and/or infarction while on these agents and their ultimate prognosis. Original concern about the first generation sulfonylureas was raised as early as the 1970s with the University Group Diabetes Study casting aspersions on tolbutamide and its worsening prognosis in macrovascular disease [5]. Several recent trials have evaluated the performance of second generation sulfonylureas for various endpoints including cardiovascular disease. The major risk of second generation sulfonylureas like glipizide, glyburide, and glimepiride are hypoglycemic episodes.

A meta-analysis in *Diabetes Care* included three studies concerning the cardiovascular effects of glyburide and found no increased association with cardiovascular events or overall mortality [6]. However, a retrospective review by Simpson et al. evaluated the dose response relationship with the sulfonylureas and mortality in type 2 diabetics using a population based cohort study. In this study, death risks were higher with glyburide compared to metformin and increased with higher doses [7].

Rao et al. reported a meta-analysis of nine observational studies in *Diabetes Care* in 2008 and reported an increased composites end point of cardiovascular hospitalizations and all-cause mortality with combination metformin/sulfonylurea therapy [8].

The Mayo Clinic reported results on 2,189 patients (386 of whom had type-2 diabetes) who had experienced a myocardial infarction to evaluate the effects of sulfonylureas on survival in January 2009. Patients who were taking first generation sulfonylureas, biguanides or TZD's were excluded from the study. In this study, patients taking the second generation sulfonylureas actually had a lower risk of death that diabetic patients taking insulin, although the diabetic patient population had greater mortality rates than the non diabetics.

In general all sulfonylureas are equally effective in terms of their hypoglycemic potency, although a recent trial has indicated that glimepiride (Amaryl) may be slightly more efficacious than the others. One can expect a 1.5–2% drop in hemoglobin A1C with entry hemoglobin A1C's greater than 9.0 in most patients. In general, the greater the fasting plasma glucose on initiation of therapy the greater the benefit [9].

Of course these agents depend upon good beta-cell function for their efficacy and the absence of any glutamic acid decarboxylase or islet cell antibodies. Many patients, particularly those with an entry hemoglobin A1C's greater than 8.0, will require the addition of a second oral agent, usually a sensitizer or insulin. Somewhat disappointing has been the fact that patients on oral agents, although they achieve an initial drop in hemoglobin A1C, over a period of 2–4 years, experience progressive hemoglobin A1C and fasting glucose elevations due to progressive beta-cell deterioration.

Despite their efficacy in causing insulin release from the pancreas, these agents have not been shown to preserve beta-cell function. Weight gain, lack of exercise, and dietary indiscretion are also associated with failures on sulfonylureas. Side effects with these medications are generally mild and reversible with discontinuation of therapy, with less than 2% of patients discontinuing therapy because of adverse affects. The major problem is hypoglycemia which is more common in agents with longer duration like glyburide and chlorpropamide [10].

It is also important to keep in mind that these agents are metabolized hepatically and excreted renally, hence any patients with renal insufficiency may run into trouble with hypoglycemia with all of these agents except for glipizide whose hepatic metabolites are not active, and hence there is no dosage decrease necessary in patients with renal insufficiency and taking this product.

In some studies, glyburide has been shown to have increased amounts of hypoglycemia due to its significant suppression of hepatic gluconeogenesis and its long duration of action. The frequency of hypoglycemia requiring hospital admission is 0.2–0.4 cases per 1,000 treatment years for sulfonylurea therapy, although there were somewhat higher levels in the United Kingdom Prospective Diabetes Study (UKPDS) trials.

In those patients with a risk for hypoglycemia, the shorter acting agents, like glipizide, may be more efficacious particularly as glomerular filtration rates begin to decline, and also in elderly patients.

Most instances of hypoglycemia with these agents are occurring, however, because of variations in patients' diet and progressive renal insufficiencies. Patients must be cautioned while taking oral agents about avoiding alcohol ingestion, which may promote an antabuse-like reaction and irregular eating habits which can cause havoc with glycemic consistency.

Ischemic preconditioning, as shown in animal models, indicates that brief period of ischemia with intermittent perfusion may protect the myocardium from the effect of a major ischemic episode. Some sulfonylureas used in the treatment of type-2 diabetes may have adverse effects on cardiovascular outcomes because they close the potassium channels that are necessary for ischemic pre-conditioning protection. Glimepiride appears to have less of an effect on the potassium channel than other sulfonylureas.

Despite the concerns about potassium channel interference with these agents, their benefit in achieving tighter glycemic control is important in reducing microvascular complications of the disease, but not in statistically significantly reducing the risks of macrovascular disease-particularly myocardial infarction. Subsequent long term trials covering over 10 years of therapy did not show an increased incidence of cardiovascular complications with the use of these agents.

The Diabetes Mellitus Insulin-Glucose Infusion in Acute Myocardial Infarction (DIGAMI) Trial showed a significant difference in mortality between the sulfonylurea treated group and the insulin treated group in terms of sudden death and fatal re-infarction [11]. This may in part be related to the beneficial effects of insulin in these acute settings. The UKPDS trial did not include patients with significant coronary artery disease, and hence the issue of postinfarction prognosis in these patients was not evaluated in these trials.

Although glimepiride, in general, has less effect on the cardiac potassium channel, no head to head trials have actually confirmed a cardiovascular benefit with this agent over other sulfonlureas. These secretogogues been reported to cause rash, nausea, and abnormalities in liver enzymes with a pattern most consistent with cholestatic injury.

Chlorpropamide can cause significant hyponatremia, particularly in elderly patients, due to increased sensitivity of the renal tubule to endogenously produced antidiuretic hormone. Although some weight gain can occur with the sulfonylureas, this is not as prominent as the weight gain we see with the TZD's. It is to be noted that these agents are sulfa drugs and are contraindicated in patients with *bona fide* allergies to sulfa products [10].

Drugs that undergo protein binding like the beta-blockers, warfarin, and nonsteriodal anti-inflammatory drugs may compete with sulfonylureas exacerbating hypoglycemia. However, the second generation sulfonylureas are non-ionically bound to plasma proteins and hence there is less of a risk of this potential drug interaction when compared to the first generation agents [9].

First generation sulfonylureas include

1. Acetohexamide (Dymelor) which has a duration of action of 12–18 h
2. Chlorpropamide (Diabinese) which has a duration of action of 48 or more hours
3. Tolazamide (Tolinase) with a duration of action of 12–24 h
4. Tolbutamide (Orinase) with a duration of action of 6–12 h

Second generation agents include:

1. Glyburide (Micronase, Glynase, or Diabeta) with a duration of action of 12–24 h
2. Glipizide (Glucotrol, Glucotrol XL) with a duration of action of 12–18 h and up to 24 h with Glucotrol XL
3. Glimepiride (Amaryl) with a duration of action of 24 h

These agents should be taken approximately 15–30 min before meals except for Glucotrol XL. The lowest effective dose should be started and titrated up slowly every 3–4 weeks. Of the class only acetohexamide and tolbutamide are primarily renally cleared, the rest are metabolized hepatically and cleared renally.

The Meglitinides (Glinides)

These agents are more properly referred to as the "Glinides" since technically repaglinide and nateglinide are not members of the same chemical class. Repaglinide is a benzoic acid derivative and nateglinide is a phenylalanine derivative. These agents specifically target postprandial hyperglycemia with less risk of hypoglycemia compared to sulfonylureas and less continuous stimulation of the beta cells.

These are designed to return insulin levels to baseline between meals while stimulating insulin secretion when needed at meal time. These agents, in general, are rapidly absorbed and quickly eliminated and are ideally positioned for those patients with primarily postprandial hyperglycemia with modest elevations of hemoglobin A1C less than 8.0. Both of these agents stimulate insulin secretion only in the presence of glucose, and hence these agents exert their primary and major effect at meal time [12]. They act by binding to the sulfonylurea receptor and closing the adenosine triphosphate (ATP) sensitive potassium channel. They should not be used with sulfonylureas.

Repaglinide (Prandin) was approved by the FDA in 1998 and Starlix (nateglinide) was approved by the FDA in December 2000.

Nateglinide has the shortest duration of action of all the insulin secretagogues with the least specific inhibition of the cardiac potassium channel. This agent possesses the least risk for hypoglycemia of any of the secretagogs along with lower insulin levels and more physiologic insulin release at meal time [13].

When used alone, repaglinide can be as effective as the sulfonylureas in reducing hemoglobin A1C and appears to be slightly more potent in that effect than nateglinide. Occasionally, patients can be switched off sulfonylureas and switched to repaglinide with better control. This has not been the case with nateglinide. A risk of hypoglycemia with repaglinide appears to be comparable to and occasionally slightly decreased compared with sulfonylureas. This risk can be mitigated by giving the glinides before meals rather than without eating.

Although these agents have minimal effect without having a meal, they can still increase the risk of hypoglycemia when taken in this fashion. No adverse cardiovascular toxicity has been associated with the glinides and there has been no subsequent demonstration of hepatic or renal toxicity with these medications.

Repaglinide is metabolized by the cytochrome P450-3A4 system and a warning has been instituted against the concomitant administration of gemfibrozil and repaglinide with an increased risk of hypoglycemia due to inhibition of metabolism of repaglinide secondary to inhibition of 3A-4 by gemfibrozil. Nateglinide is metabolized predominately through cytochrome P450-2C9 with both glinides being significantly bound to plasma proteins and hence minimally affected, if at all, by dialysis.

The hypoglycemic action of the glinides can be potentiated by nonselective beta-blockers, salicylates, monoamine oxidase inhibitors, and NSAIDS whereas steroids, thyroid hormones, sympathomimetic agents, and thiazide diuretics may reduce the effects of the glinides.

These agents are contraindicated in patients with type-1 diabetes or patients with known hypersensitivity to these agents or their ingredients. Caution should be exercised when used by the elderly or in patients with adrenal and pituitary insufficiency because of the increased risk of hypoglycemia as well as exacerbation of hypoglycemia with alcohol ingestion, strenuous physical exercise, and irregular dietary habits.

The glinides are not contraindicated in patients with renal insufficiency, but should be used cautiously in patients with liver disease with a slower titration schedule and lower doses being initially attempted. These agents are not indicated for concomitant use with sulfonylurea therapy since the sulfonylureas also inactivate the potassium channel rendering the glinides ineffective if used together [14].

The glinides are ideally suited for early diabetics, where the predominant and occasionally only abnormality is postprandial hyperglycemia, the elderly, and in patients with mild elevations of hemoglobin A1C with irregular dietary habits and or busy work schedules. They are now approved for use with the insulin sensitizers – metformin and the TZD's [12].

The Biguanides

In the USA, metformin is the only available member of this class. The previous biguanide, phenformin, was withdrawn from the United States market in the 1970s because of episodes of severe recurrent lactic acidosis and death. Metformin also comes in an extended release preparation and is approved for use in patients at least 10 years of age with the extended use preparation also approved for patients 17 years of age or older.

In the UKPDS trials, metformin use was associated with a reduced risk of macrovascular complications and is ideal for use in the obese patient and in any patient in whom weight gain is a concern. Any therapeutic regimen, especially patients on insulin, in which weight gain is a concern, can experience an attenuation of weight gain with the use of this product [15].

In the BIGPRO trial in 1994, non-diabetic patients were shown to lose weight with this product although it is not approved for use in this setting. Metformin has also been shown to be efficacious in patients with polycystic ovaries and in patients with impaired glucose tolerance although the product does not have official endorsement for these indications at this time [16].

The biguanides act by enhancing the sensitivity to insulin at the hepatic tissue level, decreasing hepatic gluconeogenesis, while having some effect in the peripheral tissue as well. By inhibition of insulin receptor tyrosine kinase activity, metformin has also been shown to reduce glycogenolysis, enhance glycogen sensitivity, increase glycogen synthesis and augmenting GLUT-4 glucose transporter activity. This product has also been shown to reduce insulin secretion since it enables the insulin to operate in a more efficient manner.

Metformin has not been shown to increase adiponectin levels as has been seen with the TZD's; however, it has been shown to reduce free fatty acid secretion while decreasing intestinal absorption of glucose and enhancing peripheral glucose utilization [17]. Unlike the sulfonylureas, metformin will not produce hypoglycemia in patients with type-2 diabetes. Food can decrease the extent of and delay the absorption of the product with 40% lower mean peak plasma levels following administration with food compared to taking the same medication on a fasting basis. Clinical relevance of this, however, has not been determined.

Metformin is excreted unchanged in the urine and does not undergo hepatic metabolism or biliary excretion. Renal clearances of this product are approximately 3.5 times greater than creatinine clearance indicating that tubular secretion presents the major route of metformin metabolism, hence this drug needs to be used very cautiously in patients with renal insufficiency and is not indicated for creatinine clearances less than 60 or serum creatinines greater 1.4 mg/dl in women and 1.5 mg/dl in men [18].

Metformin has been shown to decrease fasting sugars by 60–70 mg/dl and hemoglobin A1C by up to 2% in patients with poorly controlled diabetes and at times be equivalent to that seen with sulfonylureas. In addition, combination with sulfonylurea therapy has been shown to be synergistic as a result of the subsequent reduction in insulin resistance.

Metformin vs. placebo has been shown to lower total cholesterol up to 5%, triglyceride 16%, and LDL of 8% with modest improvements of HDL of 2–5%. These values are not significantly changed when used in combination with sulfonylureas. The major adverse effects of metformin are gastrointestinal including abdominal bloating, cramping, diarrhea, anorexia, and nauseousness being reported in up to 20–30% of patients. These are usually mild and can occasionally be mitigated by dosing with food.

Despite this, the discontinuation rate with this product is about 5%. Other reported side effects include diminished B-12 levels, metallic taste, and decreased appetite. Lactic acidosis is a rare but catastrophic complication with metformin therapy with mortality rates as high as 50%, although the incidence has been described as 3 cases per 100,000 patient years, it nonetheless remains a dreaded complication.

Therapeutic levels of this product have not been shown to increase serum lactate levels although adherence to contraindications should be practiced. These include renal disease and renal dysfunction as previously mentioned, congestive heart failure requiring pharmacologic therapy, known hypersensitivity to metformin and any metabolic or respiratory condition that can make the patient prone to acidosis including respiratory failure, chronic liver disease, alcohol ingestion, previous episodes of lactic acidosis from whatever cause [13].

Metformin should be temporarily discontinued in patients undergoing radiologic procedures involving intravascular administration of iodinated contrast materials because these products can interfere with renal function. Metformin should only be re-instituted within 48 hrs after these procedures or the return to baseline renal status has been assured. The subsequent risk of developing lactic acidosis can be decreased by regular monitoring of renal function when patients are taking this particular product.

The onset of lactic acidosis can certainly be accompanied by non-specific symptoms such as malaise, respiratory distress, abdominal distress, shortness of breath, or even myalgias with associated hypotension, hypothermia and cardiac arrhythmia with more severe cases. Prompt withdrawal of the product should be accomplished when these symptoms present themselves. It is important to understand that lactic acidosis can be suspected in any diabetic patient who presents with a metabolic acidosis in the absence of ketonuria, ketonemia, and ketoacidosis.

Lactic acidosis is a medical emergency and requires prompt medical attention. Cimetidine is the only known drug shown to reduce the renal clearance of metformin, although other products can have the potential to decrease its renal excretion, namely amiloride, digoxin, quinidine, vancomycin, procainamide, morphine, ranitidine and quinine. Metformin is also available in a combination product with glipizide (Metaglip) and glyburide (Glucovance) as well as pioglitazone (Actoplus MET), rosiglitazone (Avandamet), and repaglinide (Prandimet). Metformin is also available as a liquid preparation for those patients who have trouble swallowing pills and an extended release preparation (Glumetza). This extended release preparation may have less gastrointestinal side effects (diarrhea) than the shorter acting preparations by utilizing a unique polymer-based type delivery system, depositing the drug in the upper gastrointestinal tract where metformin is primarily absorbed. This decreases peak concentrations and slowly increases during contractions to the maximum level. In clinical trials, once daily metformin extended release was as effective as twice daily intermediate release metformin.

The Alpha-Glucosidase Inhibitors [19]

These non-systemic agents are used primarily to control postprandial hyperglycemia by delaying the absorption of polysaccharides and disaccharides in the intestinal brush border and can be used as initial agents or in combination therapy. Recent trials have indicated that patients placed on acarbose can reduce their risk of developing cardiovascular events.

Acarbose (Precose) was approved for use in the USA in September of 1995 and miglitol (Glyset) was approved for use in December 1996. It is to be understood that these products do not decrease, but delay the overall absorption of carbohydrates producing a smaller peak in serum glucose concentrations postprandially resulting in a more prolonged carbohydrate absorption curve. This allows the beta cell to have greater opportunity to match insulin responses to subsequent glucose demands enabling the available insulin to metabolize circulating glucose better in the postprandial state.

Miglitol has been shown to inhibit sucrase and alpha-amylase in the lumen of the small intestine which are responsible for the metabolism of sucrose and starch respectively. Alpha-amylase facilitates the breakdown of starch into dextrins, maltotriose, and maltose while sucrase inhibits the breakdown of sucrose. Miglitol's inhibition of the enzymes delays subsequent carbohydrate degradation attenuating postprandial plasma glucose elevation by delaying glucose uptake.

These agents are modestly effective in treating diabetes with hemoglobin A1C reductions of 0.5–1% and can be particularly effective in patients who consume significant carbohydrate diets. Adverse effects of these products are gastrointestinal and include abdominal bloating, pain, diarrhea, and flatulence in up to 70% of patients. Although these effects tend to dissipate in 4–6 weeks they tend to be a major reason for discontinuation of medications.

High doses of acarbose have been shown to elevate transaminases, while miglitol has been shown to be less irritating hepatically. Miglitol has been shown to decrease the bioavailability of propranolol and ranitidine. Their activity can be impaired with concomitant administration of intestinal absorbants such as cholestyramine and digestive enzyme preparations – particularly those containing carbohydrate splitting enzymes.

Acarbose is contraindicated in patients with cirrhosis, while miglitol is not contraindicated in patients with liver disease. Alpha-glucosidase inhibitors are not indicated in patients with severe renal insufficiency or in patients with inflammatory bowel disease or pre-existing bowel obstruction.

It is important to understand that patients experiencing hypoglycemia with these agents on board are to be given pure glucose. The administration of more complex carbohydrates may not be effective.

The Thiazolidinediones

These insulin sensitizers bind to the peroxisome proliferator activated receptor (PPAR) gamma (pioglitazone binds also to the PPAR-alpha). PPAR-gamma is a transcription cofactor that modifies expressions of various genes responsible for the encoding of proteins that are involved in lipid and glucose metabolism in homeostasis.

Those in this class include pioglitazone (Actos) and rosiglitazone (Avandia). The first TZD in this class troglitazone (Rezulin) was withdrawn from the market in March of 2000 because of significant hepatocellular injury.

Both of these agents at the present time are indicated for treatment of type-2 diabetes although recent studies have shown preservation of beta-cell function and regeneration of beta cells in animal models, and the potential efficacy for use of these products in patients with impaired glucose tolerance, as well and non-alcoholic steatohepatitis (NASH) is undergoing investigation.

These agents act predominately on the adipocyte decreasing tumor necrosis factor alpha, interleukin-6, and resistin while increasing adiponectin and GLUT-4 glucose transporter activity. The result is decreasing cytokine levels that reduce insulin resistance not only in liver tissue but muscle as well.

TZD's have also been shown to act directly at tissue level to redistribute fatty acids away from muscle, liver, cardiac, pancreatic tissue, and into the subcutaneous fat. This redistribution of fat results in less intramuscular and intra-abdominal fat with subsequent accumulation in the subcutaneous tissue [20].

In addition, TZD's may also have a direct effect on vascular smooth muscle enhancing endothelial function inhibiting arteriosclerotic vascular disease. Both pioglitazone and rosiglitazone have been shown to reduce high sensitivity CRP and other inflammatory markers such as interleukin-6 and plasminogen activator inhibitor 1 (PAI-1).

These agents have been shown to be efficacious in monotherapy and demonstrate synergistic glycemic effects when used with biguanides as well as sulfonylureas, glinides, and exogenous insulin.

Pioglitazone is metabolized by hydroxylation and oxidation with the metabolites partly converted to glucouronide or sulfate conjugates. These metabolites are pharmacologically active. This product is metabolized by CYP2C8 (39%) and CYP3A4 (17%). This may reduce the effectiveness of oral contraceptive agents containing ethinylestradiol and norethindrone. No other significant drug interactions have been reported to date.

Rosiglitazone is predominately metabolized by cytochrome P450-2C8 (and to a lesser extent 2C9) and has not been reported to have any significant drug interactions. The major routes of metabolism are N-demethylation and hydroxylation followed by conjugation with sulfate and glucouronic acid. All the circulating metabolites are considerably less potent than the parent product [20].

It should be kept in mind that the TZD's are contraindicated in patients with class III or class IV congestive heart failure and should be used with extreme caution in patients with significant valvular heart disease, borderline ejection fractions, significant diastolic dysfunction and are not indicated in patients with moderate hepatic dysfunction or in patients in whom entry transaminases that are 2.5 times greater than normal [21].

These products can enhance the formation of edema by increased sodium reabsorption at the tubular level due to enhanced insulin activity at these sites as well as arterial dilatation. The sodium retention effect can be somewhat attenuated by administration of diuretics and aggravated by concommitant use of any other products that increase the risk of edema formation such as the dihydropyridines, rofecoxib, and alpha-blockers or in patients with pre-existing severe venous disease.

Weight gain and edema is increased in patients on concommitant insulin therapy and care should be exercised in administering the TZD's in type-2 diabetics on insulin therapy with the lowest possible dose of the sensitizer being more prudent in these situations. It is always prudent to start with the lowest clinical effective dose and gradually titrate upward [22].

Hypoglycemic effects of the TZD's have been demonstrated as early as 2–4 weeks from initiation of therapy with maximum effects usually reached in approximately 4–6 weeks. When used concommitantly with sulfonylureas, hemoglobin A1C levels tend to remain consistent over extended periods of time up to 4–5 years, while progressively rising after the 1-year period using sulfonylurea therapy alone or even in combination with metformin. This effect may be due to the preservation of beta-cell function and perhaps even regeneration of beta-cell activity that has been shown to be experimentally demonstrated in animals.

In clinical trials with monotherapy and in combination, pioglitazone has been shown to have a triglyceride lowering effect that has not been demonstrated by rosiglitazone.

In addition, LDL levels tend to rise with rosiglitazone with both products causing a shift from the more atherogenic, small, dense LDL to the less atherogenic, large, fluffy LDL [23].

Reductions of hemoglobin A1C, anti-inflammatory factors, and fasting sugars are similar with both products with major difference being in triglyceride handling. Curiously both products tend to increase triglyceride production in the liver, while only pioglitazone enhances triglyceride disposal. This results in reductions of serum triglycerides with pioglitazone.

When used in monotherapy, reductions in glycosylated hemoglobin have been reported up to 1.5% in patients given 8 mg/day of rosiglitazone, especially when given in two doses with fasting glucose levels decreasing by 58–78 mg/dl [22]. Although approved for once a day, rosiglitazone appears to achieve better hemoglobin A1C reductions with BID administration than once daily. Glucose lowering potency of these two agents appears to be equivalent. When used in triple agent therapy, reductions in hemoglobin A1C of up to 1.3% have been reported.

From a physiological point of view, the TZD's offer some significant advantages at the cellular level due to their anti-inflammatory and anti-atherogenic effects in addition to their benefits in enhancing insulin sensitivity within the muscle cell and also within the liver. The small adipocytes are responsible for the production of adiponectin which decreases insulin resistance, while the large adipocytes produce leptin releasing free fatty acids which can enhance insulin resistance. Both rosiglitazone and pioglitazone have been shown to reduce free fatty acid concentrations, while increasing adiponectin levels.

Pioglitazone is the only available TZD with effects on both PPAR-gamma as well as PPAR-alpha [24].

The weight gain with these products primarily results from an increase in subcutaneous fat content with a decrease in intra-abdominal fat along with a subsequent decline in triglycerides and free fatty acid concentrations. These products also result in decrease in intramuscular fat content. Animal models have indicated that TZD's will help preserve beta-cell function.

Significant drug induced hepatoxicity has been reported with both products, but these cases are rare and usually confined to those individuals who are consuming alcohol or taking other hepatoxic drugs such as acetaminophen in large quantities. When taken as directed these products are far safer to the liver than their precursor, troglitazone.

Due to concerns regarding hepatotoxicity, liver function tests should be performed before starting TZD therapy and every 2–3 months during the first year of therapy thereafter.

If liver function tests rise to greater than three times the upper limit of normal, the TZD should be stopped. Also reported has been a slight decrease in hemoglobin and hematocrit due to fluid retention and the dilutional effect resulting from expansions in plasma volume.

Edema occurs in 2–4% of patients with monotherapy and 4–6% of patients receiving combination therapy, while the incidence of edema can be as high as 10–15% in individuals taking insulin. The TZD's are contraindicated in diabetic individuals with New York Heart Association Class III and Class IV cardiac status.

Pioglitazone is strictly a once a day drug, while rosiglitazone can be administered twice daily.

Rosiglitazone and pioglitazone are both highly protein bound, but differ in their metabolism within the cytochrome P-450 system, drug interactions of any significance have not been reported. Since beta-cell deterioration and insulin resistance may begin long before the onset of type-2 diabetes, overcoming enhancing insulin sensitivity and preserving beta-cell function remain strong considerations for the use of these agents first line. However, the clinician must be aware of the warnings concerning precipitation of heart failure in those individuals with vavular heart disease, impaired systolic function or even significant diastolic dysfunction that would place these patients at increased risk for congestive heart failure. In addition, patients on TZD's should be regularly monitored for a change in clinical status or cardiac function. Recently, however, several clinical trials have shed light on other significant benefits from TZD's – especially pioglitazone.

The Carotid Intima Media Thickness in Atherosclerosis Using Pioglitazone (CHICAGO) Trial evaluated 361 patients with type-2 diabetes over an 18 month period time to randomization of treatment with glimepiride 1–2 mg or Pioglitazone 15–30 mg [25]. All patients were titrated to achieve a fasting glucose of less than 140 mg/dl. hemoglobin A1C values at baseline were 6.5–9.0%.At the conclusion of the trial, mean posterior wall carotid intima thickness had decreased in the pioglitazone group and increased in the glimepiride group. HDL-C rose in the pioglitazone group and declined in the glimepiride group creating a statistically significant difference of 6.4 mg/dl. The statistically significant difference between triglycerides between the pioglitazone group and the glimepiride group was 45.6 mg/dl. The trial provided surrogate data to appreciate the possible benefits of TZD therapy.

Nissen et al. reported a coronary artery intravascular ultrasound study, The Pioglitazone Effect on Regression of Intravascular Sonographic Coronary Obstruction (PERISCOPE) trial on 543 patients from 97 academic and community hospitals throughout North and South America, to determine the effect of oral anti-diabetic agents on the progression of coronary artery disease [26]. Prior to this study, no antidiabetic regimen had been successful in reducing the progression of coronary arteriosclerotic disease. This double blinded randomized trial evaluated patients with type-2 diabetes and known coronary artery disease. Patients were randomized to receive 1–4 mg of glimepiride or 15–45 mg of pioglitazone, while receiving baseline coronary intravascular ultrasound and a follow up study in 18 months. At the end of the trial, patients on pioglitazone had significantly lower progression of coronary atherosclerosis than their counterparts on glimepiride. In addition, mean fasting insulin levels dropped with pioglitazone and rose with glimepiride. The percent of atheroma volume increased by 0.73% in patients on glimepiride and decreased by 0.16% with pioglitazone. In addition, when compared with glimepiride, HDL levels increased by 5.7 mg/dl.

The Prospective Pioglitazone Clinical Trial in Macrovascular Events (PROACTIVE) trial was a randomized double blinded study of 5,238 patients to determine the impact of pioglitazone on reducing macrovascular events in patients with type-2 diabetes [27]. This study randomized patients to placebo or treatment with 45 mg of pioglitazone in addition to an existing regimen of beta-blockers, ace-inhibitors, metformin, sulfonylureas insulin, aspirin, statins, and fibrates. Mean follow-up period was 2.8 years and showed a non-statistically significant reduction in primary end points (non-fatal myocardial infarction, stroke, major leg amputations, acute coronary syndrome, leg revascularization, coronary bypass surgery, and percutaneous vascular intervention. However, reduction in secondary end points (death, myocardial infarction, and stroke) was statistically significant at 16%. Also noted was a 50% less progression to insulin, blood pressure and hemoglobin A1C reduction, increases in HDL and a higher incidence of heart failure events, edema and weight gain with pioglitazone compared to placebo. This study has generated much debate about the results – particularly the utility regarding the results of secondary outcomes in a study that did not achieve its primary outcomes. Clearly, however, this study, once again, underscores the importance of risk stratification of patients for heart failure before considering TZD therapy.

The DREAM (Diabetes Reduction Assessment with Ramipril and Rosiglitazone). Trial was conducted to prospectively assess the ability of rosiglitazone to prevent type-2 diabetes in those patients at risk for developing the disease [28]. The study was conducted in individuals 30 years of age or older with impaired fasting glucose or impaired glucose tolerance and no previous cardiovascular disease. About 5,269 individuals from 21 countries participated. In this trial, rosiglitazone halted the progression to type-2 diabetes in this group with a higher incidence of heart failure in those on this TZD with 50.3% of individuals reverting to euglycmeia compared to 30.3% on placebo. The DREAM (Diabetes Reduction Assessment with Ramipril and Rosiglitazone).

This data, combined with the beneficial effects on preserving pancreatic beta-cell function and restoring beta-cell insulin content, while preventing loss of beta-cell mass provide encouraging support for the use of TZD's in patients who are not at risk for heart failure. TZD's have also been shown to decrease free fatty acid concentrations, which is another important cause of insulin resistance. This effect has not been demonstrated to any significant degree with metformin.

Type-2 diabetics have been shown to possess an increased proinsulin/insulin ratio, another marker for beta-cell dysfunction with elevated pro-insulin levels enhancing the possibility of producing smaller, dense, more atherogenic LDL molecules. Reduction in both systolic and diastolic blood pressure has been demonstrated in clinical trials with rosiglitazone, while both TZD's have shown reductions in microalbuminuria, a known indicator of glomerular damage and precursor of renal dysfunction and failure.

TZD's have also been shown to reduce inflammatory markers. PAI-1 attenuates endogenous intravascular hemolysis. Individuals with diabetes, insulin resistance, those with polycystic ovary syndrome, and those at risk for cardiovascular disease will possess elevated PAI-1 levels. Addition of rosiglitazone to a sulfonylurea regimen had a more demonstrative effect in decreasing these levels than the sulfonylurea alone. By inhibiting macrophage activation, suppressing matrix metalloproteinase production, inhibiting cytokine production, and attenuating smooth muscle cell proliferation, TZD's have been shown to reduce inflammatory markers like interleukin-6 and hs-CRP [29].

Physicians should also be aware that both men and women who take TZD's may be at increased risk of fractures. Randomized trials involving TZD's indicated a risk that was doubled in women with no change in men [31]. However, a prospective cohort study published in the *Archives of Internal Medicine in 2009* by Dormuth et al. indicated that both men and women may be at increased risk [30]. The basis of this concern centers around the effects of TZD's on bone metabolism – accelerating bone loss and decreasing bone formation. Further study is needed to determine fracture risk with greater certainty.

DPP-IV Inhibitors (Gliptins)

Dipeptylpeptidase 4, a type-2 integral membrane protein widely distributed throughout the body is a serine protease whose gene is positioned along the long arm of chromosome 2. DPP-IV inactivates GLP-1 by 50% within 1–2 min by cleaving the N-terminal acid.

The deactivation of GIP is somewhat longer, taking approximately 7 min to inactivate 50%, resulting in an inactive metabolite. DPP-IV circulates freely throughout the plasma and rapidly inactivates several biologically active peptides, while being located at the surface of endothelial cells [32].

GLP-1, as measured in the plasma, represents a small amount of the protease that actually exists in the gut. Since closer to 50% of the secreted GLP-1 has already been degraded before it reaches the general circulation, greater than 40% is degraded before it reaches the beta cells. GLP-1 is stored essentially as the active amide in the subsequently cleaved GLP-1 molecule residue at position 2 of the alanine terminal end. The action of GLP-1 is somewhat different from the sulfonylureas, which predominantly stimulate insulin release.

Within the beta cell, both GIP and GLP-1 bind to two specific receptors resulting in the activation of proteinase A, increasing cyclic AMP, subsequently stimulating G protein coupled adenyl cyclase, enhancing pro-insulin synthesis, and subsequently potentiating insulin secretion. GIP receptors have been described in the adrenal gland, brain, pituitary, adipose tissue, stomach, duodenum, alpha and beta islet cells; whereas GLP-1 receptor distribution has been found in the liver, brain, skeletal muscle, kidney, lungs, as well as the alpha and beta islet cells.

It should be kept in mind that islet-cell function represents a complex response regulated by not only incretin hormones, but also by the direct effects of blood glucose concentration, which increases insulin secretion and also decreases glucagon secretion. The physiologic actions of GIP and GLP-1 are not identical although both proteases stimulate insulin secretion. GLP-1 inhibits glucagon secretion and reduces food intake as well as gastric emptying while both proteases promote beta-cell proliferation.

In patients with type-2 diabetes, GIP secretion is normal, but the response to GIP is impaired; whereas GLP-1 secretion and release is reduced while the response to GLP-1 is essentially preserved. In the alpha cell, GLP-1 enhances glucose sensing while suppressing glucagon release in a glucose dependent manner with no effect on glucagon release in response to hypoglycemia. These effects are alleviated by specific G protein coupled receptors located on the alpha cells [33].

Plasma insulin levels increase following oral glucose ingestion exceeding levels produced with intravenous glucose administration. This incretin effect is responsible for more than 70% of the response to an oral glucose challenge! [34] GIP is produced mainly by the K cells of the duodenum, with carbohydrates and fats serving as the main stimulators for its release. GLP-1 is produced mainly by the small intestinal L cells and can be stimulated by proteins as well as fats and carbohydrates.

The first DPP-IV inhibitor, sitagliptin, received approval from the FDA in October, 2006 and has been approved for mono therapy as well as combination therapy with metformin, a TZD or a sulfonylurea at a standard dose of 50–100 mg daily with dose reduction required in individuals with renal dysfunction. Following a single dose, sitagliptin has been shown to double the level of postprandial GLP-1 and subsequently reduce DPP-4 activity by 80%. These effects appear to be dose related with reduction of DPP-4 activity ranging from 80 to 96% with dose ranges from 25 to 200 mg of sitagliptin. In addition, it has been demonstrated that GLP-1 levels increased by 1.3–1.9-fold following all glucose tolerance testing of individuals pre-treated with DPP-IV inhibition by sitagliptin in a dose range from 25 to 200 mg, while lowering hemoglobin A1C by 0.6–1.2% compared to placebo in 12–24 week trials [35].

In patients poorly controlled on metformin, the addition of sitagliptin 100 mg daily for 24 weeks reduced the hemoglobin A1C by 0.65% compared to placebo. When 100 mg was used with long term efficacy in 52 week trials with combination therapy, the hemoglobin A1C was 6.7% lower compared to baseline metformin monotherapy. Interestingly there were similar reductions reported with glipizide and metformin. When used as initial therapy, combination of sitagliptin and metformin had a more powerful effect, with hemoglobin A1C levels being reduced by 2.07% from baseline in patients receiving sitagliptin 100 mg and metformin 2,000 mg vs. 1.20% for the placebo group [36].

In patients suboptimally controlled with pioglitazone, the addition of 100 mg daily of sitagliptin for 24 weeks reduced the hemoglobin A1C by 0.7% compared to placebo, and 45% of patients with TZD and DPP-IV inhibitor combination had hemoglobin A1C's of less than 7% compared to 23% of those on pioglitazone alone. Fasting blood glucose was reduced by 17.7 mg/dl [37].

In all these studies, the effects on weight with sitagliptin appear to be neutral with some reporting weight losses of 1.5 kg, while there was weight gain of 1.8 kg compared to placebo. Data with another DPP-IV inhibitor, vildagliptin, demonstrates similar improvement in glycemic control compared to sitagliptin. In addition, 12 week studies of vildagliptin 50 mg in patients with impaired fasting glucose and impaired glucose tolerance demonstrated increased levels of gastric inhibitory peptide and GLP-1 postprandially with improvement in both alpha-and beta-cell function, decreased hemoglobin A1C, and reductions in post prandial glucose when compared to placebo. This short term study may indicate that the DPP-IV inhibitors and vildagliptin may play a role in preventing progression of type-2 diabetes in patients in the pre-diabetic state [38].

In phase I and phase II clinical trials in healthy male volunteers, alogliptin has been shown to be rapidly absorbed reaching peak concentrations in 1–2 h and an elimination half life varying with the dosage from 12.5 to 21 h. This peptidase is metabolized hepatically, but it is excreted primarily unchanged in the urine with the blood levels increasing from 1.7 to 3.8-fold in patients varying in degrees of renal insufficiency from mild to end stage [39].

Despite the fact that the drug is 25–30% hepatically metabolized, hepatic dysfunction was not associated with clinically significant changes in kinetic patterns. Alogliptin has a wider base range than sitagliptin. Twelve week studies have shown that patients who had been newly diagnosed with diabetes not controlled with exercise and diet and who were given alogliptin 6.25–100 mg daily vs. placebo demonstrated significant reductions in hemoglobin A1C as well as fasting glucose [40].

In phase III clinical trials, enhanced response was seen when the drug was used in combination with metformin, glyburide, and pioglitazone. When used in combination with insulin, 26-week trials have also shown the significant reductions of hemoglobin A1C at 26 weeks in patients inadequately controlled with insulin monotherapy or insulin plus metformin. Although currently not approved in the pre-diabetic state, these encouraging clinical trials may point to more expanded use of the DPP-IV inhibitors in the future [41].

The most recently approved DPP-IV inhibitor, saxagliptin (Onglyza), has demonstrated its efficacy in several recent clinical trials. In monotherapy with type-2 diabetics naive to therapy, a 24-week study showed that saxagliptin reduced hemoglobin A1C 0.6% compared to placebo in patients with baseline hemoglobin A1C levels of 7.9% for the 2.5 mg dose and 8.0% for the 5.0 mg dose. Using combination saxagliptin with metformin as initial therapy for 24 weeks in patient with baseline hemoglobin A1C levels of 9.4%, demonstrated a 0.5% reduction in hemoglobin A1C compared to metformin alone using 5.0 mg of the DPP-IV inhibitor and titration to 2,000 mg of metformin with more patients achieving an hemoglobin A1C level less than 7.0% with combination therapy compared to metformin alone. When saxagliptin was added to a submaximal dose of glyburide 7.5 mg in 768 adult patients with type-2 diabetes, reductions in hemoglobin A1C of 0.6% was observed compared to an uptitration of glyburide at the 24-week period. When added to metformin therapy in 192 type-2 diabetics, saxagliptin reduced the hemoglobin A1C by 0.7 and 0.8% in the 2.5 and 5.0 mg doses respectively [42].

In patients with moderate or severe renal impairment or with end stage renal disease requiring hemodialysis, the once daily 2.5 mg dose is recommended. A dose related decrease in lymphocyte count of 220 cells/μl compared to placebo has been reported with this product. The clinical significance of this remains to be determined and has not been associated with adverse clinical events; however, in clinical cases of unusual or prolonged infections, lymphocyte counts should be measured. The effects of saxagliptin in patients with human immunodeficiency virus are not known. Safety and efficacy of this product in pediatric patients has not been established and the drug should be used only if clearly needed in pregnancy (Category B). The secretion of this drug into breast milk is unknown. Saxagliptin is metabolized via cytochrome P450-3A4, and therefore the dose should be decreased to 2.5 mg when coadministered with a strong 3A4 inhibitor like, ketoconazole, clarithromycin, nefazodone, or atazanavir [43].

Bile Acid Sequestrants (Colesevelam)

It is well known that the gastrointestinal tract plays a critical role in lipoprotein and triglyceride regulation. Essential in this process is the role of steroid and bile acids which function by activating the farnesoid X receptor (FXR). Recent evidence indicates that this receptor also plays an important role in glucose metabolism. Hence, by inhibiting the absorption of bile acids, these sequestrants function as FXR antagonists.

This diminished activity of the FXR receptor can indirectly increase liver X receptor activity, which reduces plasma glucose levels as well as enhancing reverse cholesterol transport. Other proposed mechanisms of the glucose lowering effects of colesevelam include alterations in the hepatocyte nuclear factor 4 alpha expression, an inhibition of cholecystokinin release, or interactions with the G protein coupled receptor TGR5, which has been reported to enhance insulin secretion by virtue of its effects on GLP-1 [44].

Combined glucose and lipid effects were elucidated in the Glucose Lowering Effect of Welchol Study (GLOWS). This randomized double blinded, placebo controlled pilot study enrolled 65 patients and showed that colesevelam treatment resulted in reductions of fructos-amine (−29.0 μmol/l), postprandial glucose (−31.5 mg/dl), and HbA$_1$C of −1.0%. The LDL decreased by 9.6% and the total cholesterol was 7.35 lower than the placebo group. Adding colesevelam to an existing regimen of metformin monotherapy resulted in a significant reduction of hemoglobin A1C levels of 0.47% compared to placebo with reductions of 0.54% shown when compared to metformin combination therapy. Similar data resulted when this drug was added to insulin or sulfonylurea based therapy with reductions in hemoglobin A1C of 0.54% compared to placebo at 26 weeks. Hence, this unique bile acid sequestrant can be of value to enhance glycemic and lipid control during the entire course of the type-2 diabetic continuum. Since this agent is not systemically absorbed, there are no direct hepatic, cardiac or renal effects and should not be used in patients with triglycerides greater than 200 mg/dl [45].

ORAL AGENT COMBINATIONS [*12*]

Less than 20% of type-2 diabetics presenting to primary care physicians offices with an initial glucose of 200–240 mg/dl (Hemoglobin A1-C's of 9–10) will be able to reach a hemoglobin A1C of less than 7.0 if treated with maximal doses of a sulfonylurea alone or metformin alone.

With the new guidelines lowering the bar for hemoglobin A1C, the majority of patients seen in primary care offices with this degree of hyperglycemia will require combination therapy to achieve the desired goal of 6.5. Even those with initially good response to a single agent will subsequently require a second or even a third agent in the future due to the progressive nature of type-2 diabetes, dietary indiscretion, and non-compliance

Let's look at some of the various combinations of oral agents.

Metformin and Sulfonylurea

This most popular combination provides additive glucose and lipid lowering effects with metformin preventing weight gain, while reducing triglyceride and LDL cholesterol concentrations. This is particularly important since close to 80% of type-2 diabetic patients are overweight and almost all have some type of dyslipidemia. Metformin was the only oral agent shown to reduce myocardial infarction, stroke and cardiovascular mortality in the United Kingdom Prospective Diabetes Study (UKPDS) [*46*]. A combination of metformin and glyburide (Glucovance) and metformin and glipizide (Metaglip) are currently available in the USA for glycemic control. These products provide a unique opportunity to begin combination therapy with one pill for those poorly controlled type-2 diabetics with fasting blood glucoses greater than 200 mg/dl or hemoglobin A1C's greater than 8.0%.

These combination drugs should be given with meals, splitting the dose equally between breakfast and dinner. Caution should be exercised in treating patients with lower plasma glucoses at fasting glucoses less than 150 mg/dl due to the increased risk of hypoglycemia. It is always better to start with a lower dose of the sulfonylurea in these combination products, because of the profound effect of the combination of sulfonylurea and metformin on glucose lowering.

It is important to keep in mind that these combination products, since they contain metformin, are not indicated with serum creatinines greater than 1.4 mg/dl in women and 1.5 mg/dl in men, or creatinine clearances less than 60 ml/min, or in congestive heart failure, respiratory conditions prone to acidosis, chronic alcoholism, significant hepatic disease, and any history of significant hypoxia or lactic acidosis. The same restrictions for withholding this product before any dye studies previously mentioned are applicable.

These combination products enhance patient compliance by providing two agents acting synergistically in one pill, but also raise the added caution of increased potency and the potential for hypoglycemia or hypoglycemic reactions [*12*]. Combination pills include Glucovance (glyburide and metformin), Duetact (glimepiride and pioglitazone), Avandaryl (rosiglitazone and glimepiride), and Metaglip (glipizide and metformin)

Metformin and Thiazolidinediones

When pioglitazone or rosiglitazone is added to metformin the decline in hemoglobin in hemoglobin A1C is 0.8–1.0%. When used as triple agent therapy with metformin and a sulfonylurea, troglitazone use actually lowered the hemoglobin A1C by 1.3%. Similar results can be seen with the other TZD [47].

Weight gain normally seen with TZD use is attenuated with the addition of metformin. Synergistic effects on triglyceride lowering and increases in HDL are seen when metformin and pioglitazone are combined. The combination of a biguanide and a TZD has become increasingly popular since the former primarily inhibits hepatic gluconeogenesis and the latter primarily enhances insulin sensitivity in the muscles. In addition, the biguanides will also improve peripheral insulin sensitivity, while the TZD's inhibit gluconeogenesis [48]. Combination pills include Actoplus MET and Avandamet.

Metformin and Repaglinide

Combination therapy with these two agents has shown additive effects with reductions of hemoglobin A1C of 1.4% with a combination compared to 0.4% with repaglinide alone and 0.3% with metformin alone. Since repaglinide is metabolized in the cytochrome P450-3A4 enzyme system, drugs that are metabolized through this system (Rifampin, barbiturates, carbamazepine, certain statin drugs, amiodarone, benzodiazepines, sildenafil (Viagra), theophylline, and certain SSRI's) may increase repaglinide metabolism [49].

Although in vitro data indicate that repaglinide metabolism may be inhibited by antifungal agents such as ketoconazole and miconazole along with antibacterial agents such clarithromycin, systematically acquired data is not available on increased or decreased plasma levels with other 3A4 inhibitors or inducers.

Risk of hypoglycemia is increased with this combination compared to either agent alone. Repaglinide should be avoided in elderly, debilitated or malnourished patients and in those with adrenal or pulmonary insufficiency, and is not indicated for combination use with any sulfonylurea. Repaglinide should not be used in patients with severe liver disease and used only with caution in those with impaired hepatic function. A combination pill is available (Prandimet) for these two drugs.

Metformin and Nateglinide

Nateglinide is metabolized in the liver primarily by cytochrome P450-2C9 (70%) and 3A4 (30%) with its metabolites excreted renally. No dose adjustment is therefore necessary in patients with renal or hepatic insufficiency. This agent is indicated for combination therapy with metformin in those patients whose diabetes has not been adequately controlled with either agent alone. Patients whose diabetes has not been controlled by sulfonylureas or metformin should not be switched to nateglinide alone.

Although this agent is not appropriate in patients with advanced diabetes, especially with fasting blood glucose levels greater than 200 mg/dl, it can be used very effectively in combination with metformin to enhance insulin sensitivity. A recent trial presented at the American Diabetes Association Scientific Sessions showed that nateglinide reduced postprandial glucose levels from 195 to 150 mg/dl in monotherapy and from 209 to 160 mg/dl in patients in combination with metformin and nateglinide. Hemoglobin A1C levels dropped an additional 0.8% when nateglinide was given to patients inadequately controlled on metformin monotherapy [50].

Other trials have shown more robust reduction of hemoglobin A1C levels to 1.4% with the nateglininde/metformin combination with fasting glucose reductions of 40 mg/dl. This combination is ideal for those overweight patients whose primary disturbance is postprandial hyperglycemia with hemoglobin A1C 's less than 8.0% [51].

Repaglinide and Thiazolidinedione

This combination demonstrated a reduction in hemoglobin A1C of 1.3% when repaglinide was added to Troglitazone (Rezulin). Current studies with pioglitazone and rosiglitazone have demonstrated a synergistic effect that reduced hemoglobin A1C levels by 1.3% after 6 months. Since repaglinide and pioglitazone, and to a certain extent, nateglinide, are metabolized in cytochrome P450-3A4, a potential for drug interaction exists although none has yet been described [12].

Sulfonylurea and Thiazolidinedione

Clinical trials evaluating the addition of pioglitazone or rosiglitazone to poorly controlled sulfonylurea treated type-2 diabetics have shown synergistic effect with decreases in hemoglobin A1C levels of 1.2–1.4%, slightly greater than when the glitazones are combined with metformin. When used in monotherapy or in combinations, pioglitazone therapy reduces triglyceride up to 15% and increases HDL up to 19% with essentially no significant effects on the LDL [52].

Alpha-Glucosidase Inhibitors and Sulfonylurea

Introduced in 1996, miglitol and acarbose are currently approved for monotherapy and in combination with sulfonylureas, insulin, metformin, and the TZD's. These agents do not cause malabsorption, but delay the digestion of carbohydrates with subsequent absorption shifted to the more distal parts of the small intestine and colon. These agents can be very effective in blunting postprandial plasma glucose elevations allowing the beta cells significant enough time to increase insulin secretion.

These are most effective in patients who are on a sulfonylurea and require an additional 25–30 mg/dl reduction in fasting glucose concentrations or those individuals who need enhanced postprandial control. One study demonstrated reduction of 0.65% in hemoglobin A1C levels when acarbose was added to metformin with reductions of 0.5% in hemoglobin A1C levels in patients on insulin in addition to a reduction in total daily insulin dose of 8.3% [53].

Alpha-glucosidase inhibitors should be taken with the first bite of food. Gastrointestinal effects of bloating, flatulence, diarrhea, and stomach pain can occur early in therapy and diminish with time. These agents are ideally suited for those patients who ingest significant amounts of complex carbohydrates as adjunctive therapy to sulfonylureas and insulin sensitizers. Although working on two different mechanisms in controlling postprandial sugar, significant data does not exist as of the present time to give a formal recommendation on concomitant use of alpha glucosidase inhibitors and glinides [12].

DPP-IV Inhibitors and Metformin and/or Thiazolidinediones

Combination therapy with sitagliptin and metformin has been shown to be particularly effective. In a review of 701 patients with type-2 diabetes for 24 weeks, sitagliptin, in combination with metformin at a dose of 1,500 mg a day, provided significant improvement in hemoglobin A1C, FPG, and 2 hr PPG compared to placebo and metformin, with the hemoglobin A1C being reduced by 0.7; FPG's by 17 mg/dl, and 2 hr postprandial reduced by 62 mg/dl. Similar encouraging results were seen when sitagliptin was combined with pioglitazone. In a 24-week study of 354 patients, hemoglobin A1C 's were reduced by 0.9 and fasting sugars by 17 mg/dl. The recent approved of use of sitagliptin and sulfonylureas have significantly expanded the options for primary care physicians when using DPP-IV inhibitors. A recent study combining sitagliptin with glipizide over a 52-week period of time in patients with type-2 diabetes demonstrated that hemoglobin A1C 's decreased by 0.67 in patients with a baseline hemoglobin A1C of 7.5 with this combination and also demonstrated that sitagliptin was not inferior to glipizide in hemoglobin A1C lowering over 52 weeks in the predefined patient population [54]. The combination pill, here, is Janumet (sitagliptin and metformin).

Combinations with Bile Acid Sequestrants

The approval of colesevelam for glycemic control provides another intriguing option for using oral agents in patients with type-2 diabetes. This product has been used in clinical trials with sulfonylureas, metformin and insulin with modest, but significant hemoglobin A1C reductions [30].

Combination medications provide the physician a unique opportunity to use combination therapy with fewer pills. Glimepiride has been used as a combination pill with both rosiglitazone and pioglitazone. Sitagliptin can also be prescribed in a pill with metformin (Janumet). Both rosiglitazone and pioglitazone are available in a combination tablet with metformin (Avandimet and Actoplus MET). This allows the physician the opportunity of providing the patient with quadriple therapy using only two different pills, combining sensitizers with a DPP-4 inhibitor and a secretagogue. Even the glinide, repaglinide is now available in combination with metformin (Prandimet).

MULTIPLE ORAL AGENT THERAPY

Although this approach is effective when all three agents are used synergistically, little data exists with regard to multiple agent therapy. The addition of troglitazone before its withdrawal from the market to type-2 diabetics poorly controlled with a sulfonylurea and metformin, produced an additional 1.3% decrease in hemoglobin A1C. Similar results have been reported with pioglitazone and rosiglitazone [24].

Adding an alpha-glucosidase inhibitor to metformin and a secretagogue has also been found to be an attractive regimen. Due to the availability of combination drugs (sulfonylurea plus metformin, or sulfonylurea plus a TZD, or metformin plus TZD, or DPP-IV inhibitor plus metformin), the physician has the opportunity of using three drugs all with synergistic activity in two different medications, using either a combination of sulfonylurea and metformin or a combination of two sensitizers and/or DPP-IV inhibitor and/or sulfonylurea. Keep in mind, however, that the glinides should not be used with secretagogues and have not been evaluated in combination with DPP-IV inhibitors.

Table 2
Determinants of glucose control

Fasting glucose

   Reflects hepatic gluconeogenesis

   Increased when evening post-prandial glucose is elevated

   Increased with basal insulin deficiencies

Postprandial glucose

   Reflects effectiveness of bolus insulin secretion/incretin release

   Affected by preprandial glucose level

   Major contributor to the HbA_1C with levels ≤8.5%

HbA_1C=fasting glucose+postprandial glucose

From DeFronzo [10]

With the availability of multiple agents and various combinations, the physician can make use of quadruple and even quintuple therapy with the use of a sensitizer or sensitizers, secretagogue, bile acid sequestrant, alpha-glucosidase inhibitor, and DPP-IV inhibitor – all of which addressing various aspects of the type-2 diabetes paradigm. With the cost restraints that exist today, fitting all of these into a patient's budget is a constant challenge and continuous work in progress, however.

Regardless of the combination used, Table 2 lists some general principals to keep in mind.

1. Fasting (pre-meal) hyperglycemia is caused by increased hepatic glucose production, decreased basal insulin secretion, reduced insulin sensitivity, and high sustained postprandial glucose levels. For those individuals with AM fasting hyperglycemia, be aware of supper time postprandial excursions and bedtime snacks. All oral agents are effective in lowering fasting or pre-meal glucose, although the glinides and alpha-glucosidase inhibitors specifically target postprandial excursions. Metformin can be particularly effective in reducing pre-breakfast hyperglycemia due to its inhibition of hepatic gluconeogenesis and enhanced hepatic insulin sensitivity.

2. Levels of postprandial glucose are regulated by preprandial glucose levels, insulin sensitivity, and bolus or first phase insulin release. Those oral agents effective in reducing postprandial hyperglycemia include the glinides (repaglinide and nateglinide), alpha-glucosidase inhibitors, DPP-IV inhibitors, and to some extent, TZD's and biguanides.

Physicians, care providers and patients should familiarize themselves with the advantages and disadvantages of the various medications listed in Table 3.

The following is a recommended treatment strategy [10]:

1. For fasting glucoses that are slightly elevated (126–160 mg/dl., hemoglobin A1C 's less than 8%), insulin resistance predominates and plasma insulin levels are usually elevated. A rational approach would be to use the insulin sensitizers alone or in combination, DPP-IV inhibitors or sulfonylureas as initial therapy with diet and exercise.

2. For fasting glucoses of 160–180 mg/dl (hemoglobin A1C 's 8–9%) combination therapy with a DPP-IV inhibitor and/or secretagog, (sulfonylurea, nateglinide, or repaglinide) and a

Table 3
Differences among current therapies – effects and limitations

Agent	Mechanism of action	Metabolism/ excretion	Limitations	Special populations	Comments
Sulfonylureas Glimepiride Glyburide Glipizide	Enhance insulin secretion by predominantly increasing basal insulin production by binding to a pancreatic beta-cell receptor, closing potassium dependent ATP channel (K-ATP)	Hepatic/renal	Hypoglycemia Weight gain	Dose reduction with renal insufficiency with glimepiride and glyburide but not glipizide	Dependent on satisfactory beta-cell function and do not preserve beta-cell mass or deter progressive beta-cell deterioration
Glinides (Meglitinides) Nateglinide Repaglinide	Improve bolus insulin secretion when taken prior to meals and return insulin levels to baseline between meals. Effects are glucose dependent. Highly selective pancreatic potassium channel blockade	Repaglinide (cytochrome P450-3A4) Nateglinide (cytochrome P450-2C9)	Hypoglycemia/ weight gain	Repaglinide has an increased risk of hypoglycemia compared to nateglinide; avoid in those with hepatic disease, caution with gemfibroziil and with other 3A4 agents	Extremely effective in early stages of diabetes Repaglinide contraindicated with gemfibrozil
Biguanides Metformin	Enhances insulin sensitivity, inhibits glycogenolysis and hepatic gluconeogenesis, enhancing glucose uptake in muscle and fat, increasing tyrosine kinase activity Decreases intestinal glucose absorption	Renal clearance with tubular secretion	GI adverse effects Lactic acidosis (rare)	Avoid in patients with: GFR <60 serum creatinine >1.5 (men) and >1.4 (women) Dehydration states, CHF Chronic liver disease Metabolic or respiratory acidosis	When indicated will attenuate weight gain with any combination used, especially TZDs and insulin. Reduce triglycerides (16%), LDL cholesterol, (8%), and hsCRP

Drug class	Mechanism	Metabolism	Side effects	Contraindications/Precautions	Comments
Alpha-glucosidase inhibitors Acarbose Miglitol	Delay absorption of carbohydrates in the mid- and distal intestine, compensating for impaired early phase insulin release	Miglitol is renally excreted while acarbose is metabolized exclusively within the GI tract	GI adverse effects	Avoid with cirrhosis or significant liver disease; Severe renal insufficiency; Inflammatory bowel disease or pre-existing bowel problems; Lactose intolerance	Use is limited due to flatulence, abdominal discomfort, and diarrhea due to non-absorbed disaccharides. Give glucose for hypoglycemic episodes
Thiazolidinediones (TZDs) Rosiglitazone Pioglitazone	Enhance insulin sensitivity in adipocyte and muscle tissue, suppressing hepatic gluconeogenesis mediated through PPAR-γ stimulation	Pioglitazone: Oxidation and hydroxylation in cytochrome P450-2C8 and 3A4; metabolites partially converted to glucuronide or sulfate conjugates; Rosiglitazone: Cytochrome P450-2C8, minimal 2C9	Weight gain Edema Anemia Potential for liver toxicity CHF Concerns of CV events	Class III or IV CHF; Regurgitant valvular disease; Borderline injection fractions or Significant diastolic dysfunction; Moderate hepatic dysfunction with liver enzymes >2.5 normal	Decrease triglycerides with pioglitazone, increase HDL, decrease hsCRP and decrease small dense LDL
Dipeptidyl peptidase-4 inhibitors Sitagliptin Saxagliptin Alogliptin	Slow the inactivation of GLP-1 and GIP through inhibition of DPP-4; suppress glucagon secretion, suppress hepatic glucose output, and enhance glucose-dependent insulin release	Metabolized in the liver and excreted renally; 50–75% dose reduction in patients with renal insufficiency	Headache upper respiratory tract infection Pruritus serious hypersensitivity (sitagliptin, rare)	One-step reduction with renal impairment (sitagliptin)	Approved for use in combination with TZDs, sulfonylureas, and metformin

(continued)

Table 3 (*continued*)

Agent	Mechanism of action	Metabolism/ excretion	Limitations	Special populations	Comments
Bile acid sequestrants Colesevelam	Binds bile acids in the intestine	Water-insoluble polymer not hydrolyzed by digestive enzymes and not systemically absorbed	GI adverse events	Avoid with bowel obstruction and with triglycerides >300 mg/dl GI motility disorders, dysphagia, or other swallowing disorders	Reduces LDL (11.7%), apolipoprotein B (11.8%), and LDL particles (209 nmol/l)

From Inzucchi [51]

Table 4
Glycemic effects of oral agents

Drug	Hemoglobin A1C (%)	FPG	PPG
Sulfonylurea	1–2	↓↓↓	
Metformin	1–2	↓↓↓	
TZD	1–2	↓↓	↓
AGI	0.5–0.8		↓↓↓
DPP-4 inhibitor	0.7–1.4	↓	↓
Nateglinide	1		↓↓↓
Repaglinide	1.5	↓	↓↓↓

Hemoglobin A1C glycosylated hemoglobin; *AGI* alpha-glucosidase inhibitors; *FPG* fasting plasma glucose; *PPG* postprandial plasma glucose; *TZD* thiazolidinediones
From Inzucchi [*51*]

sensitizer (metformin and/or TZD) will usually be necessary. Combination drugs involving a sulfonylurea or DPP-IV inhibitor and biguanide can be ideal for this purpose starting with the lowest dose 1.25 mg of sulfonylurea or DPP-IV inhibitor (2.5 mg for saxagliptin and 50 mg of sitagliptin) and 500 mg of metformin and titrating up.

3. Patients with fasting glucose levels in excess of 180–200 mg/dl (hemoglobin A1C levels greater than 9%) will require a combination with a sulfonylurea, DPP-IV inhibitor, and a sensitizer either alone or in combination with another sensitizer. Those patients failing to achieve an hemoglobin A1C less than 6.5% may require multiple oral agents with different, but synergistic mechanisms of action, usually including a sulfonylurea, DPP-IV inhibitor, metformin, and a TZD. These patients may also respond to the addition of a bedtime long acting insulin. Table 4 lists the relative potency of the various oral agents.

SUMMARY

The multiple oral agents available provide the physician with various options in achieving glycemic control. Key principles to be kept in mind are using these agents in a complementary manner, addressing insulin secretion, insulin resistance, and preservation of beta-cell function.

Ultimately, the majority of type-2 diabetics will require insulin either alone or in combination with oral agents or other insulin. The next chapter will deal with insulin use as well as the use of insulin with various oral agent combinations.

REFERENCES

1. Hurst RT, Lee RW. Increased incidence of coronary atherosclerosis in type-2 diabetes mellitus: mechanism and management. Ann Intern Med 2003;139(10):824–834.
2. Wallace TM, Matthews DR. Poor glycemic control in type-2 diabetes. QJM 2000;93(6):369–374.
3. Mudaliar S, Henry RR. New oral therapies for type 2 diabetes mellitus: the glitazones or insulin sensitizers. Annu Rev Med 2001;173:54–57.

4. Luna B, Feinglos MN. Oral agents in the management of type-2 diabetes mellitus. Am Fam Physician 2001;63:1747–1756.
5. Feinglos FM, Bethel MA. Therapy of type-2 diabetes, cardiovascular death and the UGDP. Am Heart J 1999;138:S346–S352.
6. Sutton MS, Rendell M, Randona P. A comparison of the effects of rosiglitazone and glyburide on cardio-vascular function and glycemic control in patients with type-2 diabetes. Diabetes Care 2002;25(11):2058–2064.
7. Simpson SH, Majumdar SR, Tsuyuki RT. Metformin reduces cardiovascular mortality risks vs. placebo and other oral diabetes drugs in type-2 diabetes. N Engl J Med 2007;356:2457–2471.
8. Rao A, Kuhadiya N, Reynolds, K, Fonseca V. Is the combination of metformin and a sulfonylurea associ-ated with increased risk of cardiovascular disease and all cause mortality? Diabetes Care 2008;31(8):1672–1678.
9. Ahmann AJ, Riddle MC. Oral pharmacological agents. In: Medical Management of Diabetes Mellitus. New York, NY: Marcel Decker, CRC press 2000;267–283.
10. DeFronzo RA. Pharmacologic therapy for type 2 diabetes mellitus. Ann Intern Med 1999;131:281–303.
11. Malmberg K, Ryden L, Efendic S. Randomized trial of insulin glucose infusion followed by subcutaneous insulin treatment in diabetic patients with acute myocardial infarction (DIGAMI study). J Am Coll Cardiol 1995;26:57–65.
12. Codario R. A guide to combination therapy in type 2 diabetes. Patient Care 2003;37(4):16–24.
13. Dude DS, Peiris AN. Concise update to managing adult diabetes. South Med J 2002;95:4–9.
14. Horton ES, Clinkinbeard C, Gatlin M, et al. Nateglinide alone and in combination with metformin improves glycemic control by reducing mealtime glucose levels in type 2 diabetes. Diabetes Care 2000;23:1660–1665.
15. United Kingdom Pospective Diabetes Study Group (UKPDS). Effect of intensive blood glucose control with metformin on complications in overweight patients with type-2 diabetes. Lancet 1998;352:854–865.
16. Fontbonne A, Charles MA, Juhan-Vague I, Bard MM, Andre P, Isnard F. The effect of metformin on the metabolic abnormalities associated with upper body fat distribution. BIGPRO Study Group. Diabetes Care 1996;19:920–926.
17. Reaven GM, Johnston P, Hollenbeck CB, et al. Combined metformin-sulfonylurea treatment of patients with non-insulin dependent diabetes in fair to poor glycemic control. J Clin Endocrinol Metab 1992;74:1020–1026.
18. Dailey GE. Improving oral pharmacologic treatment and management of type-2 diabetes. Manag Care 2004;13:41–47.
19. Kuritsky L, Samraj G, et al. Improving management of type 2 diabetes mellitus: alpha glucosidase inhibi-tors. Hosp Pract 1999;34:43–46.
20. Parulkar A, Pendergrass M, et al. Non hypoglycemic effects of thiazolidinediones. Ann Intern Med 2001;134:61–71.
21. Singh S, Loke YK, Furberg CD. Thiazolidinediones and heart failure. Diabetes Care 2007;30:2148–2153.
22. Malinowski JM, Bolesta S. Rosiglitazone in the treatment of type-2 diabetes mellitus: a critical review. Clin Ther 2000;22:1151–1168.
23. Goldberg RB, Kendall DM, Deeg MA, Buse JB, Zagar AJ. A comparison of lipid and glycemic effects of pioglitazone in patients with type-2 diabetes and dyslipidemia. Diabetes Care 2005;28:1547–1554.
24. Bell DS, et al. Long term efficacy of triple oral therapy for type 2 diabetes mellitus. Endocr Pract 2002;8:271–275.
25. Davidson M, Meyer P, Haffner S, Feinstein S, Kondos G, D'Agostino R. Increases in HDL-C in the CHICAGO Study explain the benefits of pioglitazone for reducing CMT progression in patients with type-2 diabetes. 43rd Annual Meeting of the European Association for the Study of Diabetes, 2007. Abstract 0864.
26. Nissen S, Nicholls S, Wolski K, Nesto R. Comparison of pioglitazone vs. glimepiride on progression of coronary atherosclerosis in patients with type-2 diabetes. JAMA 2008;299(13):1561–1572.
27. Dormandy JA, Charbonnel B, Eckland DJA. Secondary prevention of macxrovascular events in patients with type-2 diabetes in the PROactive study. Lancet 2005;366(9493):1279–1289.
28. Gerstein HC, Yusuf S, Bosch J. Effect of rosiglitazone on the frequency of diabetes in patients with impaired glucose tolerance or impaired fasting glucose: the DREAM trial. Lancet 2006;368:1096–1105.

29. Ovalle F, Bell DSH. Lipoprotein effects of different thiazolidindiones in clinical practice. Endocr Pract 2002;8:406–410.
30. Dormuth C, Carney G, Carleton B. Thiazolidinediones and fractures in men and women. Arch Intern Med 2009;169(15):1395–1402
31. Grey A. Skeletal consequences of thiazolidinediones. Osteoporos Int 2008;19(2):129–137.
32. Holst JJ, Deacon CF. Glucagon like peptide-1 mediates the therapeutic actions of DPP-4 inhibitors. Diabetologia 2005;48:612–615.
33. Drucker DJ. Enhancing incretin action for the treatment of type-2 diabetes. Diabetes Care 2003;26:2929–2940.
34. Aschner P, Kipnes MS, Lunceford JK, Sanchez M, Mickel C. Effect of the dipeptidyl peptidase-4 inhibitor sitagliptin as monotherapy on glycemic control in patients with type-2 diabetes. Diabetes Care 2006;29:2632–2637.
35. Charbonnel B, Karasik A, Liu J, Wu M, Meininger G. Efficacy and safety of sitagliptin added to ongoing metformin therapy in patients with type-2 diabetes. Diabetes Care 2006;29:2338–2643.
36. Rosenstock J, Brazg R, Andryuk PJ, Lu K, Stein P. Efficacy and safety of sitagliptin added to ongoing pioglitazone therapy in patients with type-2 diabetes. Clin Ther 2006;28:1556–1568.
37. Bosi E, Camisasca RP, Collober C, Rochotte E. Garber AJ. Effects of vildagliptin on glucose control in patients with type-2 diabetes inadequately controlled on metformin. Diabetes Care 2007;30:890–895.
38. Feng J, Zhang Z, Wallace MB. Discovery of alogliptin: a potent, selective, bioavailable and efficacious inhibitor of dipeptidyl peptidase IV. J Med Chem 2007;50(10):2297–2300.
39. Anduri R, Drincic A, Rendell M. Alogliptin: a new addition to the DPP-IV inhibitors. Diabetes Metab Syndr Obes 2009;2:1–3.
40. Rosenstock J, Rendell M, Gross J. Alogliptin added to insulin therapy in patients with type-2 diabetes reduces A1C without weight gain. Presented at the 68th Session of the ADA, June 6–10, 2008, San Francisco, CA. Abstract 444-P.
41. DeFronzo R, Hissa M, Garber A, Gros JL. The efficacy and safety of saxagliptin when added to metformin therapy in type-2 diabetic patients not adequately controlled on metformin alone. Diabetes Care 2009;32(9):1649–1655.
42. Augeri D. Discovery and pre-clinical profile of saxagliptin. J Med Chem 2005;48(15):5025–5037.
43. Chiang JY, Kimmel R, Weinberger C, Stroup D. Farnesoid X receptor responds to bile acids and represses cholesterol 7 alpha-hydroxylase gene transcription. J Biol Chem 2000;275:10918–10924.
44. Zicvc FJ, Kalin MF, Schwartz SL, Jones MR, Bailey WL. Results of the glucose lowering effect of WelChol study (GLOWS). Clin Ther 2007;29:74–83.
45. United Kingdom Prospective Diabetes Study. 13. Relative efficacy of randomly allocated diet, sulfonylurea, insulin or metformin in patients with newly diagnosed non-insulin dependent diabetes followed for three years. BMJ 1995;310:83–88.
46. Mudaliar S, Henry RR. New oral therapies for type-2 diabetes mellitus: the glitazones or insulin sensitizers. Annu Rev Med 2001;52:239–257.
47. Fonseca V, Grunberger G, Gupta S. Addition of nateglinide to rosiglitazone monotherapy suppresses mealtime hyperglycemia and improves overall glycemic control. Diabetes Care 2003;26(6):1685–1690.
48. DeFronzo RA, Goodman AM. Efficacy of metformin in patients with non-insulin dependent diabetes mellitus. The Mutilcenter Metformin Study Group. N Engl J Med 1995;333:541–549.
49. Moses R, et al. Effect of repaglinide addition to metformin monotherapy on glycemic control in patients with type 2 diabetes. Diabetes Care 1999;22(1):119–124.
50. Hanefield M, Bouter KP, et al. Rapid and short acting mealtime insulin secretion with nateglinide controls both prandial and mean glycemia. Diabetes Care 2000;23:349–353.
51. Inzucchi SE. Oral antihyperglycemic therapy for type-2 diabetes. JAMA 2002;287:360–372.
52. Rosenstock J, Brown A, Fischer J, Jain A. Efficacy and safety of acarbose in metformin treated patients with type-2 diabetes. Diabetes Care 1998;21(12):2050–2055.
53. Miller S, St. Ange E. Sitagliptin: a dipeptidyl peptidase IV inhibitor for the treatment of type-2 diabetes. Ann Pharmacother 2006;40(7):1336–1343.
54. Bays H, Goldberg R, Truitt K, Jones M. Colesevelam hydrochloride therapy in patients with type-2 diabetes mellitus treated with metformin. Arch Intern Med 2008;168(18):1975–1983.

SUPPLEMENTARY READINGS

Buse J. Combining insulin and oral agents. Am J Med 2000;108(suppl 6a):23S–32S.

Bloomgarten ZT. Gut hormones and related concepts. Diabetes Care 2006;29:2319–2324.

Dunn CJ, Faulds D. Nateglinide. Drugs 2000;60:607–617.

Evans A, Krentz AJ. Benefits and risks of transfer from oral agents to insulin in type 2 diabetes mellitus. Drug Saf 1999;21:7–22.

Glucovance (glyburide and metformin HCL tablets) Package Insert. Bristol Myers Squibb Company, Princeton, NJ. July 2000.

Heinemann L. Hyperglycemia and insulin analogues: is there a reduction in the incidence. J Diabetes Complications 1999;13:105–114.

Kabadi M, et al. Efficacy of sulfonylureas with insulin in type 2 diabetes mellitus. Ann Pharmacother 2003;37:1572–1576.

Kirpichnikov D, et al. Metformin, an update. Ann Intern Med 2002;137:25–33.

Kudlacek S, Schernthaner G. The effect of insulin treatment on HbDPP-IV, body weight and lipids in type-2 diabetic patients with secondary failure to sulfonylureas. Horm Metab Res 1992;24:478–483.

Motz R. Metformin associated lactic acidosis: fact, fiction or both. CV&R, March–April 2004, 74–75.

Palumbo PJ. Glycemic control, mealtime glucose excursions, and diabetic complications in type 2 diabetes mellitus. Mayo Clin Proc 2001;76:609–618.

Starlix Package Insert. Novartis Pharmaceuticals Corp., Basel, Switzerland. 2001.

Sherwin RS, et al. The prevention or delay of type 2 diabetes. Diabetes Care 2002;25:743.

Unger J. Targeting glycemic control in the primary care setting. Female Patient 2003;28:12–16.

Yki-Jarvinen H, Ryysy L, Nikkila K, et al. Comparison of bedtime insulin regimens in patients with type 2 diabetes mellitus. A randomized, controlled trial. Ann Intern Med 1999;130:389–396.

7 Insulin Use

CONTENTS

Key Words: Insulin therapy, Human insulin preparations, Insulin analogs, Intermediate-acting insulins, Pre-mixed insulins, Biphasic insulins, Multiple daily injections (MDI), Infusion pumps, General therapeutic principles

INTRODUCTION

Several clinical trials covering thousands of patient cohorts have clearly demonstrated the correlation between the long-term macro and microvascular complications of diabetes and poorly controlled blood glucose with the subsequent benefits of tighter glycemic control. This data has made us all much more aware that insulin, used even in the early stages of diabetes, to insure proper control, can be invaluable in reducing mortality and morbidity. In fact, earlier insulin use reduces glucose toxicity, allows endogenous insulin to function more efficiently and reduces the strain on the deteriorating beta cell [1].

From: *Current Clinical Practice: Type 2 Diabetes, Pre-Diabetes, and the Metabolic Syndrome*
Edited by: R.A. Codario, DOI 10.1007/978-1-60327-441-8_7
© Springer Science+Business Media, LLC 2011

Table 1
Indications for insulin therapy in type-2 diabetes [2]

Pregnancy

Severe hyperglycemia with ketonuria and/or ketonemia

Uncontrolled hyperglycemia on maximum oral agent doses

Hyperglycemia and decompensation due to infection, surgery, and injury

Hyperglycemia with severe liver disease

Hyperglycemia with steroid therapy

Severe hyperglycemia at diagnosis

Allergic or serious reactions to oral agents

Inpatient glycemic control

Latent, autoimmune diabetes

For many years the concept of insulin resistance really referred to the patient's resistance to take insulin because of preconceived prejudices and the physician using insulin as a hammer threatening the patients with insulin use if sugars were not appropriately controlled. It is important for primary care providers to consider insulin therapy an important part of the therapeutic strategy and not as a burden or a stigma, but a benefit and valuable therapeutic weapon that can help patients maintain better control and reduce their risk of subsequent complications. Table 1 lists the indications for insulin use in patients with type-2 diabetes.

It is vital to remember that based on data from the United Kingdom Prospective Diabetes Study (UKPDS) over 50% of beta-cell function has been lost with the onset of fasting hyperglycemia in the diabetic range. The most recent American Diabetes Association/ European Association for the Study of Diabetes (ADA/EASD) treatment algorithm assigns a prominent role for insulin therapy in type-2 diabetic patients [3].

Critical to making insulin use more acceptable, however, is picking an insulin that works best for the patient's life style and glycemic requirements. Table 2 illustrates the onset, peak, and duration of action of the various insulins. For some patients it is better to give insulin at bed time, for others a once a day long acting insulin is superior. Still others like the flexibility of controlling postprandial sugars, if needed, with insulin injections based upon postprandial glucose self monitoring or using bolus insulin prior to eating.

Such approaches make good sense in view of the fact that the diabetic spends most of the day (approximately 17 h) in the postprandial state and with many patients eating food at various times and in different quantities during the course of the day; a more flexible regimen for different patients should certainly improve the accessibility and availability of this important therapeutic modality.

Premixed insulins have gained great popularity because of their ability to deliver two varieties of insulin, a bolus type for more immediate postprandial concerns and a basal type for prolonged control and fasting sugar reductions. These types do have the disadvantage of not being able to be tweaked sufficiently in patients who eat irregularly.

Table 2
Onset, peak, and duration of various insulins [2]

Insulin	Onset (min)	Peak (h)	Effective duration (h)	Maximum duration (h)
Bolus insulin				
Aspart (NovoLog)	5–10	1–3	3–5	4–6
Lispro (Humalog)	15	0.5–1.5	2–4	4–6
Regular (Humulin R) (Novolin R)	30–60	2–3	3–6	6–10
Basal insulin				
NPH (Humulin N) (Novolin N)	2–4	4–10	10–16	14–18
Lente (insulin zinc suspension)	3–4	4–12	12–18	16–20
Ultralente (extended Insulin zinc suspension)	6–10	None	18–20	20–24
Glargine (Lantus)	1–2	Peakless	24	24
Detemir (Levimir)	1–2	Peakless	18–20	20–22

Clearly though since type-2 diabetes is a progressive disease, these patients will suffer continued beta-cell deterioration and eventually all type-2 patients will require insulin. It is estimated that currently approximately 25% of type-2 diabetics are taking insulin in some fashion [5].

In the normal physiologic state, insulin secretion progresses in two distinct phases. A basal or fasting phase and a postprandial phase. In the basal state insulin is secreted during the course of the day at a constant low rate between 0.25–1.5 units hourly. When one is consuming a meal, the pancreas is stimulated to secrete insulin in a bolus fashion biphasically. This insulin peaks approximately 40–45 min after a meal returning to baseline within 3–4 h. It is this constant basal-bolus insulin secretion pattern that we are attempting to mimic with our therapeutic endeavors [5]

Recently, designed insulin analogs make it possible to reduce hyperglycemia both on a basal and on a bolus level. The shorter acting analog of insulins make it possible to increase the amount of insulin administered without prolonging the duration of action, reducing the risk of hypoglycemia, and thus functioning more efficiently with less hypoglycemia than the human insulins.

It is important for primary care physicians to understand the concept that enough insulin will always overcome insulin resistance and that there is no evidence of increased cardiovascular risks in individuals taking insulin. It is especially important for patients undertaking insulin therapy to set and understand glycemic goals, while appreciating the importance of outcomes data supporting these goals. Medical nutrition therapy and an exercise plan for all are critical along with regular visits to a diabetic educator if and when available.

The administration of insulin on a temporary basis to overcome glucose toxicity is one the most neglected aspects of the management of type-2 diabetes and one that we will be addressing in later chapters.

In general, when a patient has plateaued on maximum oral diabetic agent therapy and is unable to get the hemoglobin A1C less than 7.0 in association with appropriate exercise program and dietary modification, insulin therapy must be utilized to achieve glycemic goals One may also consider insulin therapy as an adjunct to glycemic control for significant postprandial excursions particularly in those patients who have a tendency to be erratic with their dietary habits, but once again these fears can be allayed when we understand that delaying the institution of insulin in a patient with an elevated hemoglobin A1C and not being as aggressive as possible to achieve these goals could accelerate the progression of both macro and micro vascular disease. Clearly tighter control reduces the risk of microvascular complications [6].

INDICATIONS FOR INSULIN THERAPY

The indications for insulin therapy in type-2 diabetes are: [7]

1. Decompensation due to intercurrent events like acute injury, stress, infection, and steroid therapy
2. Development of severe hyperglycemia with ketonuria and/or ketonemia
3. Uncontrolled weight loss, pregnancy, progressive renal or hepatic disease
4. Patients who are pre-operative for surgery
5. Patients who have developed idiosyncratic or allergic reactions to various oral medications
6. Latent autoimmune diabetes in adults

An estimated 10% of patients who appear to have clinical type-2 diabetes actually have a slower more delayed onset form of type-1 diabetes, which is referred to as latent autoimmune diabetes [4]. These patients experience, faster progression to insulin dependency, lower insulin secretion, autoantibodies to islet-cell antigens, and may have similar HLA genetic susceptibility to individuals with type-2 diabetes.

The diagnosis is established by demonstrating antibodies to insulin, islet cells, and especially glutamic acid decarboxylase. Any individuals who have a low C-peptide level with rapid progression to insulin deficiency could be considered candidates for this syndrome. It is important to understand that this appears to be a less aggressive form of the autoimmune type-1 diabetes and, indeed, insulin may not be needed for a period of time in these types of patients.

Use of insulin in patients, who are not controlled with oral agents, overcomes glucose toxicity, corrects decompensation, and will aid the patient in meeting glycemic targets. The concept of glucose toxicity is also an important one to understand because hyperglycemia begets more insulin resistance which causes further increased glucose. As the glucose rises above 150 mg/dl for greater than 24 h, insulin resistance begins to increase making it more difficult to achieve tight control and making whatever agents are used to control diabetes less effective [8].

This is seen, for example, in a newly diagnosed patient with severe hyperglycemia with blood glucose levels greater than 300 mg/dl and A1C levels >8.0. This patient is unlikely to receive sufficient and timely benefit from an oral agent, certainly not monotherapy. Many of these patients have already experienced polyuria, polydypsia, numbness, visual disturbances, or even weight gain. These patients may benefit by being started on insulin immediately to achieve better and quicker control. This will reduce glucose toxicity and subsequently decrease insulin resistance enhancing endogenous insulin effectiveness.

This concept can certainly be applied to acutely ill patients who will also require rapid control of their blood glucose with insulin especially, since recent outcomes data have supported better prognosis in acutely ill patients with hyperglycemia than those in whom hyperglycemia is casually treated. However, hypoglycemia should be avoided – particularly in those with cardiovascular disease where outcomes can be worsened with low glucose levels and tighter control.

Be aware that thin patients with type-2 diabetes tend to be less sensitive to oral regimens because these individuals tend to have primarily insulin secretion problems rather than insulin resistance. A trial of dietary therapy, exercise, and oral agents can be acceptable as long as the patient is not in the glucose toxic range on a consistent basis.

Even patients with latent autoimmune diabetes can remain controlled for short periods of time on oral agents. Weight gain is always a big patient concern with use of insulin, which has also been another major factor in their resistance to taking this particular product. In the UKPDS, weight gain was more common with patients on insulin, gaining an average of about 4 kg compared to 2.6 kg for those on sulfonylurea therapy [9].

As mentioned previously, the use of metformin will tend to attenuate weight gain in any treatment modality whether it be insulin or oral agents.

Another concern has been the incidence of hypoglycemia with the use of insulin. In the DCCT trial, in type-1 diabetics, tighter control did increase the risk of hypoglycemia three fold over conventional therapy [10]. One must understand, however, that there was a significant improvement in microvascular events and neurological complications.

In the Kumamoto study with type-2 diabetics, average hemoglobin A1C values were 7.1 and 9.4 for tightly controlled and conventional groups, respectively, with only mild hypoglycemic reactions resulting in similar rates in both groups. In the UKPDS trial, the rate of hypoglycemic episodes was increased in patients taking insulin 2.3% compared to less than 1% with other agents [11].

It should be understood that with tighter glycemic control will come an increased risk of hypoglycemia, but nonetheless, aggressive therapy is extremely important in order to minimize risks. As we will see later on in this chapter, newer insulin analogs tend to mitigate the risk of hypoglycemia and better mimic natural insulin patterns.

There are other strategies that physicians can use in having patients accept insulin use including turning fears into motivators, asking the patient about family history of diabetes and its complications. Ask the patient about employment issues relative to common diabetic complications, ask them about their work duties, their vision problems, personal concerns, responsibilities, sexual dysfunction, exercise capacity, and symptoms.

It is critically important to make patients understand that improving the hemoglobin A1C with tighter control will reduce their risk of complications and whether tighter control means more medication and/or the use of insulin, it is certainly worthwhile on a long term basis. Making the transition from oral agents to insulin is often a great challenge when patients are very resistant.

It also is important to view insulin as a critical therapeutic modality to enhance glycemic control allowing oral agents or endogenous insulin to work in a more efficient way, reducing the risk of overall complications from this disease.

Initiating therapy must be achieved by individualization to fit the patient's needs. The primary objective of insulin therapy is to replace the lack of or the progressive deficiency of insulin. This should be done in a physiologic way in a pattern that follows the normal insulin secretion physiology in the body.

Thirty-five to fifty percent of type-2 diabetics, regardless of ethnicity, have hemoglobin A1C levels greater than 8% [12]. It is important for primary care physicians to understand that their role can be critical in improving these statistics. With the progression from impaired glucose tolerance to type-2 diabetes, it is the early first phase insulin response that is diminished and is ultimately lost. This diminution of first phase insulin results in a shift from the peak endogenous insulin action time of about 60 min, which is normal, to 120 min and finally to a severely impaired state. Subsequently, the patients lose their ability to handle a glucose load causing both postprandial and fasting hyperglycemia.

Postprandial contributions of hyperglycemia can be as much as 70% when the hemoglobin A1C is increased. So it is important for us to understand that tight diabetic control begins with not only controlling the fasting sugar or basal insulin, but giving proper attention to controlling the postprandial glucose or bolus insulin. So physicians and patients alike must not ignore the importance of measuring postprandial hyperglycemia [13].

Unlike patients with type-1 diabetes, type-2 diabetics retain some insulin secretory capacity and although these patients are not dependent upon insulin to prevent ketoacidosis and preserve life; the progressive nature of the disease reflects the continuous deterioration and pancreatic beta-cell function that eventually causes the type-2 diabetic to require insulin to maintain glycemic control.

Basal insulin replacement meets about half of the body's total daily insulin needs, and regulates hepatic glucose production to correspond to tissue glucose uptake nocturnally and between meals. Bolus insulin is responsible for the other 50% and primarily regulates postprandial excursions.

Insulins that are used in the USA can be divided into three categories: human insulin, analog insulin, and beef and pork preparations. The beef and pork preparations are no longer commonly used.

The four human insulins that are used are:

1. Regular insulin – has an onset of action in 0.5–1 h, peaks in 2–4 h, and lasts for 6–12 h.
2. Neutral protein Hagedorn (NPH insulin) – has an onset of action of 1–4 h, peaks in 4–12 h, and lasts for 10–24 h.
3. Lente insulin – has an onset of action of 1–3 h, peaks in 4–8 h, and duration of action of 10–20 h.
4. Ultralente insulin – has an onset of action of 2–4 h, is unpredictable in terms of its peak, and has a duration of action of 16–20 h [14].

The analog insulins include:

1. Lispro (Humalog), which has an onset of action of 5–15 min, peaks in 1 h, and a duration of action of 4–5 h.
2. Aspart (NovoLog), which has and onset of action of 5–15 min, peaks in 1 h, and a duration of action of 4–5 h.
3. Glulisine (Apidra), which has an onset of action of 5–15 min, peaks in 1 h, and a duration of action of 4–5 h.

4. Glargine (Lantus) which has an onset of action of 1–2 h, is essentially peakless, and a duration of action of 24 h.
5. Detemir (Levimir), which has an onset of action of 1–2 h, is relatively peakless, and a duration of action of 18–20 h.

The time periods listed here are general guidelines, since these time courses can vary among individuals and even at different times in the same individual.

In addition, mixed insulins are now available that include NPL/Lispro combinations (Humalog Mix) in 75/25% and 50/50%, NPL/Aspart (NovoLog Mix) in 70/30% combinations, and NPH/regular insulin (70/30% and 50/50%) combinations. These will all be addressed separately.

Human regular insulin and the short acting analogs, lispro, glulisine, and aspart, are better used to control postprandial sugars, while the intermediate-and long-acting insulins like NPH, Lente, ultralente, detemir, and glargine supply basal insulin.

HUMAN INSULIN PREPARATIONS

Although undergoing some major improvements over the past several years, human insulin still has some limitations. The variable and inconsistent absorption rates of these insulins, which are reflected in the erratic and unpredictable blood glucose lowering effects, reflect the varying onset of actions, peak, and duration of action of these products. This is because when regular insulin is administered subcutaneously, its absorption into the circulation is slow with a subsequent slow onset of action. Because of this situation, regular insulin should be administered 30–40 min prior to a meal in order to avoid a physiologic potential mismatch with subsequent hypoglycemia.

This becomes inconvenient and somewhat hazardous at times particularly if the patient is unable to eat and has insulin on board, or if the meal becomes surprisingly delayed, or for some reason is not palatable to the patient. In addition, when larger doses of regular insulin are given subcutaneously, the duration of action is prolonged. This prolonged duration of action may result in an increased risk of hypoglycemia.

Intermediate human insulins such as NPH and Lente are usually used in daily, once a day, or BID regimens, or even at bedtime. These agents usually have a gradual onset of action and a pronounced effect, usually 4–8 h after injection. The problem is that, once again, these agents demonstrate significant variations both within each patient and from patient to patient. Administration of these products still requires a strict schedule for meal intake in order to take advantage of the onset of action of the particular products [15].

As a result of their prolonged effects, postprandial hypoglycemia may occur along with overlapping of peak effects contributing to recurrent episodes of hypoglycemia and Somogyi phenomena. The Somogyi phenomena can be demonstrated in those individuals who exhibit weight gain with less than 5% glucose spillage in their urine in the face of elevated glucoses. In this setting, the patient should be treated with a reduction of insulin for better control and less hypoglycemia [16].

Ultralente has a long duration of action, but unfortunately once again demonstrates substantial day to day variability with broad and erratic peaks, which makes its use more difficult.

Ultralente is usually given before the evening meal or at bedtime, has a duration of action that is quite variable at 13–18 h, and variable peaking times between 8–14 h. This has fallen into disfavor because of the peaks and valleys with its coverage.

INSULIN ANALOGS [17]

By switching amino acids in the primary structure of the insulin molecule, insulin analogs have been produced that are characterized by a more favorable insulin replacement pattern, a lower variability of effect, better absorption profiles and the same onset and duration of action despite increasing doses.

The three rapid acting insulin analogs Lispro (Humalog), Glulisine (Apidra), and Aspart (NovoLog) have absorption profiles that mimic more closely physiologic replacement patterns of mealtime insulin secretion. Each possesses fast absorption patterns, which reduces their tendency to dissociate into hexamers or dimers and exhibit increased absorption rates. This allows the insulins to be given closer to mealtime and even on occasion shortly after eating. This makes these insulins very popular and ideal from a patient point of view because of the relative proximity to meal consumption. Indeed, in head to head studies with human insulin, these products have been shown to produce less hypoglycemia, lower postprandial glucose levels with comparable hemoglobin A1C control [18]. These types of insulins are ideal add-ons for regimens that include long and intermediate-acting insulins, or patients maximized on oral therapy who need coverage for intermediate postprandial hyperglycemia due to stress, dietary, irregularities, or medication adjustments [19].

Glulisine, a very rapidly acting analog of insulin, differs from human insulin in the B chain of the molecule with the analog having lysine at the B3 position instead of asparagine, and glutamic acid replacing lysine at the B29 position. Aspart insulin features a substitution of aspartic acid at the B28 position, while Lispro is formed from a switch of lysine and proline at the B28 and B29 positions (from PRO-LYS to LYS-PRO). Due to their rapid onset of action, these analogs can be administered within 15 min of a meal (before or after) and even as soon as 5–10 min before a meal with Aspart.

Glulisine, humalog, and aspart insulins have been shown to be equally potent to human insulin on a molar basis. This means that 1 unit of humalog or aspart has the same glucose lowering potency as 1 unit of human regular insulin. They differ, however, in terms of speed of onset and duration when given subcutaneously.

When lispro, glulisine, aspart, or human regular insulin is given intravenously, however, the glucose lowering capabilities, onset, and duration of action are the same. The bioavailability of lispro, glulisine, aspart, and regular insulin are similar, ranging between 55–77% with doses between 0.1–0.2 units/kg [20].

The absorption of glulisine, lispro, and aspart has shown to be quicker than human regular insulin. For example, when volunteers were given subcutaneous doses of lispro ranging from 0.1 to 0.4 units/kg, peak serum levels were seen 30–90 min after dosing in contrast to equivalent doses of human regular insulin which peaked between 50–120 min after dosing.

The analog insulins are absorbed at consistently faster rates regardless of the subcutaneous injected site tested and have been shown to have less intra- and interpatient variability compared to human regular insulin although their metabolism is similar to that of human regular insulin. When short acting analogs are injected subcutaneously, their half lives are shorter than that of human regular insulin, but the analogs and human insulin possess identical half lives when given intravenously.

Earlier onset of activity of lispro, glulisine, and aspart are directly related to their more rapid rate of absorption. The time course of action of insulin with the analogs make these drugs ideally suited for administration at mealtime or shortly thereafter. Rapid acting insulin analogs better mimic the body's insulin dynamics allowing for slow, safe, and simple titration with better postprandial glucose control and less weight gain [21].

As a direct result of their rapid onset and shorter duration of action, the shorter acting insulin analogs represent a significant upgrade of human insulin. These insulins are also ideally suited to control postprandial excursions in those patients with erratic glycemic levels after a meal by self monitoring and administering a short acting insulin analog on a graded scale designed by the physician.

Postprandial hyperglycemia can be addressed if and when it occurs, reducing the likelihood of glucose toxicity and providing the patient with a "go to" regimen when these postprandial excursions occur (the post-emptive approach). A convenient regimen is to give 2 units of a short-acting analog of insulin for every 50 mg/dl elevation in postprandial glucose. This would be as follows for postprandial glucoses:

1. 150–200 mg/dl – 2 units
2. 201–250 mg/dl – 4 units
3. 251–300 mg/dl – 6 units
4. 301–350 mg/dl – 8 units
5. 351–400 mg/dl – 10 units
6. >400 – 12 units (and call the physician)

This regimen has the advantage of being a practical way of reducing postprandial excursions, particularly effective in those patients who cannot or will not count carbohydrates before the meal. It is also ideal for those individuals who frequently eat "on the run" or at various restaurants where the exact carbohydrate amounts may be unknown. It is totally dependent, however, on the patient checking their glucose 1–2 h postprandially. I have found that non compliance increases when the interval for glucose checking is greater than 1 h.

The other option for postprandial excursion control is to administer insulin before the meal (the preemptive approach). This method is preferred by most endocrinologists and requires carbohydrate counting. This method directs the patient to administer short-acting insulin (15 min prior to the meal for analog or 30–45 min with human regular). For this method, 1 unit of insulin is used to cover 10–15 g of carbohydrates as directed by the physician.

The disadvantages of this method are:

1. Inaccuracies in estimating the carbohydrate content of a meal
2. Increased risk of hypoglycemia if the patient finds the meal unpalatable or is unable to eat for various reasons

The advantages of this method are:

1. It is more physiological. Insulin use prevents postprandial surge and closely mimics in vivo insulin release

The option still remains for the patients to check glucose postprandially and administer another dose if the glucose still remains elevated at that time.

Glargine (Lantus) represents the first insulin analog with a flat and prolonged duration of action. This analog features a substitution of glycine for asparagine at the A21 position along with the addition of two arginine molecules at the C-terminus of the B chain. By changing the amino acid sequence in the alpha chain and attaching two arginines to the end of the beta chain of human insulin, a shift in the isoelectric point of the molecule occurred which resulted in an acidic insulin analog soluble only at a PH of 4. The neutralization of this acidic solution at the injection site results in the formation of microprecipitates which allow for a smooth and continuous release into the circulation [22].

The glargine molecule will show a tendency to dissociate into hexamers and dimers following subcutaneous administration. The dissociation time of these hexamers to subsequent dimers and monomers had been a major obstacle in affecting absorption into the systemic circulation and thereby affecting the time-action profile of standard insulin preparations.

The reduced solubility of glargine allows this insulin to precipitate after subcutaneous injections, stabilizing the hexameric form of insulin, and delaying its subsequent dissociation into monomers and dimers. This prolongs its absorption into the systemic circulation, providing glargine with a long biological effect that truly lasts 24 h.

A surprising benefit of this drug has been an attenuation of postprandial glycemic excursions, despite not being a bolus insulin. Patients taking glargine tend to have tighter glucose control with less hypoglycemia than patients who are given NPH. This analog represents an ideal replacement basal insulin for regulating glucose fluctuations during the night and between meals, while lowering A1C's [23].

Similar to the effect seen with intermediate-acting insulins (neutral protamine Hagedorn and neutral protamine Lispro), the addition of glargine at bedtime to patients poorly controlled on oral agents has been shown to be an effective strategy in reducing A1C levels. Glargine has been shown to have a lower incidence of nocturnal hypoglycemia than NPH, which is given at bedtime or before supper. The smooth peakless action of glargine may be insufficient in some patients to handle significant postprandial glycemic excursions or the early morning hyperglycemia that is associated with insulin resistance [24].

Glargine (Lantus) is an analog of insulin with significant advantages over the Ultralente preparation. This has an onset of action of 1–2 h and is virtually peakless with a duration of action of 24 h. This is produced by recombinant DNA technology utilizing a nonpathogenic strain of *Escherichia coli* as the principal organism.

This product differs from human insulin, in that the amino acid asparagine at position A21 on the alpha chain is replaced by glycine with two arginine molecules added to the C-terminus of the beta chain [25].

Insulin glargine is then dissolved in a clear aqueous fluid that has a pH of approximately 4.0 when adjusted by the aqueous solutions of hydrochloric acid and sodium hydroxide. After glargine is injected into the subcutaneous tissue, neutralization of the acidic solution is achieved. This leaves the formation of microprecipitates from the small amounts of glargine that are slowly released and result in a consistent concentration time profile over 24 h with essentially no peak, and thus allowing for once a day dosing as the patient's basal insulin. This insulin has shown an equivalent glucose lowering effect on molar basis to human insulin. The longer duration of action of this product is directly related to its slower absorption rate.

Glargine insulin cannot be diluted or mixed with other insulins or solutions. This newer long-acting analog of insulin also has lower inter and intra subject variability than NPH and Ultralente. It closely mimics continuous subcutaneous insulin infusion, which still remains the gold standard for insulin replacement.

Studies by LePore in 2000 confirm glargine's close comparison with continuous subcutaneous insulin infusion. In head to head comparisons with NPH insulin, glargine insulin had a lower incidence of nocturnal hypoglycemia in both type-1 and type-2 diabetics than NPH (31 vs. 40% in type-2's and 18 vs. 27% in type-1's), while fasting plasma glucoses were reduced from baseline to a greater extent in type-2's than type-1's with insulin glargine (32–22% for type-2's and 31–6% for type-1's) [25].

In these studies, final hemoglobin A1C's were comparable with A1C's achieved with NPH insulin of 7.9% and glargine 8.2%, and in type-2's 7.49% with NPH and 7.54 with glargine. Studies published in *Diabetes Care* in 2000 by Hinella Yki-Jarvinen et al. have shown less nocturnal hypoglycemia and better postprandial dinner glucose control with a bedtime insulin glargine regimen compared to bedtime NPH insulin for type-2 diabetics [15].

This consistent absorption allows for less risk of mistakes and bedtime administration to do a better job at controlling the dawn phenomenon without risking hypoglycemia. This phenomenon, characterized by pre-breakfast hyperglycemia, can sometimes occur in response to nocturnal hypoglycemia (due to excess insulin therapy or the Somogyi effect), which provokes a surge of counterregulatory hormones that result in hyperglycemia from 5:00 a.m. to 7:00 a.m. However, in about 75% of patients with type-1 and type-2 diabetes, the morning catecholamine and growth hormone surge that occurs during the early morning hours decreases insulin sensitivity resulting in elevated blood glucose levels. Longer acting insulin preparations like glargine permit greater flexibility of lifestyle and less worry about glycemic variability.

Table 3
Using glargine (Lantus) in patients with type-2 diabetes [27]

Initial dose

Not on insulin previously: 10 units or 0.15 units/kg at same time daily

On once daily insulin: give total daily dose at same time daily

On twice daily or multiple daily doses: give 2/3 total daily dose at same time daily

Suggested titration schedule

Adjust dose weekly to achieve fasting glucose <100 mg/dl

FBG	Increase glargine dose (units/day)
100–120 mg/dl	0–2
120–140 mg/dl	4
140–180 mg/dl	6
>180 mg/dl	8

When combined with short acting insulins to cover postprandial hyperglycemia, the ideal basal/bolus therapeutic concept can be achieved. A large randomized controlled clinical study compared a basal/bolus regimen of glargine once daily at bedtime vs. Humulin NPH insulin is administered once or twice daily along with regular human insulin before meals as needed in both groups. Glargine had similar effectiveness as NPH (which was given once or twice daily) in reducing A1C and fasting glucose with less hypoglycemia [26].

Dosage of glargine should always be individualized with lower starting dose required if oral agents are retained. Patients maxed out on oral agents can usually be started on low dose once a day administration of glargine (5–10 units initially and titrated up slowly increasing by 2 units weekly to achieve a fasting blood sugar less than 100 mg/dl).

This approach must always be individualized with each patient. The key principal is to start low and go slow when using glargine. Table 3 outlines a strategy for initiating glargine therapy. In patients who are switched from once daily, mixed or intermediate insulins, a 1:1 conversion can be used. If intermediate or mixed insulins are administered on a twice-daily basis, then two-thirds of the total daily dose of the mixed insulins can be used as a starting dose for glargine. Due to its true 24 h duration of action, glargine can be used at any time of the day, as long as the next dose is given 24 h later [28].

In 2009, the first of four studies was submitted to evaluate the association of increased cancer risk with glargine compared to human insulin. These four studies were published in the journal *Diabetologia* and were conducted by German, Swedish, Scottish, and Welch groups – all involving substantial cohorts from 36,254 in the Scottish study to 127,031 in the German analysis [29].

The German study followed individuals from a national health insurance database who had received aspart (4,103), lispro (3,269), human insulin (95,804), or glargine (23,855) exclusively for 1.63 years. In this study, the unadjusted risk of developing a malignancy was lower in those using the three analogs. When, however, the data was adjusted for the daily dose, the risk was significantly increased for glargine compared to human insulin. This dose response relationship was not seen with the short-acting analogs.

The Scottish analysis followed people initially over a 4-month period of time from a national database and a subsequent 4-year follow-up of 3,959 patients exclusively on glargine. The overall group of glargine users did not show an increased incidence of all cancers compared to non users. However, a subset of 447 patients who used only glargine as their insulin treatment had a higher incidence of all cancers than 32,295 patients who used other insulins exclusively. Curiously, in those individuals who used glargine with another insulin, the risk of cancer was reduced compared to the glargine-only group. It is important to also keep in mind that the treatments groups were not homogeneous, however. The glargine-only group was much older (68 years) than the glargine/other insulin group (41 years), and the other insulin group (60 years).

The Swedish data analyzed 114,841 individuals by linking prescription insulin with cancer registry data. Here, there was no increased incidence of cancers in the glargine treated group overall, although breast cancer incidence was higher in women who took glargine compared to those who took other insulins.

The Welsh study divided 62,809 people from the UK, all over 40 years of age into four groups: insulin, combination therapy with two oral agents, monotherapy with metformin, and monotherapy with sulfonylurea. The insulin users were further categorized into human biphasic insulin, analog biphasic insulin, glargine, and long acting human insulin. In this analysis, the incidence of malignancy was highest in the insulin treated group (hazard ratio of 1.42) and lowest for metformin treated group (hazard ratio of 1.08). The hazard ratio was reduced to 0.54 when metformin was added to insulin.

No increased incidence of cancer was noted when glargine was compared with other insulins. Insulin has the ability to bind to two receptors — an insulin like growth factor-1 receptor (IGF-1) which induces cell proliferation, and an insulin receptor which promotes glucose lowering. Insulin binds much stronger (500 times) to its insulin receptor site than the IGF-1 site. Changes in insulin structure have the potential of altering affinity for these receptors. This carcinogenic concern has been raised because of the greater affinity of glargine (compared to human insulin) for the IGF-1 receptor site, which has been associated with tumor growth promotion.

Taken collectively, the data are not conclusive in this association. Although the German data is of interest, further study will be needed to determine the validity of a dose response relationship to malignancy developments. The Welsh data showed increased cancer incidence in all insulin treated patients, while the Swedish analysis raised concerns about enhanced breast cancer risk in glargine users. The decreased cancer incidence in metformin users also merits further study. A meta-analysis of all randomized trials in type-1 and type-2 diabetics showed no cancer relationship and neither did a 4.2 year study of 1,017 patients with type-2 diabetes treated with NPH insulin and glargine.

Insulin detemir (Levemir) differs from its human counterpart due to the attachment of lysine at the B29 position of myristic acid (a C14 fatty acid chain) along with the omission of threonine at the B30 position. This formulated as a neutral solution that remains soluble in the subcutaneous tissue, while its reversible binding to albumin molecules allows for its prolonged action, buffering the alterations in absorption rates and limiting pharmacodynamic variations. This long acting analog has a relatively flat action profile with duration of action shorter than glargine and dose related. Mean duration of action with this type of insulin can range from 5.7 h at the lowest dose to 23.2 h with the highest dose. In doses of 0.2–0.4 unit/kg, detemir will exert its maximum effect from 3 to 14 h following injection, with a maximum concentration reached between 6–8 h after injection with 98% bound to albumin. Detemir (Levimir) can be given once or twice daily. In a comparison study with 6,004 patients (3,724 with type 1 and 2,280 with type 2 diabetes) A1C levels were similar to patients using glargine, once or twice daily NPH. In another study, detemir administered once or twice daily in addition to patients on oral agents was compared to NPH insulin given once or twice daily in 476 patients over 24-week period. Once again, similar reductions in A1C levels from baseline were seen. A 52-week multinational treat to target trial in 319 type-2 diabetics comparing detemir with glargine in a basal-bolus regimen with mealtime aspart demonstrated no significant differences between the two analogs in mean A1C or mean decrease in A1C compared to baseline [30]. Interestingly, in this study, the reduction in A1C was similar with once or twice daily with detemir.

In insulin naïve patients, glargine and detemir provided comparable glycemic control in a retrospective analysis of 306 patients with type-2 diabetes, who initiated basal therapy with detemir ($n=48$) or glargine ($n=258$). During the 6-month follow-up period the mean dose of the two insulins were essentially the same (detemir 29.9 units daily vs. 29.5 units daily for glargine) with no significant changes between the two groups post treatment (A1C of 8.4 in detemir vs. 8.0% with glargine) [31] while 27.1% of patients in the glargine group vs. 22.9% in the detemir group achieved an A1C less than 7.0%. The PREDICTIVE

303 Trial was a 26-week randomized trial in which patients were instructed to adjust their dose of detemir insulin every 3 days (up or down) depending upon fasting glucose levels (up three units for levels greater than 110 mg/dl and down three units if less than 80 mg/dl) or had the physicians adjust the dose based on standard care with both groups showing equal efficacy in A1C reduction [32]. The TITRATE study successfully applied the same approach as the PREDICTIVE TRIAL in a 20-week randomized treat to target trial in 244 insulin naive patients with type-2 diabetes taking oral agents. In this study 54.5% of patients in the 80–110 mg/dl FPG group and 64.3% of those in the 70–90 mg/dl group achieved an A1C less than 7.0% with once daily detemir [33].

With regard to the controversy concerning a possible increased cancer risk with glargine, detemir has an affinity for the IGF receptor that is similar to or less than human insulin. Thus far no increased cancer signals have been identified with detemir. A recent meta-analysis in a population of 8,693 patients with type-1 or type-2 diabetes treated with insulin detemir, glargine, or NPH insulin showed that patients treated with insulin detemir had a lower or similar incidence of cancer compared to patients with NPH insulin or glargine [34].

INTERMEDIATE-ACTING INSULINS

These include human NPH, neutral protein Lispro (NPL), and lente insulin. All of these are similar in their pharmacokinetics and work best when given twice daily or ideally at bedtime when patients are on oral agents and not yet at goal.

When given at bedtime, these insulins peak in the early morning when, in many patients, the nocturnal surge of growth hormone increases insulin resistance. However, these insulins can cause recognized or unrecognized hypoglycemia if they peak before the morning surge. The intermediate-acting insulin Humulin NPH is synthesized by a non-disease producing genetically altered *Escherichia coli* by the addition of the gene for human insulin production. Humulin N exists as a crystalline suspension of human insulin with protamine and zinc providing an intermediate acting molecule with a slower onset of action and longer duration of activity than human regular insulin.

NPH insulin has a duration of action of 13–18 h with a peak onset of action of 5–7 h with Lente being similar, having a duration of action of 13–20 h and a peak onset of 4–8 h. These insulins are designed to provide basal insulin coverage when given either at bedtime in association with oral agents or on a twice daily regimen, usually at breakfast and supper.

PRE-MIXED (BIPHASIC) INSULINS

Mixtures of short acting and intermediate-acting insulins have become a convenient method for primary care physicians to manage the basal bolus problem with one vial or one pen. Various mixtures currently exist:

1. Humulin or Novolin 70/30 (70% insulin isophane suspension-NPH/30% regular insulin)
2. Novolog mix 70/30 (70% protamine aspart and 30% aspart)
3. Humulin 50/50 (50% insulin isophane suspension-NPH and 50% regular insulin)
4. Humalog mix 75/25 (75% lispro protamine and 25% lispro)

Of these, the 70/30 and 75/25 preparation seem to be the most popular. Patients with A1C levels in the ranges greater than 9.5% may benefit from premixed preparations. All the intermediate moieties in these mixtures have similar onset and duration of action. There major differences lie in the short acting portion which, as stated previously, will provide quicker onset, shorter duration of action, and will not have a prolongation of duration of action with increased doses.

The analog mixes provide better postprandial control and less hypoglycemia in head to head comparisons with the NPH based mixes.

One of the criticisms of fixed dose combinations is the question of inconsistent blood glucose readings increasing the risk of hypo and hyperglycemia compared to regimens that segregate and vary the intermediate and short acting insulin doses based on dietary needs and irregularities. The mixes are not as easy to titrate as varied doses of just the shorter acting analog insulins adjusted according to daily needs.

This is why patient selection is extremely important before committing an individual to a fixed mixture preparation. The biggest advantage of these mixes seems to be convenience in supplying basal and bolus insulins. Both aspart and lispro containing mixtures have shown superiority in head to head trials with comparable doses of NPH/human insulin mixes for postprandial glucose control despite similar overall Hemoglobin A1C reductions [35].

The NPH of the human insulin and the NPL of the analog insulins have virtually identical onsets of action and duration of activity. Most mixed insulins are ideally used in twice daily regimens consisting of a morning and an evening dose. The bolus insulin has its major effects postprandially, while the intermediate acting effects of the NPH or NPL moieties extend until dinner time.

When administered with the evening meal the second mixed dose regimen provides insulin coverage between dinner and bedtime usually eliminating the need for supplemental overnight coverage.

Of course the dosage of these various insulins depends upon the patients needs and some patients respond better to a 75/25 or 75/30 mix preparation and others may respond to a 50/50 mix preparation.

The major differences as we will see in further detailed discussions between the premixed human insulins and the premixed analog insulins is less of an incidence of hypoglycemia with the analogs because progressively higher doses of the bolus human insulin results in prolonged duration of action of the shorter acting insulin, increasing the risk for hypoglycemia. The fact that premixed insulins contain fixed percentages of intermediate and short acting insulins make it impossible to adjust only one of the components and consequently work best with those patients on a consistent caloric intake.

The main benefits of the premixed analogs over the human premixes are more convenience with meal time dosing, earlier and higher peak concentration providing lowered postprandial glycemic excursions, and quicker onset of action. These advantages allow the analog mixes to be dosed up to three times daily, if necessary, whereas human premixes should not be used more than twice daily due to peak action overlapping.

Premixed insulin analogs can also be given once daily before dinner to achieve glycemic control in greater than 40% of type-2 diabetics. The analog mixes should not be given at bedtime due to the increased risk of nocturnal hypoglycemia from the rapid acting moiety. Human mixes need to be injected 30–60 min prior to meals which may be impractical for many patients – especially children.

MULTIPLE DAILY INJECTIONS

Multiple daily injections (MDI) are used widely in the treatment of type-1 diabetes and can be employed in patients with type-2 diabetes with BID intermediate acting insulin plus two or three injections of short-acting insulin with meals. When this regimen is used, the second dose of NPH is usually given at bedtime rather than dinner in an attempt to decrease nocturnal hypoglycemia and control basal hepatic gluconeogenesis and the dawn phenomenon characterized by an early morning glycemic surge [36]. Less insulin is necessary to attenuate hepatic gluconeogenesis compared to the amount needed to drive insulin intracellularly.

Another variant of the multidose insulin (MDI) approach consists of two or three premeal injections of insulin lispro, apidra, or aspart rather than regular insulin at mealtime. This covers the post meal hyperglycemic episodes. This unfortunately requires patients to pre-estimate the amount of carbohydrates in their meals. With many patients today consuming varied diets and hidden carbohydrates found in the various foods, this can sometimes be difficult or even hazardous.

Recent studies have confirmed that an MDI regimen using premeal short acting insulins can be optimized by adding a once-daily bedtime use of insulin (glargine, detemir, or NPH).

Interestingly, the outcomes trials that have targeted postprandial control in the acutely ill patients (Van den Bergh and DIGAMI) and data in gestational diabetics have utilized the post-emptive approach. The optimal approach depends on a mutual decision between patient and physician [11].

The short acting insulins are as follows:

1. Insulin aspart (NovoLog)
2. Insulin lispro (Humalog)
3. Insuline glulisine (Apidra)
4. Regular human insulin (Humulin R, Novolin R, Velosulin BR) – onset in 30 min, peaking in 2–4 h, except Velosulin which peaks in 1–3 h, with a duration of 6–8 h
5. Regular pork insulin (Iletin II regular) – onset in 30 min, peaking in 2–4 h, and duration of action of 6–8 h

The intermediate-acting human insulins with onset of 1–3 h, peaking in 6–12 h, and duration of 18–24 h are:

1. Humulin N – insulin isophane suspension – human
2. Novolin N – insulin isophane suspension – human
3. Humulin L – insulin zinc suspension – human
4. Iletin II NPH – insulin isophane suspension – pork
5. Iletin II Lente – insulin zinc suspension – pork

Long Acting Insulins are:

1. Glargine (Lantus)
2. Detemir (Levimir)
3. Ultralente

A common dilemma in primary care occurs when a patient is maxed out on oral agents and insulin is now necessary. What is the best approach? Which oral agent should be continued and what is the thought process involved in this decision making?

Patients are considered maxed out on oral agents when they have received maximum doses of synergistically acting oral medications including secretagogues, sensitizers, and absorptive agents. Retaining sulfonylurea when insulin is added has been shown to require less insulin and subsequently less weight gain.

It is important also to understand that there are some individuals for whom insulin is indicated as initial therapy. These include:

1. Patients presenting with fasting glucoses in excess of 280 mg/dl with ketonuria or ketonemia
2. Gestational diabetes uncontrolled with diet and exercise where all oral agents are contraindicated during pregnancy
3. Latent autoimmune diabetes

Giving a modest dose of an intermediate-acting insulin like NPH or a long acting insulin like glargine or detemir at bedtime can effectively suppress hepatic gluconeogenesis and overcome insulin resistance. A meta-analysis of 16 randomized trials comparing bedtime insulin and daytime sulfonylurea (BIDS) demonstrated lower A1C, fasting glucoses and lower total insulin in the absence of weight gain with BIDS compared to a multiple split insulin regimen with intermediate-acting insulins [6].

In a large randomized controlled study of 570 patients, the long acting insulin analog glargine and human NPH insulin were evaluated in combination with oral agents including metformin, acarbose, and a sulfonylurea or combinations of these drugs [37].

Glargine administered at bedtime with oral agents was as effective as NPH at bedtime with oral agents in reducing hemoglobin A1C and fasting glucoses with lower rates of hypoglycemia. Concomitant use of insulin and thiazolidinediones (TZDs) is associated with the most weight gain of any preparation in addition to significant fluid retention properties. This should be kept in mind when insulin is added to a patient already on a TZD or when a TZD is added to a patient on insulin.

Weight gain and edema are major concerns with TZD usage in general and this should be kept in mind when tailoring an appropriate regimen for the patient. As the result of its lipogenic properties, insulin therapy alone usually results in weight gain, but it is to be remembered that insulin can cause sodium retention at the renal tubular level, which can subsequently augment the fluid retaining capabilities when adding TZD therapy. Both TZD's are indicated for use with insulin. A wise therapeutic maneuver is to use the lowest doses of the TZD to ameliorate this tendency retaining the synergistic glycemic and lipid lowering capabilities [6].

The effectiveness of adding at bedtime intermediate-acting insulin to oral agent therapy vs. switching to a multiple split dose insulin regimen was evaluated in two large well designed clinical trials. In the Finnish Multicenter Insulin Study (FINMIS), 153 type-2 diabetic patients poorly controlled on a sulfonylurea alone were randomized to (1) a sulfonylurea, (2) a sulfonylurea plus NPH insulin given at 7 o'clock in the morning, (3) a sulfonylurea plus NPH given at 9 p.m., (4) NPH/regular insulin before breakfast and dinner, (5) NPH insulin at 9 p.m. and regular insulin with each meal. All regimens were successful in improving glycemic control, but the total insulin dose was 50–60% lower in the two groups receiving a sulfonylurea plus once a day NPH insulin. The combination of bedtime insulin plus a sulfonylurea once again resulted in significantly less weight gain and less total insulin usage [38].

In type-2 diabetics inadequately controlled with metformin alone, addition of a bedtime NPH insulin resulted in 50% less insulin and weight gain compared to a regimen that involved multiple insulin injection, producing equivalent glycemic control.

Several well designed studies have compared the efficacy of adding a second oral agent vs. adding bedtime NPH insulin in poorly controlled type-2 diabetics already on mono-therapy. The addition of bedtime insulin to sulfonylurea as well as combination therapy with metformin plus a sulfonylurea were equally effective. Advantages of any metformin containing combinations are less weight gain [6].

In general 60–70% of newly diagnosed type-2 diabetic patients with entry plasma glu-coses between 200–240 mg/dl will be controlled or maintained with a combined sulfony-lurea/metformin regimen. The Fin/Fat study evaluated 96 type-2 diabetic patients who were poorly controlled with sulfonylurea and/or metformin and randomly assigned to receive: (1) bedtime NPH plus glibenclamide 15 mg/day, (2) bedtime NPH plus metformin 2 g/day, (3) bedtime NPH insulin plus metformin plus a sulfonylurea and (4) bedtime NPH plus morning NPH insulin [39].

The group receiving bedtime insulin plus metformin achieved significantly better glycemic control after 1 year than the other group within the group, bedtime insulin plus sulfonylurea plus metformin. This was attributed to the attenuation of weight gain which allowed insulin to be titrated to a higher dose. Predictably, the group that achieved the greatest amount of weight gain was the group on bedtime insulin and morning insulin. Clearly, a decision as to which regimen will work in a particular patient depends on a joint collaboration between physician and the patient.

Once two oral agents have been prescribed the decision regarding the choice of a third agent or a switch to insulin must be determined by the likely success of the therapeutic intervention. Often insulin is prescribed in favor of a third agent to ensure better control and with the availability of the long acting, peakless glargine, better A1C reductions are now possible. Any aggressive treatment to target goal should be combined patient educa-tion and dietary counseling in order to achieve optimum results [6].

Patients must be constantly counseled and reminded that insulin use does not signify that the patient is in the end-stage of their disease and does not represent failure on their part. I have found that with the advent of the insulin pens and the increased availability of self monitoring of blood glucose devices, patients are better capable of controlling postprandial glucoses and administering a short-acting analog of insulin accordingly. This tends to allay fears and serves as a bridge to the time when insulin is needed on a more regular basis.

In addition, giving insulin on an as-needed basis seems to prolong the time interval between taking oral agents and depending on a consistent daily dose of insulin. Rosenstock and Riddle have proposed a convenient insulin titration schedule for insulin naïve patients currently on oral medication [10]. This involves starting with 10 units/day at bedtime basal insulin, either NPH or glargine and adjusted weekly, with self monitoring of fasting blood glucose for two consecutive days assuming no episodes of severe hypoglycemia or plasma glucose is less than 72.

The weekly adjustments are as follows:

1. For fasting sugars between 100–120 mg/dl an increase in 2 units is recommended
2. Between 120 and 140 mg/dl – 4 units
3. 140 and 180 mg/dl – 6 units
4. Greater than 180 mg/dl – 8 units

Decreases of 2–4 international units per day are recommended if fasting sugars are less than 56 or a severe hypoglycemic episode occurs. Insulin mixes can be used effectively because of their availability of providing both a basal and bolus insulin in one preparation. The analog mixes allow for injection closer to meal time and can be transferred unit for unit with human mixes. They also can be used in type-2 diabetics new to insulin, patients who are unable to freely mix insulins, and patients who are maxed out on oral medications and would prefer a more convenient method of mixture.

The fixed percentages, however, can cause some concerns that are not ideally suited for those patients with variability in diet. A rapid acting mixture preparation before dinner involving analog or human insulin can control those patients who tend to have one meal a day or the majority of their calories at dinner time. This provides the advantage of bolus insulin to cover postprandial hyperglycemia and a basal insulin to control insulin needs after supper and during the early evening. Split mix doses are usually given at breakfast and supper with two-thirds of the total insulin dose administered before breakfast and one-third before supper. This works best in those patients consistently consuming meals with consistent caloric content [35].

Various multidose preparations can also be used, but a popular and common regimen is to use a long-acting analog of insulin (detemir or glargine) with pre or postprandial administration of an analog of insulin. Keep in mind that there is no perfect combination regimen or magic formula that can be used universally in all type-2 patients. Treatment must be individualized to achieve glycemic goals of hemoglobin A1C less than 6.5%, a postprandial glucose less than 140 mg/dl, and fasting sugars less than 100 mg/dl subsequently reducing the likelihood of end-organ damage and minimizing weight gain by using the least amount of insulin.

CONTINUOUS SUBCUTANEOUS INSULIN INFUSION PUMPS [40]

Continuous subcutaneous insulin infusion via the external insulin infusion pump is an alternative to MDI for those patients with labile glucose levels and frequent episodes of hypoglycemia. These pumps attach to the body through flexible plastic tubing with a needle inserted subcutaneously in the abdominal area.

Weighing 4–6 oz, 2–3 in. wide by approximately 4 in. long, these can be easily worn on a belt or slipped into a pocket. The patient needs to clean the needle and tubing apparatus every 2 days with refillable cartridges holding enough insulin for about a 48 h period. These pumps provide greater flexibility in life style, meal schedules, and travel. Continued subcutaneous infusion still supplies state of the art and best coverage because insulin pumps can deliver short acting insulin continuously and specifically according to glucose patterns. The ability to supply a bolus insulin injection at the touch of a button according to elevated blood glucose results due to varied carbohydrate and caloric intake, physical activity, and other factors provides an added benefit to this form of insulin delivery [40].

Compared with multidose injections, continuous subcutaneous infusions show more flexibility and have the potential for better hyperglycemic control. When used in continuous infusion pumps, lispro, apidra, and aspart have proved highly compatible and shown a more optimal bolus dose action than regular insulin because of their rapid subcutaneous absorption. When used in these pumps, the total amount of insulin used is less when analogs are employed because of their shorter duration time, quicker onset of action, and better efficiency.

Obviously the continuous infusion pump is not suitable for all patients and this approach requires a significant amount of patient cooperation, motivation, education, and involvement to continually monitor glucose status.

Blood glucose should be determined frequently to ascertain the correct insulin dose being delivered. The patient sets the pump to deliver a basal level of insulin during a period of time during the day. This can be varied for periods of time depending upon insulin use by setting the pump at different rates. The pump also has the flexibility of providing a bolus button to inject supplemental insulin for hyperglycemic episodes. The pumps should be checked frequently for interruptions in insulin delivery, while infections or inflammation at the needle site can occasionally be a complication.

Careful hygiene and frequent site changes can minimize this complication. Use of the insulin pumps for type-1 diabetes first began in the late 1970s. Since then these pumps have become dramatically smaller and much easier to use.

The currently available pumps also are equipped with multiple basal rates, several bolus options, a safety block-out feature, electronic memory, and even remote control. In the DCCT trial (type-1 diabetics), 42% of subjects used this technology in their last 4 years of treatment observing a decrease of 0.2–0.4% in Hemoglobin A1C's as well as improvement in life style [41].

Indications for continuous subcutaneous insulin pump infusion are:

1. Inadequate glycemic control defined as Hemoglobin A1C above the target level of 6.5%
2. Marked variability in glucose levels with history of hypoglycemic unawareness or hypoglycemic events requiring assistance
3. Persistent dawn phenomenon with glucose levels 140–160 mg/dl (8–9 mM/l in the morning)
4. Need for flexibility in life styles, people who work in a safety sensitive job, varying hours, business travelers, pregnant diabetics, etc.
5. Those individuals with daily insulin requirements that may fluctuate

The most important aspect of glycemic control in patients with insulin pumps is self monitoring of blood glucose. Of 106 patients who self monitored glucose levels five or more times a day, 62% had an average hemoglobin A1C of less than 7%. Subsequent recording of blood glucose values and insulin doses in a log book are helpful to the patient to give them an understanding of their fluctuation in levels [42].

Use of the analog insulins has resulted in overall less insulin use in a 24 h period with even less episodes of less hypoglycemia. In the DCCT trial on type-1 diabetics, the incidence of severe hypoglycemia was three times greater in the group receiving intensive therapy than those on conventional therapy, but less than those on multiple dose injections. This is probably due to reduction in insulin requirements and better pharmacologic delivery of insulin and minimal weight gain with insulin pump [17].

GENERAL THERAPEUTIC PRINCIPLES

There are some general principles to keep in mind in an attempt to achieve optimal basal-bolus therapy to achieve glycemic goals with insulin therapy [43]:

1. Measure the A1C at the initiation of therapy. Keep in mind that as the A1C exceeds 8.0%, it is the preprandial glucose that becomes the major driving force. So address

basal insulin management. When the A1C is less than 8.0%, the postprandial glucose is the driving force, so make certain that post meals excursions are controlled with a bolus regimen. In general, 50% of the total daily insulin dose should be bolus and 50% basal insulin.

2. Determine the total daily dose of insulin – this is 70% of the weight in kilograms. Thus, a 100 kg person would require 70 units of insulin (100×0.7).
3. Determine the insulin to carbohydrate ratio. This is sometimes referred to as the rule of 450. This determines the grams of carbohydrates that can be covered by 1 unit of insulin to control postprandial glucose and is dependent upon the total amount of insulin used daily (basal + bolus). Using this formula, the insulin/carbohydrate ratio is 450/total daily insulin dose. So, if a patient is taking a total of 45 units of basal + bolus insulin daily, 450/45 or 10 g of carbohydrates will be covered by 1 unit of insulin. If an individual is taking 100 units of insulin daily, then 450/100 or only 4.5 g of carbohydrate will be covered by 1 unit of insulin.
4. Determine the insulin sensitivity factor. This is also called the rule of 1700. This lets us know how much one unit of insulin will lower existing blood glucose. For example, if an individual takes a total insulin dose (basal + bolus) of 100 units, the insulin sensitivity factor is 17. Therefore, if the glucose is 310 mg/dl and the desired glucose is 140 mg/dl, then to lower the glucose to 170 mg/dl (310–140) would require 10 units of insulin (170/17). However, if an individual is taking a total daily dose of 50 units, then only 5 units would be required to achieve the same reduction.

Although formulas like these present useful guidelines it is important to keep in mind that various factors can also be involved in determining each individual patient's response to insulin including concomitant medications (steroids, anti-retrovirals, thiazide diuretics, and anti-psychotics), the duration and intensity of exercise of the patient, glycemic index of food consumed along with caffeine, alcohol and fat ingestion, the presence of autonomic abnormalities that can be responsible for hypoglycemic unawareness and gastroparesis, and the presence of any coexisting diseases (chronic or acute infections, malignancies, emotional, or physical distress), and the sight of insulin injection which can lead to insulin stacking. This accumulation effect occurs when short acting insulin is reinjected into the same site within 6 h of the previous injection. When injected subcutaneously, insulin forms a depot which results in continuous absorption for up to 6 h with about 80% of the injected dose dissipated within 4 h. By reinjecting into the same area, an additional depot is formed which can have an additive effect with the previous injected insulin remaining.

This cumulative stacking of insulin can cause significant hypoglycemia and can be a special concern in those individuals who experience hypoglycemic unawareness, since unexpected loss of consciousness can subsequently occur.

NOVEL THERAPIES

External insulin pumps provide continuous subcutaneous infusion (CSII) delivery. These devices make use of rapid-acting analogs (aspart, lispro, and glulisine) or regular human insulin allowing the patient to deliver bolus and basal insulin therapy. The needles that are inserted into the subcutaneous space should be changed every 72 h along with the site of insertion to prevent infection. These pump systems achieve better glycemic control with lower A1C levels, requiring less insulin when compared to multiple injection therapy. CSII can be used with many patient types and also used with increasing frequency in type-2 diabetics. The disadvantages of pump therapy rest in device malfunction and infection. Crystallization of insulin may cause catheter obstruction, although this occurs less frequently with the analogs and progressive improvements in pump technology.

A novel insulin delivery system, the OmniPod, contains a built-in insulin reservoir, automatic inserter, pumping mechanism, single disposal infusion set that weighs 1.2 oz, has no tubing and attaches to the skin by an adhesive, and can be worn in the shower, in the pool and even in the ocean. This device delivers insulin subcutaneously via wireless transmitted instructions from a digital remote controlled programmer. The device comes with a built-in blood glucose monitor that eliminates the need for carrying a separate glucometer. This disposal device needs to be changed every 3–5 days depending on total daily insulin requirements.

When pump therapy is initiated, the total daily insulin dose should be reduced by 25–30% in adults with ½ of the total daily dose being used as the basal dose and ½ as the total bolus dose. Dividing the basal doses by 24 allows the units per hour that can be given as a single basal rate. Both bolus and basal doses are adjusted according to the patient's blood glucose measurements taken preprandially, postprandially, and at bedtime. Clinical trials have demonstrated that patients using rapid acting analog insulins had lower A1C levels with better postprandial glucose control using less insulin than human regular insulin.

The basal rate is adjusted to avoid glucose excursions greater than 30 mg from baseline. The basal rate should only be adjusted during the day if there are significant glucose excursions more than 2 h after a meal bolus. Bolus doses are adjusted according to glucose measurements which can be taken either preprandially or postprandially. Using the preprandial approach, patients are given guidelines as to their carbohydrate insulin ratio.

This may vary among individuals from 1 unit per 5 g of carbohydrate up to 1 unit per 30 g of carbohydrate with an average being 1 unit for every 10–15 g of carbohydrate. Due to this inter-person variability and because of the unknown carbohydrate content of various foods, postprandial glucose measurements particularly with the use of rapid acting insulin analogs may be more practical.

When the patient still does not achieve A1C goals, the clinician must examine the frequency of the patient's monitoring and recording the patient's diet and knowledge of food intake, and determining whether the basal rate is set properly, whether the patient is using the proper correction bolus factor to treat blood sugars, and if the patient is preemptively counting carbohydrates in appropriate fashion. For some people, a post-emptive or post meal approach may be more convenient, practical, and effective.

It is important to remember that as the A1C level exceeds 8.0%, attention should be given to adjusting the basal rate since the contribution of the pre-prandial glucose becomes increasingly significant at these levels. For A1C levels between 6.5–8.0%, attention should be directed at controlling the bolus infusion since the contribution of the postprandial glucose is more significant at these levels.

Clearly the future is bright for insulin pump therapy as newer designs with remote control devices and even machines that can administer insulin according to measured levels of glucose with minimal patient interference appear to provide some important breakthroughs for future endeavors.

Implantable insulin pumps deliver insulin directly into the abdominal cavity closely resembling normal insulin physiology and production even better than subcutaneous injections. This technology, along with an implantable glucose sensor, may provide an important breakthrough and advance in pump technology.

Pancreatic transplantation is becoming another option at several medical centers for restoring insulin secretion in selective patients. Patients who undergo simultaneous kidney and pancreas transplantation have a 92% chance of renal graft survival and an 85% chance of pancreatic graft survival after 1 year. Solitary pancreatic transplantations should be used only in those individuals who are not controlled with all other insulin options.

Islet-cell transplantation in lieu of whole pancreas organ donations has been attempted by some investigators. This minimally invasive procedure uses cells from multiple donors and steroid free immunosuppression, percutaneous transhepatic portal vein transplantation of islets have been performed. However, supplemental insulin usually becomes necessary after 2 years. This technique has been limited to type-1 diabetics and requires the use of multiple donors and long term immunotherapy.

Further research is ongoing to genetically engineer beta cells, along with use of fetal islet cells, and isolation of transplanted cells from the body in special tubes sutured to the liver with semipermeable microholes to keep destructive white cells out [44].

Other alternatives to injectable insulin are currently being explored including transdermal, buckle, oral, and nasal inhalation systems. Of these, orally inhaled forms of insulin appear to have the most potential. This is because the lungs have certain advantages for insulin delivery. The epithelium is very thin, the surface area is very large making it very attractive for drug uptake.

Inhaled insulin has been shown to be equally efficacious as regular human insulin in reducing postprandial glucose, but has a slower metabolic effect and longer duration of action than rapid acting insulin analogs. However, the only FDA approved insulin for inhalation (Exubera) was withdrawn from the U.S. market after reports of decreased lung function and lung cancer, resulting in its production being stopped in October 2007.

SUMMARY

It is important for physicians and patients alike to be aware of not only the multifaceted approach of diabetic management, but the advantages and disadvantages of each of the products to be used as well as their subsequent combinations. The more familiar a physician and patient are with the product options, along with the best way they can be utilized in each individual patient, will facilitate management.

Early insulin therapy with subsequent tighter glucose control can preserve, delay, or even restore beta cell function. This is of great importance since beta cell function progressively declines in type-2 diabetics as inherited and dietary factors, and insulin resistance beget beta cell depletion while elevated free fatty acids, glucose, lipids, and inflammatory cytokines exert direct toxic effects on the beta cells.

New insulin analogs, with their more beneficial and favorable pharmacological onsets and duration of action compared to human insulin makes them more attractive and physiological in diabetic management.

We should not let patient fears or preconceived misconceptions about insulin deter us from encouraging our patients to be more aggressive to achieve tighter, optimal glucose control. Various monitoring devices, delivery systems, and proper patient education can be invaluable in overcoming these hurdles.

The goal of early insulin therapy is quicker glucose control to prevent the microvascular and possibly the macrovascular complications that we will discuss in the next chapter.

Let's apply some of these principals with case presentations.

CASE 1

A 65-year-old white male diabetic for 5 years on glimepiride 4 mg twice daily, sitagliptin 100 mg, and metformin 850 mg TID presents with an A1C of 7.8%, fasting glucose of 157 with postprandial glucoses at supper time of 195–205. He admits to sporadic eating patterns, has been known to have fatty liver with transaminases 1.5–2 times normal and is reluctant to take insulin. What do we do now?

This case is a dilemma often encountered in primary care practice. Although troglitazone (Rezulin) was used effectively to reverse fatty changes in experimental study, the glitazones are not indicated for steatohepatitis and should be avoided with these transaminase levels. Alpha-glucosidase inhibitors may give us an extra 0.8% reduction in A1C, but this will not likely get us to goal. This patient could benefit from the addition of a short acting insulin analog pen administered on an as-needed basis.

The pens tend to be better accepted by the needle insulin phobic patient and the "as needed" method allows this patient more flexibility for his erratic diet knowing that he has the capability of lowering his glucose if it rises postprandially. This also allows the patient to avoid the glucose toxicity and subsequent insulin resistance promulgated by postprandial excursions and this type of patient might not actually require the insulin every day using this regimen.

This can be a very valuable method of improving compliance in achieving glycemic goals as long as the patient can be relied upon to regularly (either once or twice daily) self monitor his glucose. If the patient cannot be relied upon to do this, then bedtime NPH, detemir or glargine should be used to increase basal insulin and lower fasting glucose. Once fasting and preprandial glucoses are at goal, postprandial glucoses should be lower especially if glargine or detemir are used. If the postprandials are still not at goal then a short-acting insulin analog can be added before meals provided that the patient can measure postprandial glucoses on a regular daily basis.

CASE 2

A 69-year-old African American female with a 10 year history of diabetes on glipizide 20 mg twice daily, pioglitazone 30 mg daily, metformin 1,000 mg BID, and saxagliptin 5 mg daily presents with an A1C of 9.8%, a fasting glucose of 201 mg/dl, and postprandial glucoses of 280–290 mg/dl.

With glycemic levels of this degree, this patient needs to be started on insulin. We could begin with levemir, glargine, or NPH at bedtime, retaining the sulfonylurea and DPP-IV inhibitor. We could also consider using an analog mix either 70/30 (Novalog) or 75/25 (Humalog) initially once daily before the largest meal and then progress to twice daily once the patient becomes accustomed to insulin use. Ideally the secretagogues should be kept in the regimen to minimize initial insulin doses. This may not be practical where cost considerations are a problem as they usually are with most patients.

It should be kept in mind that if the TZD is kept as part of the therapeutic regimen, the potential for fluid retention exists. If the long-acting insulin regimen is chosen, this individual should be checking postprandial sugars at least once a day after the largest meal or preferably twice daily. The timing of the postprandial measurement has caused some controversy, although postprandial sugars are defined as being elevated if the glucose is equal to or greater than 140 mg/dl at the 2 h period.

Clinical trials have also shown that 1 h postprandial sugars above this level are associated with increased risk of macrovascular disease. I have found that 2 h is a long period of time following a meal and is quite often forgotten or missed or simply not convenient to measure. By measuring postprandial sugars 1 h after each meal, the patient can have a convenient time interval for administration of insulin analogs allowing for the insulin to peak during the time the postprandial sugar is at its highest level, usually 2 h after eating.

CASE 3

A 43-year-old Hispanic female with polycystic ovaries, diabetic for 2 years taking nateglinide 120 mg 3 times a day and pioglitazone 30 mg daily with an A1C of 6.0%, postprandial glucoses of 130–140 mg/dl, and fasting glucoses of 100–110 mg/dl presents with a positive urine and blood pregnancy test 10 days after expected menstrual period.

Patients with polycystic ovary syndrome can ovulate and become pregnant when placed on TZD therapy. Since oral agents are contraindicated during pregnancy, both oral agents should be stopped and the patient is placed on insulin. Clinical trials have shown that close monitoring of pregnant diabetics with postprandial glucose was superior to monitoring fasting glucose, with better A1C control and less fetal and neonatal complications. Although analog insulins have been studied in pregnancy they are currently not officially approved for this use (detemir, glargine, glulisine, and apidra are listed as Category C, while aspart is Category B), and hence postprandial glucose monitoring with administration of human regular insulin would be the optimum initial choice for this patient.

CASE 4

A 62-year-old obese African American female presents with hemoglobin A1C's consistently between 7.5–8%, and fluctuating blood sugars with episodes of hypoglycemia. Her weight gain has been progressive while using a split regimen of 75/25 insulin 30 units before breakfast and 40 units before supper on a daily basis. In addition, the patient takes metformin 1,000 mg. twice daily, pioglitazone 15 mg daily, and ramipril 10 mg once daily.

The patient has been continuously frustrated with failure to achieve desired hemoglobin A1C's as well as fluctuating blood sugars with symptomatic episodes of both hyper and hypoglycemia. This case illustrates a failure on the mixed insulins. This patient would be better controlled with once daily detemir or glargine administration than the current biphasic insulin mix. Another possibility would be an insulin pump to address both basal and bolus therapy.

Table 4
The basal/bolus insulin concept [45]

Basal insulin

Suppresses hepatic glucose production between meals and overnight

Supplies ~50% of daily needs

Levels remain nearly constant throughout the day

Bolus insulin

Reduces hyperglycemia after meals

Immediate rise and sharp peak at 1 h after meals

Supplies ~50% of daily needs (10–20% of daily requirement at each meal)

In this particular incident we would begin with glargine or detemir with two-thirds of the total dose of the mixed insulin preparation, 45 units, given once daily.

Glargine insulin should not be administered more than once daily in type-2 diabetic patients although detemir can be dosed twice daily. In this particular incident the dose of the glargine insulin can be increased every 1–2 weeks by 2 units according to the previously mentioned sliding scale until the A1C reaches the desired level (<6.5%).

One could also employ the 303 approach with detemir by adjusting the dose 3 units every 3 days until the fasting glucose is less than 110 mg/dl. Postprandial glucose excursion could be controlled if necessary with a short-acting analog of insulin administered either pre- or even post meal with the aid of glucose monitoring.

CASE 5

A 56-year-old male diabetic for 13 years was on Metformin 1,000 mg twice daily, sitagliptin 100 mg daily, pioglitazone 30 mg daily, and glimepiride 4 mg twice daily. One year ago he was given detemir 15 units nightly which had gradually been increased to 30 units.

His A1C levels have been raised to the current value of 8.4%. He occasionally checks his postprandial glucose levels and finds them elevated to 260–280 mg/dl although his prebreakfast glucose levels run from 110 to 120 mg/dl. This patient will need better postprandial glucose control. As the A1C rises from the normal level to 8.0–8.5%, it is the postprandial glucose that is the driving force behind the elevation. This could be addressed by adding an analog insulin regimen before each meal, starting with a low dose delivered by pen (5 units), and gradually increasing if necessary according to A1C levels and postprandial glucose levels by glucometer. He would also benefit from dietary counseling. Many patients are not aware of the glycemic potency of the foods they are consuming and usually gain insight with appropriate instruction. Another possibility for these patients could be to stop the long-acting insulin and substitute a biphasic analog mix given during the two largest meals of the day. Normally when switching from a biphasic insulin regime to glargine or detemir, 2/3 of the total daily insulin dose is used. In this case we are going from a long-acting insulin to a biphasic one (opposite direction) and so we would begin with 3/2 of the total levemir dose (30 units) or 45 total units daily (approximately 20–22 units of the biphasic mix twice daily).

These cases provide a practical illustration of how the various insulins can be used to achieve glycemic control in individualized patients. The availability of insulin pens has provided a significant advance in overcoming patient fears with needle use and syringes and the stigma associated with such use as well as the medicolegal liability associated with proper handling and disposable of needles and syringes.

These cases illustrate the wide variability that can be seen when managing the type-2 diabetic patient. It is important to appreciate the advantages and disadvantages of all the various medications to design a program that will satisfy the unique needs of each patient and to keep in mind the basal/bolus concepts listed in Table 4, while working as a team to achieve these goals.

REFERENCES

1. Bastyr EJ, et al. Therapy focused on lowering postprandial glucose, not fasting glucose, may be superior for lowering A1C. Diabetes Care. 2000;23:1236–1241.
2. Mudulair S, Edelman SV. Insulin therapy in type-2 diabetes. Endocrinol Metab Clin North Am. 2001; 30:935–982.
3. Nathan DM, Buse JB, Davidson MB. American Diabestes Association: European Association for Study of Diabetes. Medical management of hyperglycemia in type-2 diabetes: a consensus algorithm for the initiation and adjustment of therapy. Diabetes Care. 2006;29(8):1963–1972.
4. Mayfield J, White RD. Insulin therapy for type-2 diabetes: rescue, augmentation and replacement of beta cell function. Am Fam Physician. 2004;70:489–500.
5. Burge MR, Schade DS. Insulins. Endocrinol Metab Clin North Am. 1997;26:575–598.
6. Kudlacek S, et al. The effect of insulin treatment on HbA1C, body weight and lipids in type 2 diabetic patients with secondary failure to sulfonylureas. Horm Metab Res. 1992;24:478–483.
7. American Diabetes Assoicaiton. Standards of medical care for patients with diabetes mellitus. Diabetes Care. 2002;25(suppl 1):S33–S49.
8. Hermann LS. Optimizing therapy for insulin treated type 2 diabetes mellitus. Drugs Aging. 2000; 17:283–294.
9. United Kingdom Prospective Diabetes Study group. (1998). A randomized trial of efficacy of addition of metformin to sulfonylurea. Diabetes Care. 21:87–92.
10. The Diabetes Control and Complications Trial Research Group. The effect of intensive treatment of diabetes on development and progression of long term complications in insulin dependent diabetes mellitus. N Engl J Med. 1993;329:977–986.
11. Van den Berghe G, et al. Intensive insulin therapy in critically ill patients. N Engl J Med. 2002; 346:1587–1588.
12. Bastyr EJ, Stuart CA, Brodows RG. Therapy focused on lowering postprandial glucose, not fasting glucose, may be superior for lowereing A1C. Diabetes Care. 2000;23:1236–1241.
13. DeVeciana M, et al. Targeting postprandial glucose in gestational diabetics improves HbA1C outcomes over 6 weeks. N Engl J Med. 1995;333:1239.
14. Mudaliar S, Edelman SV. Insulin therapy in type 2 diabetes. Endocrinol Metab Clin North Am. 2001;30:935–982.
15. Rosenstock J, et al. Basal insulin therapy in type 2 diabetes: 28 week comparison of insulin glargine and NPH insulin. Duiabetes Care. 2001;24:631–636.
16. Unger J. Targeting glycemic controlin the primary care setting. Female Patient. 2003;28:12–16.
17. Heller S, Kurtzhals P, et al. Insulin aspart: promising early results borne out in clinical practice. Expert Opin Pharmacother. 2002;3:183–195.
18. Antsiferov M, et al. Within patient variability in postprandial glucose excursion with lispro insulin analog compared with regular insulin. Diabetologia. 1995;38(suppl 1):A190.
19. Home PD, et al. Insulin Aspart Study Group. Improved glycemic control with insulin aspart: a multicenter randomized double blind crossover trial in type 1 diabetic patients. Diabetes Care. 1998;21:1904–1909.

20. Rolla A. Pharmacokinetic and pharmacodynamic advantages of insulin analogues and premixed insulin analogues over human insulins. Am J Med. 2008;121:S9–S19.

21. Holleman F, et al. Comparison of Lispro and regular human insulin in the correction of incidental hyperglycemia. Diabetes Care. 1996;19:1426–1429.

22. Schreiber SA, Haak T. Insulin glargine benefits patients with type-2 diabetes inadequately controlled on oral antidiabetic treatment. Diabetes Obes Metab. 2007;9:31–38.

23. Raskin P, et al. A 16 week comparison of the novel analog insulin glargine and NPH insulin used with insulin lispro in patients with type 1 diabetes. Diabetes Care. 2000;23:1666–1671.

24. Heinemann L, Linkeschova R, Rave K. Time-action profile of the long acting insulin analog insulin glargine. Diabetes Care. 2000;23:644–649.

25. Lepore M, et al. Pharmacokinetics and parmacodynamics of subcutaneous injection of long acting human insulin glargine, NPH insulin, and ultralente human insulin and continuous subcutaneous infusion of insulin lispro. Diabetes. 2000;23:1137–1142.

26. Rosenstock J, Schwartz SL, Clark CM. Basal Insulin therapy in type-2 diabetes: 28 week comparison of insulin glargine and NPH insulin. Diabetes Care. 2001;24:631–636.

27. Rosenstock J. Treatment of target study:glargine or NPH in insulin naïve patients with type-2 diabetes on oral agents. Diabetes. 2001;50(suppl 2):A129. Abstract 520-P.

28. Kelly JI, et al. Rapid decrease in clinically significant hypoglycemia with insulin glargine. Diabetes. 2002;51(suppl 2):A123.

29. Jonasson JM, Ljung R, Talbäck M. European Association for the Study of Diabetes. Insulin glargine and malignancy. Diabetologia. 2009:1418–1440.

30. Klein O, Lynge J, Endahl L. Insulin detemir and insulin glargine: similar time action profiles in subjects with type-2 diabetes. Diabetes. 2006;55(9 suppl):325.

31. Rosenstock J, Davies M, Home PD, Larsen J, Koenen C, Schernhaner G. A randomized 52 week treat to target trial comparing insulin detemir with insulin glargine when administered as add on to glucose lowering drugs in insulin naïve people with type-2 diabetes. Diabetologia. 2008;51:408–416.

32. Meneghini L, Koenen C, Weng W, Selam JL. The usage fo a simplified self titration dosing guideline for insulin detemir in patients with type-2 diabetes – the PREDICTIVE study. Diabetes Obes Metab. 2007;357:1716–1730.

33. Luddeke HJ, Philotheou A, Horn-rosenberg K. PREDICTIVE: a global, prospective observational study to evaluate insulin detemir treatment in type1 and type 2 daibetes. Diabet Med. 2006;23(suppl 4):139.

34. Nathan DM, Buse JB, Davidson MD. Medical management of hyperglycemia in type 2 diabetes. Diabetes Care. 2009;32(1):193–203.

35. Kovisto VA, Tuominen JA, et al. Lispro mix insulin as pre-meal therapy in type 2 diabetic patiens. Diabetes Care. 1999;22:459–462.

36. Malone JK, et al. Improved postprandial glycemic control with Humalog Mix 75/25 after a standard test meal in patients with type 2 diabetes mellitus. Clin Ther. 2000;22:222–230.

37. MassiBenedetti M, Humburg E, Dressler A, Ziemen M. A one year, randomized, muldticentre trial comparing insulin glragine with NPH insulin in combination with oral agents in patients with type-2 diabetes. Horm Metab Res. 2003;35:189–196.

38. Yki-Jarvinen H, Ryysy L, Kauppila M, Kujansuu E, Lahti J. Effect of obesity on the response to insulin therapy in non-insulin dependent diabetes mellitus – The FINMIS study. J Clin Endocr Metab. 1997;82(12):4037–4043.

39. Riddle MC, Rosenstock J, Gerich J. The Treat to Target trial. Diabetes Care. 2003;26:3080–3086.

40. Cefalu WTR. Novel routes of insulin delivery for patients with type 1 or type 2 diabetes. Ann Med. 2001;33:579–586.

41. Stewart KM. Insulin delivery devices. J Pharm Pract. 2004;17:20–28.

42. Wilson M, Weintreb J, Hoo GW. Intensive insulin therapy in critical care. Diabetes Care. 2007;30:1005–1011.

43. Cook CB, Boyle ME, Cisar NS. Use of continuous subcutaneous insulin infusion/insulin pump therapy in the hospital setting. Diabetes Educ. 2006;32:130. Diabetes Educ. 2005;31:849–857.

44. Palumbo P. The case for insulin treatment early in type 2 diabetes. Clev Clin J Med. 2004;71(5):385–386.

45. Owens DR, Zinman B, Insulins today and beyond. Lancet. 2004;71(5):385–386.

SUPPLEMENTARY READINGS

Boehm BO, et al. Premixed insulin aspart 30 vs. premixed human insulin 70/30 twice daily: a randomized trial in type 1 and type 2 diabetic patients. Diabet Med. 2002;19:393–399.

Dornhorst A, Luddeke HJ, Sreenan S. Safety and efficacy of insulin detimir in clinical practice. Int J Clin Pract. 2007;61:523–528.

Hermann L. Combination therapy with insulin and metformin (The Fin-Fat Study). Endocr Pract. 1998;4(6).

Hirsch IB, et al. Role of insulin in management of surgical patients with diabetes mellitus. Diabetes Care. 1990;13:980–991.

Home P, Kurtzhals P. Insulin detimir: from concept to clinical experience. Expert Opin pharmacother. 2006;7:325–343.

Meneghini LF, Rosenberg KH, Loenen C. Insulin detimir improves glycemic control with less hypoglycemia and no weight gain in patients with type-2 diabetes. Diabetes Obes Metab. 2007;9:418–427.

Ordoubadi FF, et al. Glucose-insulin-potassium therapy for treatment of acute myocardial infarction: an overview of randomized placebo-controlled trials. Circulation. 1997;96:1152–1156.

Raslova K, Bogoev M, Raz I. Insulin detemir and insulin aspart. Diabetes Res Clin Pract. 2004;66:193–201.

Standl E. Insulin analogues-state of the art. Horm Res. 2002;57(suppl 1):4045.

Van den Berghe G, Wouters P, et al. Intensive insulin therapy in critically ill patients. N Engl J Med. 2001;345:1359–1367.

Queale WS, et al. Glycemic control and sliding scale insulin use in medical inpatients with diabetes mellitus. Arch Intern Med. 1997;157:545–552.

8 Non-Insulin Injectables

Contents

Key Words: GLP-1 analogs (incretin mimetics), Amylin analogs, Incretin, K and L cells, Glucagon like peptide 1 (GLP-1), Postprandial glucagon secretion

INTRODUCTION

The description of the incretin effect was first described in 1964 by Elwick when he observed a greater insulin secretory response if glucose was administered orally compared to intravenously despite similar elevations in plasma glucose. This incretin effect is attributed to the release of peptide hormones from the K and L cells in the intestines in the response to eating, so that approximately 60% of the insulin subsequently secreted is related directly to the effect of incretins [1]. Glucagon like peptide-1 (GLP-1) is secreted by the L cells, suppresses postprandial glucagon secretion, reduces appetite and stimulates insulin secretion in a dose dependent manner.

In addition, the K cells release glucagon-dependent insulinotropic peptide (GIP). Following a meal, GIP levels may increase tenfold compared to GLP-1 levels, with both peptides showing similar insulin stimulating effects with glucose concentrations up to 180 mg/dl [2]. However, GIP does not suppress glucagon secretion and has minimal if any effect on insulin secretion at glucose concentrations greater than 140 mg/dl with no known effects on appetite. GLP-1 is derived from the pre-proglucagon peptide and is present in two bioactive forms with 80% of the GLP-1 found in the circulation present as the 30-amino acid isoform GLP-1 amide [3]. The varied effects of these two hormones are outlined in Table 1.

The physiologic responses as the result of GLP-1 activity are due to their binding to a specific GLP-1 receptor located in several organs in the body especially the pancreas and the brain. GLP-1 peptide is then rapidly degraded by the enzyme dipeptidyl peptidase-4 (DPP-4)

From: *Current Clinical Practice: Type 2 Diabetes, Pre-Diabetes, and the Metabolic Syndrome*
Edited by: R.A. Codario, DOI 10.1007/978-1-60327-441-8_8
© Springer Science+Business Media, LLC 2011

Table 1
Comparison of GLP and GIP [1]

	GLP	GIP
Secretion	L-cells	K-cells
Effect on glucagon secretion	Decreases	No effect
Appetite	Decreases	No effect
Insulin secretion	Increases	Decreases
Gastric emptying	Decreases	No effect
Secretion in type-2 diabetics	Decreased	Normal
Sensitivity in type-2 diabetics	Not affected	Decreased

GLP glucagon like peptide; *GIP* glucose dependent insulinotropic polypeptide

resulting in a half-life in the circulation of 60–90 s with the metabolites subsequently produced functioning as GLP-1 receptor antagonists [4].

Incretin effects result in enhanced glucose dependent secretion of insulin by the pancreatic beta cell, but the magnitude of that effect is strictly dependent upon plasma glucose concentration. The incretin effect on insulin secretion subsides considerably as glucose concentration approaches normal range. GLP-1 has been shown to have other important effects which ultimately influence glucose disposal, stimulating the transcription of proinsulin, and stimulating the proliferation of beta cells from precursor ductal cells, increasing beta cell mass in animal models, and promoting beta cell neogenesis. GLP-1 has also been shown to enhance glucose uptake by insulin sensitive tissues as a result of its enhanced insulin stimulating effect regulating postprandial glycemia in a glucose dependent matter, diminishing appetite thereby regulating food intake in animals, slowing and regulating gastric emptying and suppressing postprandial glucagon secretion.

Hepatic glucose output represents the principle contributor of glucose to the body in the fasting state. While also having an effect on tissue glucose uptake, fasting glucose is regulated in the narrow range between 70–100 mg/dl, with the euglycemic state achieving balance between peripheral glucose uptake and hepatic glucose output. Glucagon is released from the pancreatic alpha cells when plasma glucose concentrations decrease in the fasting state causing a rise in plasma glucose maintained at normal levels. In the postprandial state food in the gut and neurohormonal signals stimulate the secretion of GLP-1 and GIP stimulating the beta cells to secrete insulin and amylin [5].

The glucose dependent secretion of insulin in GLP-1 enhances glucose uptake in the hepatocyte and skeletal muscle decreasing postprandial glucose, while inhibiting hepatic glucose output and glucagon secretion. GLP-1 has also been shown to enhance insulin synthesis by the beta cells increasing their ability to respond to hyperglycemia. This has been demonstrated in mice with impaired glucose tolerance and in isolated rat pancreatic beta cells which secrete insulin and become glucose sensitive decreasing their fasting postprandial glucose levels when they are treated with GLP-1. Glucagon suppression in the pancreatic alpha cells reduces hepatic glucose production in a glucose dependent matter. Hence the overall effect of GLP-1 is the regulation of fasting and postprandial glucose levels by directly affecting glucagon and insulin secretion with subsequent glucose homeostasis being controlled in both the fasting and postprandial states by the interaction of insulin and glucagon [6].

Glucagon like peptide 1, synthesized in the enteroendocrine L cells located in the distal end of the colon, not only act on the alpha cells to decrease glucagon secretion and the beta cells to enhance insulin secretion, but also have an effect on the gamma cells enhancing somatostatin secretion, while promoting the synthesis of pro-insulin, increasing the regeneration, neurogenesis and growth of the beta cell, and decreasing apoptosis. It is important to understand that the rapid stimulation of GLP-1 secretion is generated by a combination of neuro and endocrine signals even before digested nutrients are in contact with the L cell in the ileum and the colon. Although L cells have been found in the duodenum and jejunum, their contribution to GLP-1 increase is uncertain at this time [7].

In the central nervous system, GLP-1 receptor is significantly expressed while the GIP receptors are somewhat decreased although the exact effects, here, remain to be elucidated. GLP-1 has been shown to affect the hypothalamus, decreasing water and food intake, enhancing satiety and decreasing appetite. Effects on gastric motility and pancreatic secretion are mediated by vagal pathways as well as GLP-1 levels in the hepatic portal region. Both intravenous and intracerebral ventricular administration of GLP-1 has been shown to suppress appetite with long term use associated with weight loss in type-2 diabetics. Interestingly, 0.5 kg weight loss and 15% reduction of caloric intake in nondiabetic obese individuals was demonstrated with 5 just days of GLP-1 administration preprandially [8].

Thus far, short term infusion of GLP-1 has not decreased insulin resistance in diabetic patients, but GLP-1 has been shown to reduce free fatty acid levels and reduce hyperglycemia and regulate glucagon secretion from the liver, indicating that hepatic glucose uptake and glucose production may be directly regulated.

Glucose dependent insulinotropic polypeptide (GIP) was actually the first incretin to be identified. This hormone contains 42 amino acids synthesized in the entero- endocrine K cells of the duodenum and jejunum in the proximal small bowel. Circulating plasma levels of GIP, as with GLP-1, increase within minutes of eating stimulating insulin secretion. GIP has not been demonstrated to have any significant effect on gastric emptying, glucagon secretion, or food intake unlike GLP-1 [9].

In type-2 diabetics, GIP secretion is generally normal, while GLP-1 secretion is reduced. While glucagon response to GIP has been shown to be impaired in type-2 diabetics, GLP-1 activity is relatively preserved. Both of these incretins affect the G protein coupled receptors in the ileal beta cells. However, the GIP receptor is expressed to a lesser extent in the central nervous system and adipose tissue. GLP-1 receptor is expressed in the gastrointestinal tract, lung, heart, kidney, central and peripheral nervous systems, peripheral tissues, and pancreatic islet alpha and beta cells. Disruption of GLP-1 action has been shown to enhance gastric emptying, increase glucagon levels and reduce glucose clearance, while decreasing insulin secretion, indicating that GLP-1 plays an essential role in glucose control. In addition, inhibition of GLP-1 action results in fasting hyperglycemia, a phenomenon that has not been demonstrated with GIP inhibition. Once released from the L cells and K cells respectively, GLP-1 and GIP are rapidly metabolized by DPP-4, a serine protease, which exists in a soluble form in plasma and located on the end of filial cells. DPP-4 action results in a substantial loss of incretin insulin atropic activity with a half-life of 1–2 min in the circulation [10].

GLP-1 RECEPTOR AGONISTS (INCRETIN MIMETICS)

Exenatide (Byetta) (Exendin-4)

This 39-amino acid dipeptide shares 53% of its amino acid sequence with human GLP-1, is produced in the saliva of *Heloderma suspectum* (Gila monster lizard) and is 550 times more potent than endogenous GLP-1 in glucose lowering. This potent peptide is a GLP-1 receptor agonist, resistant to DPP-4, with a half-life of 60–90 min, and persistence in plasma for 4–6 h after a single subcutaneous injection. Exenatide has demonstrated similar effects to GLP-1 on food intake, beta-cell function, and gastric emptying reducing post-prandial hyperglycemia in diabetic patients and persistent increased insulin secretion in nondiabetic patients for up to 180 min following infusion. As with native GLP-1, the effects are glucose dependent [11].

PHARMACOKINETICS

Exenatide reaches peak medium plasma concentrations in 2.1 h following subcutane-ous administration in patients with type-2 diabetes. The area under the curve (AUC) for this product increases proportionally in the therapeutic dose range from 5 to 10 µg. However, the C max values increase less proportionally over the same range. Concentrations appear to be similar regardless of the location of administration (arm, thigh, or abdomen). The drug is predominately eliminated by glomerular filtration with subsequent proteolytic degradation. The clearance of exenatide in humans is 9.1 L/h with a medium terminal half life of 2.4 h, independent of the dose, while concentrations are still measurable for approximately 10 h post dose [12]. In patients with mild to moderate renal insufficiency (creatinine clearance 30–80 ml/min), exenatide clearance is mildly reduced hence no adjustment is necessary. However, in patients with end stage renal disease on dialysis, exenatide clearance is reduced to 0.9 L/h. Therefore, this product is not recommended for use in patients with creatinine clearances less than 30 mg/min, with doses of even 5 µg once daily not well tolerated due to gastrointestinal side effects. Since the drug is primarily excreted by the kidney, hepatic dysfunction studies have not been performed in patients. With a diagnosis of acute or chronic hepatic insufficiency, exenatide need not be affected or dose reduced.

CLINICAL TRIALS

In phase I clinical trials, exenatide in doses greater than 0.3 µg/kg resulted in vomiting and nauseousness, and was better tolerated in subcutaneous doses of 0.1 µg/kg or less. The dose limiting adverse events of nauseousness and vomiting were minimized with initiation of therapy at 5 µg twice daily for 4 weeks with a subsequent increase to 10 µg twice daily as a maintenance dose in phase II clinical trials [13]. Phase III clinical trials evaluated the efficacy of exenatide use at 5 or 10 µg in combination therapy supplementing ongoing treatment in patients optimally controlled on oral agents including sulfonylureas, met-formin, and a combination of both or thiazolidinediones [14]. These trials were patterned after the phase II clinical trials initiating therapy with 5 μg twice daily for 4 weeks, but increasing to 10 μg twice daily. After a 30-week period of time, weight gain was attenuated or a mild weight loss of 1.5–3 kg was achieved with a reduction of A1C by 0.8–1.0%. Total weight loss was 4–5 kg after 8 weeks in an open label extension study. Once again, the common side effects were gastrointestinal, most commonly nauseousness, but occasionally vomiting and diarrhea, but these side effects dissipated with prolonged duration of therapy. The risk of hypoglycemia was increased in patients on exenatide and sulfonylureas compared to its use with metformin although the A1C reductions appeared to be similar in these trials.

It is interesting to note that antibody formation, which occurs in up to 50% of patients receiving exenatide, is not associated with impaired effectiveness in most patients treated, since the antibodies have weak binding affinity and minimal titers. The effectiveness, however, of this drug in most patients with high antibody titers are still somewhat variable and remains to be elucidated.

In phase II clinical trials in type-2 diabetics' not achieving optimal control on metformin and a sulfonylurea, postprandial glucose reduction was greater with exenatide than glargine insulin, especially at the breakfast and dinner feedings. However, the basal insulin glargine is more effective in reducing fasting glucose levels with similar reductions in A1C of 1.1% during a 20-week period of time. Discontinuation rates were higher in the exenatide treated group due to higher gastrointestinal side effects of vomiting and nausea, with a weight gain of 1.8 kg in the insulin treated group compared to a weight loss of 2.3 kg in the exenatide treated group [15].

In the phase III clinical trials done by Buse and others the efficacy of exenatide in weight reduction was clearly demonstrated with the 10 μg dose being superior to the 5 μg dose in both the metformin treated and sulfonylurea treated patients. The weight reductions were similar in patients who were on both metformin and sulfonylurea when exenatide was added to the regimen [16].

In the journal *Diabetologia*, Nauck and others reported a comparison trial of over 200 patients suboptimally controlled with sulfonylurea and metformin in a non-inferiority study with biphasic insulin aspart in patients with type-2 diabetes. In this open labeled 52-week trial, patients in the exenatide group received 5 μg twice daily for 4 weeks and 10 μg twice daily for the remainder of the study; while those in the biphasic insulin aspart comparative group received their therapy before the morning and evening meals titrated to maintain glycemic control. In this study, 24% of the insulin group achieved A1C levels equal to or less than 7% compared to 32% in the exenatide group, while 18.3% in the exenatide group received A1C levels equal to or less than 6.5% compared to 8.6% in the aspart group. The P values in both the 6.5 and 7% group were both less than 0.05 [17].

In the *Journal of Clinical Therapeutics*, Barnett and others reported on a multinational randomized open label crossover non-inferiority trial evaluating the efficacy of titrated insulin glargine compared to exenatide in adult patients with type-2 diabetes previously not controlled with a sulfonylurea or metformin [18]. In this study of 276 patients, 37.5% in the exenatide group compared to 39.8% in the glargine group achieved A1C levels less than 7.0%. The difference was not felt to be statistically significant, while 21.5% in the exenatide group compared to 13.6% in the glargine group achieved A1C equal to or less than 6.5%. However, this difference was once again not significant. Patients in the exenatide group received 5 μg twice daily for 4 weeks and 10 μg twice daily thereafter for a total of 16 weeks, while those in the insulin glargine group received titrated subcutaneous insulin injections adjusted to achieve a targeted, fasting blood glucose equal to or less than 100 mg/dl. The traditional regimens were then switched for an additional 16-week period of time to ensure the fact that both groups received 16 weeks of insulin glargine and exenatide therapy. Additional data from the completed population showed that both groups achieved a mean change of 1.4% from the baseline hemoglobin A1C of 9.0%. Exenatide was shown to achieve a greater weight reduction, while glargine caused weight gain. From baseline, the exenatide group lost 2.2 kg compared to a weight gain of 1 kg in the glargine group. When the groups crossed over, however, the insulin treated group to whom exenatide was substituted achieved a weight reduction of 2.5 kg compared to a weight gain of 2.3 kg when glargine replaced exenatide.

In the *Annals of Internal Medicine*, Heine and others reported the effects of exenatide vs. glargine in type-2 diabetics sub-optimally controlled with metformin and a sulfonylurea in a randomized trial [19]. This study compared the addition of exenatide or insulin glargine to a current therapy of sulfonylurea and metformin at maximally effective doses in an open label, randomized multicenter clinical trial lasting 26 weeks with 551 cohorts. In this trial, mean baseline A1C levels were 8.3% for the glargine group and 8.2% for the exenatide group. At the end of the 26-week period, 46% of patients in the exenatide group ($n=275$) compared to 48% of individuals ($n=260$) in the insulin glargine group achieved A1C values equal to or less than 7.0%. These differences were not clinically significant. About 57.1% of patients receiving exenatide complained of nauseousness compared to 8.6% of patients taking glargine, with vomiting occurring in 17.4% of patients on exenatide compared with 3.7% with glargine. This study demonstrated that both agents were effective in reducing A1C levels by 1% from baseline with exenatide causing more weight loss, but more gastrointestinal adverse effects than insulin glargine.

Exenatide administration at therapeutic concentrations has also been demonstrated to restore first phase insulin response in type-2 diabetics following an intravenous bolus of glucose. In addition, second phase insulin secretion was also significantly increased in those patients given exenatide compared to saline solution. This is an important therapeutic advantage and merits consideration since the loss of first phase insulin response is an early manifestation of the beta-cell defect in type-2 diabetics.

Post marketing cases of acute pancreatitis have been reported in exenatide treated patients. The cumulative spontaneous reporting rate for pancreatitis over a period of 2 years from June, 2005 to July, 2007 was 0.20 events per 100,000 patient years of exposure in over 700,000 patients who have been treated with exenatide [20]. Pre-clinical toxicology studies did not demonstrate an increased incidence of pancreatitis at plasma concentrations higher than those during clinical use. It actually was lower in exenatide treated patients, 1.7 per 1,000 subject years compared to 3.0 per 1,000 subject years. Among the post marketing reported cases of pancreatitis, a significant portion of those patients had at least one risk factor for pancreatitis such hyperuricemia, gallstone disease, and hypercalcemia, with gallstones being the most common cause followed by alcohol ingestion. Other situations like toxin exposure, hypercalcemia, hepatitis, cytomegalovirus exposure, and even treatment with the antidiabetic oral agent glyburide have been reported to increase the risk of acute pancreatitis with approximately 10% of cases being idiopathic.

In nonclinical data on exenatide, the product appeared to be well tolerated across various animal species like mice, rat, and monkeys with no target organ or dose limiting toxicities noted in these animals. Minimal to mild isolated areas of pancreatic islet cell hypercellularity were observed in monkeys with no indication of any cytotoxic, inflammatory, degenerative or any other pathological changes in the pancreas other than hypercellularity. In addition, a nonclinical trial did not demonstrate any increase in lipase or amylase activity in the pancreatic duct, pentagastrin stimulated gastric acid release and no significant effect on pancreatic exocrine function. Results from the clinical trials include nine reports of pancreatitis in the clinical developing program as of March 31, 2007 with one of those patients developing pancreatitis prior to randomization. In the remaining eight patients, six exenatide treated patients experienced pancreatitis compared to two in the placebo cohorts, with the incidence of pancreatitis across the entire exenatide development program being 1.7 per 1,000 subject years in patients given exenatide, compared to 3.0 per 1,000 subject years in patients receiving placebo, with 2.0 patients per 1,000 developing pancreatitis in the insulin comparator. The time of onset in the exenatide treated patients was variable ranging from 156 to 1,164 days. This data suggested that there is no significant increase of pancreatitis in patients given exenatide compared with the placebo or comparative group. Of the six patients who developed pancreatitis, ingestion of medications capable of producing pancreatitis was found in all of them. The pancreatitis resolved spontaneously in five patients, but remained chronic in one subject at the time of the report release in March 2007. As of July 2007, the cumulative spontaneous reporting rate for pancreatitis was 0.20 per 1,000 patient years of exposure. Resolution of the pancreatitis occurred with the appropriate support of treatment and suspension of suspect medications including exenatide. The time of onset of acute pancreatitis relative to exenatide therapy has been extremely variable ranging from 1 day to over 1 year.

Protein and peptide pharmaceuticals have the potential for producing immunogenic changes. And most patients treated with exenatide will develop antibodies; however, these antibody titers tend to diminish over time. In the 30-week controlled clinical trials of exenatide added on to metformin and/or sulfonylurea, 38% of patients had low titers of these exenatide antibodies at the end of the study with no essential change in glycemic control. An additional 6% of patients had higher antibody titers at 30 weeks. More than half of those demonstrated a mild effect on glycemic control.

In a 16-week trial of exenatide add-on therapy to thiazolidinediones with or without metformin, 9% of patients had higher antibody titers at 16 weeks with an attenuated glycemic response in patients with higher titer antibodies [21]. In a 16-week clinical placebo controlled study of exenatide added to a thiazolidinedione with or without metformin, the usual side effects were similar to that seen in a 30-week controlled clinical trial with metformin and/or a sulfonylurea, while withdrawal due to side effects being higher (16%) in the exenatide treated group than the placebo group (2%). In this trial, placebo was injected twice daily with exenatide being administered subcutaneously before the morning and evening meals. Seventy-nine percent of patients were taking metformin and a thiazolidinedione with 21% taking a TZD alone. The baseline A1C levels were similar in both groups at 7.9% with the exenatide group initiated at a dose of 5 μg twice a day for 4 weeks subsequently increased to 10 μg twice a day for 12 more weeks. At the 16-week period of time, placebo in combination with a TZD or a TZD plus metformin resulted in a weight loss of 0.2 kg compared to 1.5 in the exenatide/TZD and the exenatide/TZD/metformin group. The changes in fasting serum glucose from baseline to week 16 being significantly different compared to the placebo group, dropping 21 mg/dl for the exenatide 10 μg twice daily group compared to a slight increase of 4 mg/dl for the placebo group. In three clinical trials that reported lipid data, a small decrease in low density lipoprotein cholesterol favoring exenatide and a slight increase in HDL compared to placebo [22].

Evidence regarding the effects of exenatide on beta-cell function in patients with type-2 diabetes mellitus continues to be collected. A trial published by Bunck and others published in *Diabetes Care* assessed treatment of 69 individuals comparing insulin glargine with exenatide, showed similar reductions in A1C with weight reduction in the exenatide group and weight gain in the insulin group. Arginine stimulated C-peptide secretion during hyperglycemia increased 2.46 fold from baseline levels compared to 1.31 fold with insulin glargine after 52 weeks [23].

Long acting exenatide is a polylactide-glycolide microsphere suspension containing 3% exendin-4 peptide, which demonstrates a dose dependent control of glucose for up to 28 days after one subcutaneous injection in fatty diabetic zucker rats.

In preliminary data in 45 individuals, once weekly administration of exenatide long acting for 15 weeks compared with exenatide twice daily resulted in greater fasting glucose reductions and lower A1C's. This product is currently in phase III clinical trials, while long-term experience with the drug is still not reported.

In a study published in Lancet by Drucker and his colleagues, long acting exenatide, once weekly, demonstrated greater improvements in glycemic control than exenatide given twice daily with a lower incidence of nausea, similar reductions in body weight, and no increased risk of hypoglycemia [24]. These benefits were shown when long acting exenatide was added to a broad spectrum of glucose lowering therapies except insulin. The durability of treatment effects in this 30-week trial needs further assessment. The effect of exenatide on microangiopathy complications or cardiovascular events or the potential for a once weekly incretin mimetic to favorably and durably effect fasting and postprandial glucose control can substantially change the management of type-2 diabetes.

Potential beneficial cardiovascular effects of exenatide were demonstrated in two clinical trials with exenatide showing blood pressure reduction, increased HDL, and decreased LDL. The clinical implications of these surrogate marker reductions remain to be elucidated.

In head to head comparisons with the DPP-IV inhibitor, sitagliptin, exenatide had a greater effect than sitagliptin in reducing postprandial glucose, increasing insulin secretion, decreasing postprandial glucagon secretion, and a better effect in reducing the rate of gastric emptying. This may indicate that exenatide may generate a greater degree of GLP-1 receptor activation than the physiological concentrations of GLP-1 that are achieved with DPP-IV inhibition. The slowing of the rate of gastric emptying with exenatide, demonstrated with scintographic analysis, may also explain its greater effect in reducing postprandial glucose.

Exenatide is currently indicated as initial monotherapy or as adjunctive therapy to improve glycemic control in type-2 diabetic patients on oral agents, but has not yet been approved for concomitant use with insulin or a DPP-IV inhibitor.

Liraglutide (Victoza)

Liraglutide is a partially DPP-4 resistant GLP-1 receptor agonist which contains a glutamic acid and 16 carbon free fatty acid addition to lysine, at the 26th position, along with an arginine substitution for lysine at the 34 position, with a 97% amino acid sequence homology to endogenous human GLP-1 (7–37). This drug, by activating the GLP-1 receptor, increases intracellular cyclic AMP (adenosine monophosphate) resulting in insulin release with elevated blood glucose, while decreasing glucagon secretion. Due to its noncovalent binding to albumin, and relative resistance to dipeptidyl peptidase IV (DPP-IV), liraglutide has a half life of approximately 10–14 h after subcutaneous administration in human beings and can be given as a once daily injection with 1–2% of the product circulating as the non-albumin free peptide. In addition to preventing weight gain or inducing modest weight loss, liraglutide has been shown to reduce fasting and postprandial glucose levels up to 1.5% [25]. Thus far, liraglutide exposure has not been reported to reduce antibody formation, while nauseousness, vomiting, and diarrhea tend to be mild, transient, and only in rare instances resulted in discontinuation.

Liraglutide reduces fasting, premeal, and postprandial glucose throughout the day, lowering blood glucose by stimulating insulin secretion and lowering glucagon secretion, with insulin response increasing in a glucose dependent manner. Liraglutide also delays gastric emptying, reducing postprandial glucose excursions.

PHARMACOKINETICS

This glucagon like peptide-1 (GLP-1) achieves maximum concentrations 8–12 h post dosing with C-max and AUC increasing proportionally over the therapeutic dose range of 0.6–1.8 mg. The drug is endogenously metabolized to large proteins without a given single organ as a major route of elimination. Therefore no dose adjustment is necessary in patients with hepatic or renal impairment although caution concerning its use exists in these patients due to limited clinical testing.

TOXICOLOGY

A dose related increase in benign thyroid cell adenomas was seen in mice with treatment related malignant C-cell carcinomas occurring in 3% of females in the group tested. In addition, skin fibrosarcomas developed in male mice along the injection sites when much higher doses were used. This clustering of thyroid-cell carcinomas was also seen in male and female rats. In clinical trials of liraglutide treated patients, six cases of papillary thyroid carcinoma were reported [26]. Most carcinomas were less than 1 cm in diameter. Consequently, the FDA has placed a black box warning on the drug stating:

> It is unknown whether Victoza causes thyroid C-cell tumors, including medullary thyroid carcinoma, in humans, as human relevance could not be ruled out by clinical or nonclinical studies. Victoza is contraindicated in patients with a personal or family history of medullary thyroid carcinoma and in patients with Multiple Endocrine Neoplasia syndrome type 2 (MEN 2).

In clinical trials there were more cases of pancreatitis among liraglutide treated patients than the comparators. Hence the drug should be avoided in patients with a history of this disorder.

CLINICAL TRIALS

The Liraglutide Effect and Action in Diabetes (LEAD)-2 study evaluated the safety and efficacy of liraglutide, glimepiride, and placebo all in combination with metformin in type-2 diabetes [27]. This 26-week double blind, placebo and active controlled, parallel group trial randomly assigned 1,091 patients to once daily liraglutide (0.6, 1.2, or 1.8 mg daily injected subcutaneously) to placebo or glimepiride (4 mg once daily). All treatment arms included metformin (1,000 mg twice daily). A1C's ranged from 7 to 11%. Body weight decreased in all liraglutide groups and increased in the glimepiride group, while nausea occurred in 11–19% of the liraglutide group compared with 3–4% in the placebo and glimepiride groups. The A1C levels decreased by 1.0% in the 1.2, liraglutide,1.8 mg liraglutide and glimepiride group and 0.7% in the 0.6 mg liraglutide group, while the placebo group A1C increased by 0.1%. Hypoglycemia with liraglutide was similar to placebo, but 17% in the glimepiride group. This demonstrated that once daily liraglutide has similar glycemic control, less hypoglycemia, and reduced body weight compared with glimepiride.

The LEAD-6 study evaluated once daily liraglutide vs. exenatide twice daily in type-2 diabetes with a 26-week randomized, parallel group open label trial. This study demonstrated that once daily liragutide provided significantly larger improvements in glycemic control than exenatide twice daily and was better tolerated. Mean A1C was 8.2% in this study and liraglutide therapy resulted in a decrease of 1.12% compared to 0.79% for exenatide. Weight loss was similar in both groups with 3.24 kg for liraglutide and 2.87 for exenatide with nausea occurring less in the liraglutide group [28].

The LEAD-3 Mono study compared liraglutide (1.2 g and 1.8 mg) vs. glimepiride (8 mg) monotherapy for type-2 diabetes in a 52 week, double blinded, parallel treatment trial. This showed that liraglutide treatment lead to a greater reduction in A1C and weight than glimepiride. At 52 weeks, A1C decreased by 0.84% with liraglutide 1.2 mg and 1.14% with liraglutide 1.8 mg compared to 0.51% with glimepiride [29].

Merani and others reported on direct beta-cell effects of liraglutide in a preclinical study in the journal *Endocrinology* in 2008, demonstrating improved glucose homeostasis in marginal mass islet transplantation in diabetic mice, reducing the time to normoglycemia following islet cell transplantation [30]. Mari and others reported on the effects of liraglutide on beta-cell function in 13 patients in the journal *Diabetes Care* in 2007 [31]. In this small study, liraglutide improved beta-cell function, insulin secretion during the first meal, and lowered glucose excursions.

Liraglutide is indicated as an adjunct to diet and exercise in type-2 diabetics and is listed as a category C drug in pregnancy. It is not indicated for type-1 diabetics and not recommended as first line therapy. The drug has not been studied in combination with insulin and not approved for concomitant use with DPP-IV inhibitors.

Pramlintide (Symlin)

AMYLIN PHYSIOLOGY

In healthy adults, increases in postprandial glucose provide potent stimulation to the pancreatic beta cells causing an immediate secretory granule exocytosis. These secretory granules are composed of two glucoregulatory peptic hormones, amylin and insulin which appear in the systemic circulation following their release into the portal vein. These two beta cell hormones act in conjunction with one another to effectively limit glycemic control allowing for proper glucose utilization, while coordinating the rates of glucogenesis and glucose disposal. Insulin first stimulates glucose uptake into insulin sensitive peripheral tissues including muscle, liver, and adipocytes and subsequently inhibits hepatic gluconeogenesis directly and indirectly as a result of an inhibition of glucagon secretion from the pancreatic alpha cells.

There are several mechanisms by which amylin has been shown to compliment insulin's effects on achieving postprandial glycemic control, suppressing postprandial glucagon secretion, reducing glucagon stimulated hepatic glucose release, decreasing the rate gastric emptying, while suppressing food intake similar to cholecystokinin octapeptide. The presence of amylin allows the central glucose regulator inherent in the beta cell to coordinate rate of appearance of glucose postprandially and its subsequent rate of disappearance. Amylin, therefore, enhances postprandial glucose control by an overall reduction in the appearance of both endogenous and exogenous glucose into the circulation attenuating glycemic excursions.

Amylin deficiencies result in dysregulation of glycemic control. Type-1 diabetics have virtually no circulating amylin, while type-2 diabetics have been shown to have diminished postprandial amylin concentrations compared to healthy adults. In addition, the type-2 diabetics have an impairment in glucose regulating mechanisms responsible for maintaining physiologic balance in glucose appearance and disappearance. When the beta cell fails, in either type-1 or type-2 diabetics, chaotic glucose excursions occur throughout the day with amylin deficiencies persisting even with exogenous insulin administration. This may explain the weight gain, hypoglycemia, and postprandial excursions seen in patients given basic insulin alone. Amylin is a 37-amino acid polypeptide hormone first described in 1987 that is colocated and co-secreted with insulin in response to a glycemic load, with structural similarity to adrenomedullin, and the calcitonins [32].

High affinity binding sites present in various regions of the brain including the dorsal raphe, the nucleus accumbens, and the area postrema may play a critical role in the glucoregulatory effects of amylin. Type-1 and type-2 diabetics demonstrate an enhanced secretion of glucagon with inadequate suppression of hepatic glucose release at mealtime. Inadequate postprandial glycemic control is partially a result of a failure of exogenously administered insulin to restore postprandial insulin concentrations to the normal level within the portal vein, resulting in high glucagon/insulin ratios, which promotes hyperglycemia by enhancing hepatic glucose release. Inadequate suppression of hepatic glucose release and inappropriate hypersecretion of glucagon occur in both type-1 and type-2 diabetics resulting in postprandial glucose elevations.

Animal studies have shown that amylin will not suppress glucagon secretion in the presence of hypoglycemia. Human and rodent studies have indicated that in amylin deficient insulin treated type-2 diabetics, plasma glucagon levels increased postprandially, and remained elevated during the study period compared to non-insulin treated patients in which plasma glucagon levels increased postprandially, but declined as plasma amylin concentrations subsequently increased. In addition, data from rat studies have shown that amylin receptor antagonist administration resulted in elevated glucagon concentration relative to controls with a similar effect being demonstrated with monoclonal amylin antibodies, underscoring the physiologic role of amylin in the regulation of postprandial glucagon secretion. A common occurrence in the diabetic patient is accelerated gastric emptying, which plays an important role in the rise in plasma glucose postprandially. If gastric emptying is accelerated or insulin action is deficient, abnormal rises in plasma glucose will occur even in the presence of insulin. This accelerated rate of gastric emptying in both type-1 and type-2 diabetics is attenuated with the administration of amylin.

Accelerated gastric emptying is an important counter regulatory defense mechanism and exists as a normal physiologic response to hypoglycemia. However, it is important to realize that in hypoglycemic situations, accelerated gastric emptying still occurred in rats despite being infused with amylin indicating that hypoglycemia can override the regulation of gastric emptying. It is currently believed that amylin's effects on gastric emptying are dependent upon an intact vagus nerve and mediated by the central nervous system. This has been shown in rodent data and indicated that vagotomized rats were unable to regulate gastric emptying rates when pretreated with amylin compared to unoperated rats. The observation that intracerebroventricular infusion of amylin implanted into the fourth ventricle was three times more potent in reducing the rate of gastric emptying than subcutaneous administration or infusion into the lateral ventricle, points to central involvement, and regulation of gastric emptying rates probably in the area of the brain stem in the fourth ventricle [33].

Further localization of amylin's effect on gastric motility to the area postrema has been shown in rats having lesions in these areas, demonstrating significantly attenuated emptying effects when compared to lesion free controls. Studies in mice have shown that amylin's affect on appetite are equivalent to that produced by the peptide cholecystokinin (CCK)-8, with the reduction of food intake believed to be due to a mechanism separate from gastric emptying [34]. When GLP-1, cholecystokinin-8, and amylin were administered intraperitoneally at single injections in varying doses, CCK-8 inhibited food intake by 70% in mice fasting 18–20 h compared to 55% in the amylin treated group. GLP-1 did not significantly inhibit food intake in this model at any dose tested despite the significant inhibitions of gastric emptying. This data support the concept that suppression of food intake is not necessarily related to gastric emptying inhibition.

Amylin injected into the hypothalamus reduced food intake for up to 8 h and elevated concentrations of neurotransmitters serotonin and dopamine were demonstrated in the hypothalamus, nucleus accumbens, and the corpus striatum suggesting a critical role for these neurotransmitters in addition to amylin in the inhibition of food intake [35].

Hence, amylin is now viewed as a vital glucoregulatory hormone, partnering with insulin to regulate glucose homeostasis, adjusting the postprandial rate of glucose appearance and complementing the actions of insulin to control glucose disappearance by reducing food intake, slowing the rate of gastric emptying, and suppressing glucagon secretion.

Pramlintide is an analog (amylinomimetic) of the naturally occurring pancreatic hormone amylin, which slows gastric emptying, induces satiety, and reduces food intake while suppressing glucagon secretion and enhancing glucose lowering in the postprandial period. The product is indicated for use in type-1 and type-2 diabetics taking insulin, differing from human amylin by a substitution of proline at position 25 for alanine and positions 28 and 29 for serine [36].When used with insulin, pramlintide has been shown to enhance glycemic control greater than insulin alone and is indicated as adjunctive treatment for those patients taking mealtime insulin who failed to achieve optimal control with or without concurrent sulfonylureas, metformin, or both in addition to optimal insulin therapy. Patients who are poorly compliant with self-monitoring blood glucose, or their current insulin regimens, or those who experience recurrent severe hypoglycemia or hypoglycemic unawareness, pregnant women, confirmed gastroparesis, pediatric patients, or those patients on medications that stimulate gastrointestinal motility are not appropriate candidates for pramlintide.

It is recommended that in type-2 diabetics, doses start with 60 µg or 10 units immediately before a major meal or snack with subsequent reduction in mealtime insulin to 50%. Self monitoring of blood glucose is critical to aid in the evaluation of the effects of long acting insulin and insulin timing. Pramlintide can be advanced every 3–7 days assuming no significant nausea has occurred to a maximum dose of 120 µg (20 units). Patients with type-1 diabetes should start on a considerably lower dose of 15 µg (2½ units) advancing in 15 µg increments every 3–7 days, to a maximally tolerated dose of 60 µg. Mild and transient nausea is the most common adverse side effect of the product which has been associated with an increased rate of insulin induced severe hypoglycemia found especially in type-1 diabetics. This usually occurs within 3 h after a pramlintide injection and should not occur if the drug is used without insulin. It is recommended that the product be taken with meals or snacks that contain at least 30 g of carbohydrate or 250 calories. Nausea has also been described in patients who overeat beyond the feeling of fullness and the product does not need to be adjusted for physical activity.

Pharmacokinetics

The bioavailability of pramlintide is 30–40% with 60% of the drug bound to protein. It is metabolized renally with a half-life of 48 min with no bioaccumulation with repeated doses [37].

Clinical Trials

In a 52-week trial, Hollander and others evaluated the impact of pramlintide on 656 insulin treated type-2 diabetics given 90 or 120 µg of pramlintide twice daily. A1C levels were reduced by 0.62%, with the 120 µg dose, with a weight loss of 1.4 kg compared to a weight gain of 0.7 kg in the placebo group. Very obese type-2 diabetic patients (BMI > 35 kg/m^2) experienced a weight reduction of greater than 5% after 26 weeks with a reduction in their total daily insulin doses by 7–8%, when given this amylinomimetic [38].

Pramlintide, as an adjunct to basal insulin was evaluated by Wysham and others in a 2008 [39]. This review was a post hoc analysis of the 52-week Hollander study and another study by Karl compiled from those patients taking a basal insulin (neutral protamine Hagedorn, lente, ultralente, or glargine) to which pramlintide was added. This studied showed that the amylinomimetic reduced postprandial glucose, A1C, and reduced weight from baseline thus suggesting a role for this drug partnered with basal insulin for glycemic control.

As the result of amylin resistance, the effective dose of pramlintide is correspondingly higher in type-2 than in type-1 diabetes with nausea side effects less common. The largest trials of treatment of type-2 diabetes showed a mean weight loss of 2.1–2.5 kg after 12 months of therapy when the drug was taken two to three times daily.

In an open label clinical trial of 166 patients with type-2 diabetics for over 13 years, taking both basal and bolus insulin, mealtime insulin doses were able to be decreased by 30–50% when pramlintide was started. Patients with type-2 diabetes also achieved a reduction of A1C of 0.56% with a 2.8 kg weight loss after taking 120 μg of pramlintide with major meals for 6 months [40]. The incidence of severe insulin induced hypoglycemia was 0.04 events per patient year in this clinical practice setting. For patients taking mixed insulin preparations, a 50% reduction of total insulin dosage upon initiation of pramlintide therapy should be prescribed, while patients using 1:10 insulin to carbohydrate ratio should change that ratio to 1:20 if on pramlintide. In those patients not consuming three meals a day, some success has been achieved by administering pramlintide once daily with a large evening meal. The product should not be given or mixed in the same syringe as insulin. Thus far, the cardiovascular benefits of lowering postprandial glycemic excursions with pramlintide have not been established although data in 19 insulin using subjects with type-2 diabetes for whom pramlintide was administered demonstrated reduced markers of oxidated stress in the postprandial period with type-2 diabetes. As of this time, the FDA has not approved the use of pramlintide in patients taking basal insulin without mealtime (bolus) insulin. However, pramlintide still represents an attractive way of improving treatment options especially if basal insulin is not adequate in addition to weight loss.

Pramlintide may plan an important role in controlling postprandial hyperglycemia in type-2 diabetics with long standing disease (>12 years) who may have more severe insulin deficiency, since exenatide requires adequate beta-cell function to achieve its glucose lowering effects, while pramlintide does not.

The drug can be administered two to three times daily with meals with no dosage reduction necessary for hepatic or renal disease. It is listed as a Category C drug in pregnancy since no adequate controlled studies have been conducted in pregnant women although the drug has low potential to cross the maternal/fetal placental barrier. It is not known whether this drug is excreted in breast milk and the safety and efficacy in the pediatric population has not been established.

The mechanism of action, efficacy, and side effects of pramlintide are summarized in Table 2.

Table 2
Synthetic amylin (Pramlintide) [38]

Mechanism of action
    Reduces postprandial glucose in conjunction with insulin
    Inhibits glucagon secretion
    Slows gastric emptying
      Efficacy
        Injected with meals
        Reduces A1C by 0.5–0.7%
        Given BID-TID
    Side effects
      Nausea
      Weight loss

SUMMARY

Non-insulin injectables have provided physicians with a valuable therapeutic weapon in the fight against type-2 diabetes by their effectiveness in reducing appetite, weight reduction, and enhanced glycemic control. The promise of the GLP-1 agonists in preserving and even rejuvenating the beta cell remains an exciting frontier for future research.

REFERENCES

1. Nauck M. Unraveling the science of indretin biology. Am J Med. 2009;122(6A):S3–S24.
2. Drucker DJ, Nauck MA. The incretin system. Lancet. 2006;368:1696–1705.
3. Baggio LL, Drucker DJ. Biology of incretins: GLP-1 and GIP. Gastroenterology. 2007;132:2131–2157.
4. Eissele R, Goke R, Willemer S. Glucagon like peptide cells in the gastrointestinal tract and pancreas of rat, pig and man. Eur J Clin Invest. 1992;22:283–291.
5. Nauck MA, Baller B, Meier JJ. Gastric inhibitory polypeptide and glucagon like peptide-1 in the pathogenesis of type-2 diabetes. Diabetes. 2004;53(suppl 3):S190–S196.
6. Nauck MA, Stockman F, Ebert R, Creutzfeldt W. Reduced incretin effect in type-2 diabetes. Diabetologia. 1986;29:46–52.
7. Meier JJ, Goetze O, Anstipp J. Gastric inhibitory polypeptide does not inhibit gastric emptying in humans. Am J Physiol Endocrinol Metab. 2004:286:E621–E625.
8. Li Y, Cao X, Li LX. Beta cell Pdx1 expression is essential for the glucoregulatory, proliferative, and cytoprotective actions of glucagon-like peptide-1. Diabetes. 2005;54:482–491.
9. Meier JJ, Gallwitz B, Kask B. Stimulation of insulin secretion by intravenous bolus injection and continuous infusion of gastric inhibitory polypeptidein patients with type-2 diabetes and healthy control subjects. Diabetes. 2004;53(suppl 3):S220–S224.
10. Nauck MA. Glucagon-like peptide-1 in type-2 diabetes: the beta cell and beyond. Diabetes Obes Metab. 2008;10(suppl 3):2–13.
11. Cervera A, Wajcberg E, Sriwijitkamol A. Mechanism of action of exenatide treatment on A1C, weight and cardiovascular risk factors. Diabetes Obes Metab. 2006;8:436–447.
12. Nielsen L, Baron A, Pharmacology of exenatide for the treatment of type-2 diabetes. Curr Opin Investig Drugs. 2003;4:401–405.
13. Kolterman O, Kim DD, Shen L. Pharmacokinetics, pharmacodynamics and safety of exenatide in patients with type-2 diabetes mellitus. Am Health Syst Pharm. 2005;62:173–181.
14. Kendall DM, Riddle MC, Rosenstock J. effects of exenatide on glycemic control over 30 weeks in patients with type-2 diabetes treated with metformin and a sulfonylurea. Diabetes Care. 2005;28:1083–1091.
15. Heine RJ, Van Gaal LF, Johns D. Exenatide versus insulin glargine in patients with suboptimally controlled type-2 diabetes. Ann Intern Med. 2005;143:559–569.
16. Buse JB, Klonoff DC, Nielson LL. Metabolic effect of two years of exenatide treatment on diabetes , obesity, and hepatic biomarkers in patients with type-2 diabetes. Clin Ther. 2007;29:139–153.
17. Nauck MA, Duran S, Kim D. A comparison of twice daily exenatide and biphasic insulin aspart in patients with type-2 diabetes who were suboptimally controlled with sulfonylurea and metformin. Diabetologia. 2007;50:259–267.
18. Barnett AH, Trautmann M, Burger J, Johns D, Kim D, Brodows R, Festa A. A comparison of exenatide and insulin glargine in patients using a single oral diabetic agent. Data disclosure at the 42 annual meeting of the European Association of Diabetes. September 16, 2006.
19. Heine R, Van Gaal L, Johns D, Mihm M. Exenatide versus insulin glargine in patients with suboptimally controlled type-2 diabetes. Ann Intern Med. 2005;143(8):559–569.
20. Cure P. Exenatide and adverse events. New Engl J Med. 2008;358:1969–1972.
21. Zinman B, Hoogwerf BJ, Duran J, Garcia S. the effect of adding exenatide to a thiazolidinedione in suboptimally controlled type-2 diabetes. Ann Intern Med. 2007;146:477–485.
22. Briceno RM, Lagari-Libhaber VS. Meneghini LF. Clinical observations study of the safety, effectiveness, and tolerability of exenatide in a real world setting. Diabetes. 2007;56(suppl 1):Abstract 2147-PO.

23. Bunck MC, Diamant M, Corner A, Eliasson B, Malloy JL. One year treatment with exenatide improves beta cell function compared with insulin glargine in metformin treated type-2 diabetic patients. Diabetes Care. 2009;32(5):762–768.

24. Drucker DJ, Buse KB, Taylor K, Kendall DM. Exenatide once weekly versus twice daily for the treatment of type-2 diabetes. Lancet. 2008;372(9645):1240–1250.

25. Vilsboll T, Zdravkovic M, Le-Thi T. Liraglutide, a long acting human glucagon like peptide-1 analog. Diabetes Care. 2007;30:1608–1610.

26. Victoza (liraglutide) package insert. Princeton NJ: Novo Nordisk; 2010.

27. Nauck M, Frid A, Hermansen K. for the LEAD-2 Study Group. Efficacy and safety comparison of liraglutide, glimepiride and placebo all in combination with metformin in type-2 diabetes: the LEAD-2 study. Diabetes Care. 2009;32(1)84–90.

28. Buse JB, Rosenstock J, Sesti G. Liraglutide once a day versus exenatide twice a day for type-2 diabetes: a 26 week randomized, parallel group, multinational open label trial (LEAD-6). Lancet. 2009;374:39–47.

29. Garber A, Henry R, Ratner R. Liraglutide versus glimepiride monotherapy for type-2 diabetes (LEAD-3). Lancet. 2009;373:473–481.

30. Merani S, Truong W, Emamaullee JA, Toso C, Knudsen LB. Liraglutide improves glucose homeostasis in marginal mass islet transplantation in mice. Endocrinology. 2008;149(9):4322–4328.

31. Mari A, Degn K, Brock B. Effects of the long acting human glucagon like peptide-1 analog liraglutide on beta cell function in normal living conditions. Diabetes Care. 2007;30:2032–2033.

32. Kruger DF, Gatacomb PM, Owen Sk. Clinical implication of amylin and amylin deficiency. Diabetes Educ. 1999;25:389–398.

33. Gedulin BR, Rink TJ, Young AA. Dose response for the glucagonostatic effect of amylin in rats. Metabolism. 1997;46:67–70.

34. Beeley NRA, Prickett KS. The amylin, CGRP and calcitonin family of peptides. Expert Opin Ther Pat. 1996:6:555–567.

35. Young A. Amylin's physiology and its role in diabetes. Curr Opin Endocrinol Diabetes. 1997;4:282–290.

36. Samsom M, Szarka LA, Camilleri M, Vella A, Zinsmeister AR, Rizza RA. Pramlintide, an amylin analog, selectively delays gastric emptying: potential role of vagal inhibition. Am J Physiol. 2000;278:G946–G951.

37. Young AA, Vine W, Gedulin BR. Preclinical pharmacology of pramlintide in the rat: comparisons with human an rat amylin. Dur Develop Res. 1996;37:231–248.

38. Hollander PA, Levy P, Fineman MS, Maggs DG, Shen LZ, Strobel SA. Pramlintide as an adjunct to insulin therapy improves longterm glycemic and weight control in patients with type-2 diabetes. Diabetes Care. 2003;26:784–790.

39. Wysham C, Lush C, Zhang B, Maier H, Wilhelm K. Effect of pramlintide as an adjunct to basal insulin on markers of cardiovascular risk in patients with type-2 diabetes. Curr Med Res Opin. 2008;24(1):79–85.

40. Ryan GJ, Jobe LJ, Martin R. Pramlintide in the treatment of type-1 and type-2 diabetes mellitus. Clin Ther. 2005;27:1500–1512.

9 Macrovascular Disease

Contents

Key Words: Coronary artery disease, Peripheral vascular disease, Cerebral arteriosclerotic vascular disease, Generalized arteriosclerotic vascular disease, Hyperinsulinemia

INTRODUCTION

The hallmark of macrovascular disease in the diabetic patient comprises the ugly triad of:

1. Coronary artery disease and its complications of myocardial infarction and congestive heart failure
2. Cerebral and carotid arteriosclerotic vascular disease and its complications of stroke and cerebral ischemia
3. Peripheral vascular disease and its complications of claudication, ischemia, and amputation [1]

CORONARY ARTERY DISEASE

Type-2 diabetes, by virtue of its predisposition to generalized arteriosclerotic vascular disease, inflammatory milieu, and thrombogenesis is truly a vasculopathic state.

The role of obesity, hyperinsulinemia, and insulin resistance is a key factor in the chronic inflammatory state characterized by local tissue oxidative stress, endothelial dysfunction, activation of the sympathetic nervous system, and the rennin-angiotensin system and dysfunctional adipose tissue. The chronic inflammatory state is characterized by increased levels of plasminogen activator inhibitor-1, C-reactive protein, tumor necrosis

From: *Current Clinical Practice: Type 2 Diabetes, Pre-Diabetes, and the Metabolic Syndrome*,
Edited by: R.A. Codario, DOI 10.1007/978-1-60327-441-8_9
© Springer Science+Business Media, LLC 2011

factor-alpha, interleukin-6 and fibrinogen. Various mechanisms, including prereceptor, and postreceptor defects, have been implicated in causing insulin resistance. The alterations of signaling at the receptor level interfere with glucose transport resulting in a cascading sequence of events within the target tissues, increasing the risk of premature arteriosclerosis, microalbuminuria and dyslipidemia, and hypercoagulability.

Ischemic events are the hallmark of morbidity in the diabetic patient, with cardiovascular disease being the primary cause of demise in close to 70% of patients with the condition.

The risk of sustaining a myocardial infarction in a diabetic patient is the same as the risk of a second myocardial infarction in a non-diabetic patient, and second myocardial infarctions in diabetics are almost twice as likely as in non-diabetic patients.

When cardiovascular disease is manifested, the diabetic has a 60% chance of experiencing a cardiovascular event and a 25% chance of dying from coronary heart disease, and this risk is 50% greater than the non diabetic [2].

Over the past 10 years the number of hospitalizations as a result of cardiovascular disease has increased by 37%. Hence it comes as no great surprise that all patients with diabetes should be treated as if they have existing coronary disease and that this condition has been elevated into the top priority for risk reduction.

Haftner in the *New England Journal of Medicine* reported that non-diabetic patients with no prior history of myocardial infarction had the best prognosis for survival with diabetics and those having prior MI's having the worst prognosis. In either group, a history of previous MI foretold a worsening prognosis, but diabetics with previous myocardial infarction had approximately a 50% 8-year survival rate compared to diabetics with no previous MI having an 8-year survival rate of close to 90% [3]. The prognostic value of admission fasting glucose levels in patients presenting with acute coronary syndrome demonstrated a strong association between admission fasting glucose levels and mortality – even among the non diabetic patients with a fasting glucose of greater than 100 mg/dl associated with an increase in hospital mortality. The Monitoring Trends and Determinants of Cardiovascular Disease (MONICA)/Cooperative Health Research in the Region of Augsburg (KORA) cohort analysis also showed that elevated admission blood glucose levels were associated with enhanced mortality risk in patients with an acute myocardial infarction. In addition, persistently elevated fasting glucose levels during hospitalization were associated with an increased mortality risk [4].

Hypertension, tobacco use, obesity, sedentary life style, family history of premature coronary disease, hyperglycemia, elevated plasma lipids, all increase the likelihood of heart disease in patients with diabetes. The Multiple Risk Factor Intervention Trial (MRFIT) sought to determine risk factors for coronary vascular disease mortality. The study population looked at men with or without diabetes who had been screened for cardiovascular disease between the ages of 35–57 [5].

Risk factors included high serum cholesterol, systolic blood pressure elevation, and cigarette smoking. During a 12-year follow-up, 603 deaths of the total 1,092 deaths were attributed to coronary or cardiovascular disease among the 5,163 men studied. The absolute risk of death from cardiovascular disease was greater for men with diabetes for all ethnicities, risk factors, and ages.

Cardiac mortality is increased 2–4 times in diabetic patients compared to non-diabetic patients according to Framingham data, while 40% of deaths in renal transplant patients are the result of coronary artery disease [6].

Following myocardial infarction, 21–30% of diabetic women and 14–26% of diabetic men will die from their event. The data is also striking when these patients are followed for prolonged periods following the infarction with mortality being 60% 10 years after the event and 50% after 5 years.

There also is a strong association of coronary artery disease with the presence of cerebral vascular disease and peripheral arterial disease (PAD). Diabetic patients are more likely to have carotid arteriosclerotic vascular disease, while the condition almost doubles the risk of stroke reoccurrence, and triples the rate of mortality and stroke related dementia.

Diabetic patients are 2–4 times more likely to have peripheral arteriosclerotic vascular disease with a risk of claudication that is 3.5-fold in men and 8.6-fold in women. The risk in diabetic women may be more pronounced because diabetic women seem to have a greater risk of having small dense lipoprotein cholesterol which tends to be more atherogenic than in males. Hence, aggressive management of risk factors in women is critically important [7].

Table 9.1 summarizes the various risk factors for macrovascular disease.

In the San Antonio Heart Study, increased fasting insulin levels significantly predicted lower HDL's, high triglycerides, development of type-2 diabetes, and hypertension over an 8-year follow-up. These patients are more likely to develop multiple metabolic abnormalities that will be predicted with the additive possibility of developing each single disorder suggesting a clustering of these metabolic disorders.

The Paris Prospective Study was a long term investigation of 7,000 French working men, 43–54 years old, where cardiovascular and coronary heart disease risk factors were measured and analyzed to determine risk and the overall chances of coronary events [8].

Data has shown that coronary heart disease mortality rates are higher with those with impaired glucose tolerance than individuals with normal tolerance. Coronary heart disease is 2.5 times greater in individuals with type-2 compared to 1.9 times greater in individuals where impaired glucose tolerance with elevated hemoglobin A1C are shown to be a predictor for coronary heart disease in type-2 diabetics.

Table 9.1
Risk factors for macrovascular disease in type-2 diabetes

Smoking

Hypertension

Dyslipidemia

Hyperglycemia

Hypercoagulability

Metabolic syndrome

Microalbuminuria

Peripheral arteriosclerotic vascular disease

Coronary arteriosclerotic vascular disease

Carotid arteriosclerotic vascular disease

Vinik et al. [35]

One study looked at 1,069 diabetics evaluating the incidence of coronary heart disease mortality and all events during a 3.5-year period of time. Patients in the highest A1C tertile had a significantly higher incidence of coronary heart disease mortality than the lowest tertile. Incidence of fatal and non-fatal myocardial infarction was 3.4% for those without diabetes, but rose to 14.8% among those with diabetes. The highest tertile for coronary artery disease mortality and for all coronary heart disease events was with hemoglobin A1C's greater than 7.9% [7].

Curiously, though in both the UKPDS and DCCT trials in type-2 and type-1 diabetics respectively, tight glycemic control, although reducing the risk of myocardial infarction did not do so to a significant degree. This can be appreciated when one understands the multiple risk factors underlying vascular disease in general and coronary artery disease in particular – including dyslipidemia, hypertension, impaired endothelial function, cigarette smoking, life style, hyperinsulinemia, insulin resistance, oxidative stress, obesity, hyper-homocysteinemia, lipoprotein(a) elevations, and vascular inflammation. Only with a compressive plan addressing these risk factors can vascular disease risk be improved to more significant disease.

The presence of more than one risk factor expedentially increases cardiovascular risk. Curiously, there are some risk factors that are associated with more increased risk than others. The UKPDS showed that the most important risk factor for myocardial infarction was an LDL cholesterol level followed by diastolic blood pressure, cigarette smoking, a low high density lipoprotein, and high hemoglobin A1C. In addition to identification of risk factors, early recognition and management plays an important role as well.

Many of these factors may vary in their importance in different patients, but certainly a top priority should include blood pressure, lipid, and glucose control, while addressing coagulopathy disorders.

Cigarette smoking doubles the risk of macrovascular disease in diabetic patients and significantly increases the likelihood of developing and aggravating microvascular disease. This is because cigarette smoking promotes endothelial dysfunction, arteriosclerotic deposition, and is a source of advanced glycosylation end products, which promote diabetic vascular complications. Cigarette smoking also increases oxidation of LDL cholesterol enhancing its deposition within the intima.

Plaque instability is enhanced with cigarette smoking, which is of particular importance when we consider that 68% of all myocardial infarctions occur with less than 50% coronary artery disease stenosis. The previously mentioned MRFIT study showed that as cigarette smoking increased on a daily basis, so did coronary disease mortality. The risk of premature death in smoking diabetics was 11 times greater than non-diabetic non-smokers [9]!

Hypertension pays a particularly important contribution to cerebral vascular disease and cardiovascular survival. In the UKPDS trials, tighter blood pressure control reduced the risk of stroke by 44% despite the fact that their standards for blood pressure control were even higher than the standards that we have today. Hence even tighter blood pressure control should have even a greater impact [10].

In the UKPDS trial 1,148 of the randomized 4,297 patients had hypertension. In this particular analysis any diabetes related end point was reduced by 24% with tight blood pressure control, while diabetes related all cause mortality was reduced by 32%. The risk of stroke was reduced by 44%, retinopathy progression by 34%, and microvascular disease 37%. These values were all statistically significant [11].

Atherogenic changes in the vascular smooth muscle in the endothelium in diabetic patients are also enhanced by the dyslipidemia that is subsequently produced in the course of the disease. Decreased insulin action on lipoprotein lipase and low glucose uptake enhances the production of free fatty acids, glycerol, and PAI-1. This insulin resistance at the level of the adipose tissue leads to an overproduction of very low density lipoproteins by the liver. This is associated with decreased HDL secretion, hypertriglyceridemia, and increased preponderance of small dense LDL particles in the diabetic patient.

Results of the Framingham Study reported by Grundy in Diabetes Care showed a greater proportion of diabetic patients showing abnormalities in lipids compared to those who did not have diabetes. Of these the commonest were an elevation of the VLDL equal to or greater than 40 mg/dl in 34% of diabetics compared to 25% of diabetics, triglycerides equal to or greater than 235 mg/dl in 19% of diabetics compared to 9% of non-diabetics, and 21% HDL cholesterol less than 31 mg/dl in diabetic patients compared to non-diabetics [12].

In women, only 8% were found to have hypertriglyceridemia if they were non-diabetic compared to 17% in diabetic females. 10% of women without diabetes had HDL levels equal to or less than 41 mg/dl compared to 25% of women with diabetes. There was an increased amount of VLDL production equal to or greater than 35 mg/dl in diabetic women compared to non-diabetic women in the Framingham Heart Study.

An association between hyperinsulinemia, hypertriglyceridemia, and low HDL cholesterol was originally described in 1994. In this case study, 64 patients showed significantly lower HDL concentrations if they were hyperinsulinemic compared to subjects with normal insulin levels independent of weight, age, gender, physical activity, and cigarette smoking. A large prospective study involving 1,059 patients, 581 men and 478 women showed that the HDL concentrations were significantly and inversely related to coronary heart disease events and coronary heart disease mortality. These patients were between the ages of 45–64 and followed for a 7-year period. This study showed that as the total cholesterol increased so did the percentage of coronary heart disease, mortality, and events and conversely as the HDL decreased there was a subsequent increase in coronary heart disease events and mortality.

Several recent studies have shown the effect of lipid lowering and dyslipidemia on endothelial function. Treatment of hypercholesterolemic coronary heart disease patients with statins have clearly been shown to reduce mortality and morbidity both from myocardial infarction and stroke. Since endothelial dysfunction is a common disorder in arteriosclerotic vascular disease, therapeutic endeavors are designed to improve function at the cellular level [13].

Pioglitazone has been shown to lower triglyceride levels as well having glycemic control properties, improving endothelial function, while decreasing the levels of small atherogenic LDL. By increasing the HDL, this drug decreases oxidative stress by diminishing the levels of antioxidant enzymes, enhancing the outflow of lipid from the arterial wall, reducing coronary artery plaque burden.

The adipocyte in the type-2 diabetic is responsible for increased hepatic reductions of PAI-1 and fibrinogen thereby inhibiting clot dissolution, fibrinolysis, and shifting the hemostatic balance toward a thrombotic state. Circulating PAI-1 levels can be decreased by weight loss, lipid lowering therapy, or reduction in elevated triglycerides, reducing hypercoagulability.

Hyperglycemic control is essential in the type-2 diabetic, since hyperinsulinemia, insulin resistance, and hyperglycemia are all associated with the hypercoagulable state. Angiotensin converting enzyme therapy has been shown to be beneficial at the endothelial level as well as decreasing PAI-1 levels in diabetic patients. The inhibition of angiotensin II tends to stabilize plaque, reducing the risk of plaque rupture.

Aspirin therapy is mandatory in type-2 diabetic patients over the age of 21 because of its attenuation of vasoconstriction and platelet aggregation. Aspirin irreversibly inhibits the synthesis of thromboxane, which is responsible for these effects. The current recommendation is the use of 160–325 mg per aspirin daily for type-2 patients unless contraindicated by active ulcer disease, aspirin allergy, further anticoagulant therapy, recent gastrointestinal bleeding, or other bleeding tendencies. Seventy-five milligram of aspirin per day reduced the pooled cardiovascular risk by 15% and myocardial infarction by 36% in the HOT (Hypertension Optimal Treatment) trial [9].

Various meta-analyses have shown that in diabetic patients who have had an MI or stroke, low doses can be as effective as high doses and can reduce cardiovascular events by as much as 25%. Aspirin in doses of 650 mg daily did not increase of incidence of rectal bleeding in the early treatment of diabetic retinopathy [14].

In those patients who are aspirin allergic, Clopidogrel (Plavix) may be substituted. The recently completed CAPRIE trial (Clopidogrel vs. Aspirin) in patients at risk of ischemic events showed that this product was about as equally effective as aspirin 325 mg in reducing the risk of vascular death, ischemic stroke, or myocardial infarction. This trial was one of the largest prospective, randomized, and blinded trials ever conducted, enrolling over 19,000 patients with various manifestations of arteriosclerotic vascular disease. The majority of the patients in this trial had additional risk factors when entered into the study [15].

20.2% or 3,881 of these patients were diabetic, 51.5% had hypertension, 41.2% had hypercholesterolemia, and 29.2% were smokers. Sub-analysis of the diabetic cohort showed clopidogrel to be particularly effective in patients with peripheral vascular disease with a combined annual vascular event rate of 15.6% compared to 17.7% for aspirin.

Clopidogrel bisulfate has been shown to be a potent ADP-receptor antagonist that interferes with the ADP pathway, which ultimately is responsible for platelet activation and aggregation. The active metabolite of clopidogrel irreversibly binds to the platelet at the ADP receptor site. This low affinity receptor inhibits the binding of ADP.

The anti-platelet effects last 7–10 days (the life of the platelet) since new ADP receptors cannot be synthesized by the platelets [16]. Clopidogrel has recently been given a black box warning stating that the drug can be less effective in patients who are poor metabolizers with reduced functioning of the cytochrome P450-2C19 liver enzyme, which cannot effectively convert the drug to its active form. Examples of 2C19 drugs include omeprazole, esomeprazole, fluconazole, ketoconazole, etravir, fluoxetine, and fluvoxamine.

Various distinct sites are the targets of drug therapy during platelet aggregation to prevent thrombus formation and subsequent vessel occlusion. Each of these sites plays an important role in the ultimate formation of the platelet plug. THE ADP, TXA2, and the GPIIb/IIIa sites are the most common that are targeted by available therapy.

Intravenous prostacyclin may provide transient beneficial effects in coronary arteries, but has potent and inconsistent side effects. GPIb/vWF antagonists may inhibit platelet adhesion by blocking the interaction between von Willebrand factor and the platelet GP1B receptor in experimental models. Platelet activation may be inhibited by drugs that block various agonists, such as thrombin, serotonin, and thromboxane A2.

ADP (adenosine diphosphate) also plays a role in activating the GPIIb/IIIa receptor, which serves as the final pathway for platelet aggregation.

The subsequent synthesis of thromboxane A2 (TXA2) by the platelets is inhibited by the thromboxane synthesis inhibitors like aspirin, which can also have a paradoxical effect on platelets by virtue of its inhibition of prostacyclin formation, which can actually promote platelet aggregation.

Hyperhomocysteinemia has been shown to be an independent cardiovascular risk factor especially in diabetic patients who may demonstrate double the risk in 5 year mortality compared to non-diabetic homocysteinemic patients. Of some controversy, however, is the benefit of lowering homocysteine, with some papers showing a benefit and others failing to show a benefit. It should be understood that hyperhomocysteinemia can occur in patients with subtle B-12 deficiencies having normal B-12 levels with elevated methylmalonic acid levels. These patients may respond simply to B-12 and in these patients, hyperhomocysteinemia may simply be a manifestation of B-12 deficiency, and/or renal insufficiency, or fenofibrate therapy.

Clearly, however, hyperhomocysteinemia is one of a host of factors including tissue hypoxia, impairments in local tissue perfusion, elevated free fatty acids, systemic hypertension, dyslipidemia, hyperglycemia, and enhancing oxidative stress, which promotes and encourages the production of damaging free radicals and aggravating the imbalance between endothelial vasodilators and vasoconstrictors. The subsequent abnormality in endothelial function increases angiotensin converting enzyme, elevates angiotensin II, increasing inflammatory mediators, and decreasing nitric oxide production.

The acceleration of proteolysis promotes plaque instability and rupture, while the subsequent vasoconstriction impairs endothelial function. Elevated PAI-1 levels in homocysteinemic patients promotes thrombosis and the production of growth factors generated by angiotensin II, responsible for cardiac remodeling, vascular and even renal hypertrophy, resulting in endothelial damage, and promotion of inflammation characterized by an elevation of high sensitivity CRP.

Indeed CRP levels were shown to be the best predictor of first MI in the Physicians Health Study. Women are much more likely to have elevated CRP levels than men even when the risk factors between them are equivalent. Various medications have been shown to reduce the high sensitivity CRP including thiazolidinedione therapy, statins, metformin, fenofibrates, omega-3 acid ethyl esters, angiotensin receptor blockers, ACE inhibitors and exercise. Full dose statin therapy can reduce high sensitivity CRP to 20–40% from baseline with thiazolidinediones further reducing it by 30% [17].

It remains to be determined, however, what the relationship is between the reduction of high sensitivity CRP and the corresponding reduction in coronary artery disease events and mortality, but clearly a reduction in CRP in patients with elevated CRP appears to be beneficial.

Lipoproteins that are rich in triglycerides such as VLDL can cause the expression of extremely atherogenic proinflammatory genes, which can explain why the fenofibrates have been beneficial in reducing high sensitivity CRP and subsequent triglyceride levels.

Diabetic patients post MI should receive beta-blockers, ACE inhibitors, aspirin and statins with tight glycemic and hypertension control. Recent data from the Valsartan in Acute Myocardial Infarction (VALIANT) and Candesartan in Heart Failure: Assessment of Reduction in Mortality and Morbidity (CHARM) trial has shown a benefit in adding angiotensin receptor blockers to these patients. This will be discussed in greater detail in Chap. 14.

Beta-blockers have consistently been shown to reduce mortality in diabetic patients with extended release of metoprolol (Toprol-XL) and carvedilol (Coreg) particularly effective in reducing complications from heart failure. Reductions in up to 37% in diabetic patients have been reported with beta-blocker use. A retrospective analysis in more than 45,000 patients showed that diabetics using beta-blockers did not have increase in complications and reduced their risk of myocardial infarction by 23% [18].

The GISSI-2 trial using lisinopril after myocardial infarction showed the benefit of ACE inhibitors in improving left ventricular dysfunction and remodeling. In this study, significant reduced mortality was shown in diabetics over non-diabetic patients after 6 weeks and 6 months [19].

This was corroborated by the Survival and Ventricular Enlargement (SAVE) study, which showed the greatest benefit in high risk patients like diabetics. In the Trandolapril Cardiac Evaluation (TRACE) study, therapy with this angiotensin converting enzyme inhibitor (Mavik) reduced progression to heart failure by 62%, while reducing mortality by 36% in patients with left ventricular dysfunction. The HOPE trial showed statistically significant benefits in diabetic patients over the age of 55 given ramipril (Altace) with similar data shown for the angiotensin receptor blocker, telmisartan (Micardis) in the ON-TARGET (Ongoing Telmisartan Alone and in combination with Ramipril Global endpoint) trial. This benefit was independent of a blood pressure lowering effect or the effect of statins, aspirins or any concomitant antihypertensive or hyperglycemic therapy. These trials will be reviewed in more detail in the subsequent chapter on risk reduction [16].

The benefits of angioplasty vs. thrombolytic therapy in diabetic patients are not as crystal clear as for non-diabetic patients. The diabetics tend to experience more instant thrombosis despite having success rates that are similar immediately following angioplasty. This data may be changed with the availability of the newer tacrolimus stents, which significantly reduce post-stent complications [14].

In 2008, the *American Journal of Cardiology* published a meta-analysis of nine trials comparing outcomes with bare metal stents and drug eluting stents in patients with diabetes [20]. The review revealed that drug eluting stents were associated with a decreased risk of in-stent stenosis and target lesion revascularization compared to those diabetics treated with bare metal stents. In addition, drug eluting stents in patients with diabetes mellitus significantly reduced the risk of myocardial infarction with no change in mortality or stent thrombosis.

Recurrent myocardial infarction, revascularizations, and post stent complications with emergency surgery tend to be more common in diabetic patients. This was reduced in patients placed on fluvastatin in the recently completed (Lescol Intervention Prevention) LIPS trial. Patients placed on this statin had a decrease in post stenotic complications. The BARI trial (Bypass Angioplasty Revascularization Investigation) demonstrated a significantly lower 5-year survival rate in diabetic patients, but the (Global Utilization of Streptokinase and Tissue Plasminogen activator for Occluded Arteries) GUSTO-2B study, looking at the global use of strategies to open occluded coronary arteries, found a better 30-day trend in diabetic patients who received angioplasty compared to thrombolysis.

Meta-analyses of over 25,000 cases have shown a twofold increase in cardiac mortality after angioplasty in diabetic patients with re-stenosis rates ranging from 24 to 55% re-stenosis and correlating with microalbuminuria. In the Thrombosis in Myocardial Infarction (TIMI)-2 Trial, coronary bypass surgery and non-acute angioplasty for diabetic patients showed a higher mortality rate then when done for acute myocardial infarction alone. This was not seen in non-diabetics [*14*].

As mentioned, the newer designed coated stents, which inhibit smooth muscle proliferation and migration, may be of particular benefit in decreasing stent complications in diabetic patients.

Low molecular weight heparin has shown promise in reducing the rate of cardiac events in diabetic patients with unstable angina or non-Q-wave myocardial infarctions. In the Fragmin and Fast revascularization during Instability in Coronary artery disease 2 (FRISC-2) study, early invasive strategies were compared to early noninvasive strategies in patients with instable angina. In the data base were 2,158 patients without diabetes and 299 patients with diabetes. Coronary angiograms were performed on all patients. More patients with triple vessel and left main two vessel disease existed among the diabetic cohort with a significant difference in the severity of coronary artery disease between diabetics and non-diabetics [*21*].

In this study, the invasive strategy produced 26% reduction in the composite of death and MI at the first year. This was similar in both diabetic and non-diabetic cohorts. Although many of the risk factors and indicators for myocardial infarction and death were eliminated by this aggressive invasive approach, diabetes still remained an important risk factor in patients regardless of the approach demonstrating the importance that factors beyond coronary artery disease and myocardial injury are of considerable importance in evaluating these patients.

The Physicians Health Study noted that in patients with diabetes given 325 mg of aspirin for 5 years, there was a 60% reduction in myocardial infarction with reduction in 1-year mortality produced with beta-blockers. With this data it can be seen that control and reduction of macrovascular complications is a multifactorial task requiring a broad based therapeutic approach [*22*].

Regional left ventricular myocardial changes in functioning with diabetic cardiomyopathy demonstrate impairments in longitudinal systolic and diastolic function. The multifactorial etiology of diabetic cardiomyopathy includes not only structural changes with enhanced fibrosis in the myocardium, but also microvascular disease, altered myocardial metabolism, and inefficient mitochondrial dysfunction, associated with increased myocardial fatty acid delivery resulting in myocyte lipotoxic injury due to this overabundance of lipid supply caused by insulin resistance. The dysfunctional mitochondria (one for each myocyte) are associated with fatty acid and triglyceride accumulation within the myocardium resulting in apoptosis, cell damage, subsequent cardiac fibrosis, and contractile impairment.

PERIPHERAL ARTERIAL DISEASE

In patients with PAD (defined as an ankle brachial index or ABI less than 0.9), claudication is the most common complaint or presentation in greater than 75%. The ankle /brachial index is defined as the ratio between the doralis pedis artery (DPA) and/or posterior tibial artery (PTA)pressure and the blood pressure of the brachial artery on the same side. The most valuable physiologic test for evaluating the lower limb circulation is the ankle systolic blood pressure in these two arteries. If the pressure in either of these two arteries is less than that measured on the same side of the upper arm, occlusive disease in the arteries of the lower limb is almost always present. Medial calcification can sometimes be seen in patients with diabetes, which can create a falsely high ankle systolic pressure. Although the ABI does not differentiate occlusions at various levels in the lower extremities, usually an ABI less than 0.9 and greater than 0.5 is indicative of a single level occlusion, while an ABI less than 0.5 is consistent with multiple level lesions. Even patients with ABI's between 0.90–1.10 are more likely to have subclinical atherosclerosis compared to individuals with ABI's between 1.30–1.10. ABI's less than 0.40 are indicative of severe PAD, while ABI's between 0.70–0.90 are consistent with mild disease. The NCEP (National Cholesterol Education Program) guidelines classify ABI's less than 0.9 as a coronary artery risk equivalent. This is important for the primary care provider to consider since many of these patients may have no symptoms, and hence the ABI is an important method to risk stratify patients for lipid-lowering goals. It should also be kept in mind that individuals with ABI's greater than 1.4, consistent with non compressible lower extremity arterial disease, have an increased prevalence of diabetes and renal disease and are also at increased risk for cardiovascular mortality and morbidity.

Claudication is characterized by exertional tightness, cramping, fatigue, or aching pain with walking and is reproducible from day to day, resolving within 2–3 min of rest (sometimes up to 10 min in severe cases) and tending to reoccur at the same distance with activity resumption. These symptoms also tend to be progressive, usually causing the patient to stop walking although patients with claudication do not generally experience pain at rest, which is seen with most severe vascular disease that prohibits ambulation. Interestingly only 10–30% of patients with PAD actually have the classic symptoms of intermittent claudication. Diabetes is a significant risk factor for PAD as is dyslipidemia, cigarette smoking, hypertension, renal disease, and advancing age.

This can be differentiated from pseudoclaudication as seen with spinal stenosis because spinal stenosis is usually associated with tingling, weakness, or clumsiness and often occurs with prolonged standing and is relieved by changing body positions or having the patient sit. The discomfort with spinal stenosis tends to be variable in the most stages with the patient capable of varying walking distances.

The presence of peripheral vascular disease has been shown to be a significant risk factor equivalent to the presence of diabetes and coronary artery disease requiring LDL reductions below 100 according to the new NCEP ATP-3 guidelines. The diagnosis can be sometimes challenging because in addition to lumbar canal stenosis and degenerative joint disease, arteritis, vasculitis, arterioembolism, and atheromatous embolism, cystic adventitial disease, popliteal artery entrapment, and vasoconstrictor drugs can produce similar symptoms.

It is important for the clinician to understand that 90% of patients with symptomatic peripheral vascular disease also have concomitant coronary disease with relative 5-year mortality rates with PAD being greater than Hodgkin's disease and breast cancer according to data from the American Cancer Society.

Angiographic studies have shown that patients with PAD are 90% likely to possess coronary and 80% likely to possess carotid disease. Aggressive risk factor modification including hypertension control, lipid regulation, tight glycemic control, and judicious use of aspirin, clopidogrel, and cessation of smoking and other vasoconstrictors including caffeine have been shown to be a benefit along with an exercise walking program and the use of medication including pentoxifylline (Trental) 400 mg t.i.d. or cilostazol (Pletal) 100 mg twice daily. Cilostazol, a phosphodiesterase 3 inhibitor, is a vasodilator which inhibits platelet aggregation, arterial thrombosis, and vascular smooth muscle cell proliferation.

In head to head comparisons, cilostazol showed significant improvement when compared to pentoxifylline and placebo in lean walking distance according to Dawson's review in Circulation in 1998. It should be kept in mind, however, that cilostazol has a black box warning indicating that the drug should be avoided in patients who have any evidence of heart failure.

Diabetes and smoking have been shown to increase the absolute risk for arteriosclerotic vascular disease by 25–50% and frequently masks important presenting symptoms. Careful control of contributing risk factors is critical in managing the disease [7].

One to three percent of patients with intermittent claudication may require amputation over a 5-year period of time with a 5 year mortality rate for patients with intermittent claudication approaching 30%. A comprehensive approach is necessary and can improve symptoms. This includes lipid lowering, glycemic, and hypertension control with weight reduction diet and exercise. The use of a formal exercise program has been shown to be the most effective non surgical method of therapy. Patients are encouraged to reproduce walking in the community setting by setting treadmill settings to a grade and speed that brings on claudication pain within 3–5 min. Following a resting period, the patient resumes exercise and is reassessed on a weekly basis for progress. Typically, the rehabilitation period lasts from 3 to 6 months and usually results in 100–150% improvement in walking distance.

PAD is continuing to be underdiagnosed. In one comprehensive review, 6,979 patients, 70 years of age or older or age 50–69 years with a history of cigarette smoking or diabetes were evaluated. Forty-nine percent of the patients with a prior diagnosis of PAD were identified by the physicians treating them and 45% of patients identified with the disease in this study had gone previously undetected.

Approximately half of patients with PAD will have symptoms of intermittent claudication [23]. The percentage of patients who are symptomatic from the disease increase as patients get older peaking in the patient population over the age of 70.

Intermittent claudication is associated with several abnormalities at the cellular level including:

1. Hyperplastic mitochondria and demyelination of nerve fibers
2. Fifty percent reduction in muscle fibers compared with control
3. Metabolic disturbances stemming from reduction in flow of oxygen delivery related to local tissue ischemia and injury with angiotensin II release
4. Greater arterial ischemia with smaller type I and II muscle fibers

Inflammatory states characterized by increased circulating levels of inflammatory cytokines contribute to a decrease in muscle strength, muscle mass, and sarcopenia.

Higher levels of inflammatory markers like hs-CRP are usually associated with PAD and increased rates of restenosis after angioplasty of the lower extremities.

Smoking is the most powerful modifiable risk factor for peripheral disease with intermittent claudication being three times more common in smokers than non-smokers. The severity of the disease increases with the number of cigarettes smoked. Cessation of smoking has been reported to cause significant reductions in rest pain, myocardial infarction, cardiac deaths, and overall 10-year survival according to data published by Joneison.

The type-2 diabetic is more prone to atherogenic dyslipidemia and the metabolic syndrome and has a fourfold increased risk of developing PAD with the symptoms in diabetics not directly correlating with glycemic control. The vast majority of patients with PAD also have coronary artery disease. In a review of 381 patients from the Cleveland Clinic who presented for elective vascular surgery and underwent cardiac catheterization, only 10% had normal coronaries, with 28% having severe triple vessel disease. In addition, approximately 1/3 of patients with known coronary artery disease had PAD, while carotid duplex studies show significant disease in up to 50% of those with PAD. In addition, patients with PAD have a 2–4-fold increased mortality compared to those free of disease [24].

PAD can be associated with various vascular complications including acute vascular compromise characterized by sudden severe ischemia with paresthesia, paralysis, poor temperature, pain and palor as a result of either embolism or arterial occlusion [25].

Cholesterol emboli and/or fibrinoplatelet matter from the aorta or iliac vessels can cause a syndrome referred to as blue toe syndrome. These conditions require immediate attention. Having diabetes is a significant risk factor for mortality and morbidity along with cigarette smoking and hypertension.

The Fontaine classification of peripheral arterial occlusive disease divides it into four stages [26]:

Stage I is asymptomatic characterized by decreased pulses and ankle/brachial index less than 0.9.
Stage II is intermittent claudication.
Stage III is characterized by rest pain.
Stage IV is focal tissue necrosis and ulcer.

Common sites of claudication include obstruction in the aorto-iliac artery, which produces ischemia in the hip, thigh, and buttock. Obstruction in the femoral artery or its branches will produce ischemia in the thigh and calf, while obstruction in the popliteal artery will be manifested in the foot, ankle, and calf.

McDermott describes a cascading sequence progressing from asymptomatic PAD to disability associated with reduced muscle strength, poor walking ability, and severe cellular dysfunction by the time intermittent claudication presents itself [27].

Claudication results in significant shifts in occupational, personal and social activity, reduction in walking speed from 3 miles/h to 1–2 miles/h with significant maximal walking distance limitations. Thirty percent of patients experience difficulty in walking around the block and 65% have a great deal of difficulty walking half of a block or 150 ft.

Patients can be risk stratified according to their vascular history, physical examination and pulse palpation, ABI measurements, and noninvasive laboratory tests. Diagnosis of the condition depends clinically upon measurements of the ankle/brachial index and arterial dopplers.

The ankle/brachial index is 95% sensitive and 99% specific for PAD according to the Transatlantic Intersociety Consensus (TASC) working group. The treatment goals in all patients with PAD are [28]:

1. Improve functional status by improving symptoms
2. Preserve the limb by decreasing the need for revascularization
3. Prevent of progression of arteriosclerotic vascular disease by glycemic and lipid controls
4. Reduction in cardiovascular and cerebral vascular mortality with the aid of antiplatelet agents, vasodilators, and statin therapy.

Patients with proximal or unilateral disease, stenosis or short occlusions, no improvement after exercise or severe symptoms are candidates for aggressive intervention. Those patients who continue to smoke have severe concomitant angina or chronic obstructive pulmonary disease, have extensive multiple occlusions with distal involvement are less likely to be amenable to surgical intervention. Strategic placement of stents has provided a less invasive way of improving symptoms in some patients [28].

Peripheral vascular disease has been associated with six modifiable risk factors including:

1. Dyslipidemia
2. Diabetes
3. Hypertension
4. Obesity
5. Smoking
6. Elevated homocysteine levels

Claudication exercise programs have been shown to be effective in those patients who are well motivated in improving walking distance, exercise performance, and physical functioning. They do not work well in the non-compliant patient or the patient who has limited availability of supervised programs. These programs usually involve five sessions per week, most of which are supervised.

As of the present time Cilostazol (Pletal) seems to be the most effective with pentoxifylline (Trental) improving symptoms in some patients. Other medications like propionyl-l-carnitine, prostaglandins, angiogenic factors, and l-arginine remain to be studied. Antiplatelet therapy can provide additional adjuvant benefit in these patients decreasing the likelihood of embolization, along with statin therapy and hypertension control [26]. Curiously enough, glycemic control does not necessarily decrease the risk of PAD, in addition although there is a strong association between diabetes and peripheral atherosclerosis, the degree of hyperglycemia does not predict severity. Although the American Diabetes Association recommends reducing A1C to 7.0% or less, it is still not clear what impact this reduction has on attenuating peripheral vascular disease.

Cilostazol and several of its metabolites are inhibitors of phosphodiesterase-3, so this medication is contraindicated in those individuals who can have congestive heart failure or have any known or suspected hypersensitivity to any of its compounds. Although there is no direct evidence that this product causes or exacerbates congestive heart failure, other PDE-3 inhibitors have been known to increase mortality in patients with class III or class IV congestive heart failure. This is why this product should not be taken by these patients as of the present time. Cilostazol can also be potentiated by drugs that inhibit CYP3A4 or CYP2C19.

Patients who are good candidates for angioplasty and stenting are those with:

1. Non-calcified lesions
2. Concentric stenoses
3. Larger vessel involvement
4. Short segment disease
5. Non concomitant coronary co-morbidity
6. Treated coronary disease with normal renal function
7. Patent vessels distal to the treated lesion and no evidence of diabetes

Revascularization is usually indicated for life limiting complaints, acute severe symptoms associated with pain, immobility and loss of sensation, non-healing ulcers, gangrene, and continued disability despite appropriate nonsurgical intervention. Aggressive early diagnosis and management can prevent many of the major complications associated with this condition [28].

The availability of stenting has provided an added option to identify these patients earlier. In addition, MRA (magnetic resonance angiography) has been an important noninvasive tool in some patients to further evaluate the use of dye in the peripheral vascular system.

CEREBRAL ARTERIOSCLEROTIC VASCULAR DISEASE

Diabetic patients with cerebral vascular arteriosclerotic disease should be on ACE inhibitors or angiotensin blockers, statins, and platelet antagonists. Stroke is the third leading cause of death in this country, with more than 160,000 deaths occurring per year, with diabetic patients being at significant increased risk. The fatality rate from an acute stroke can be as high as 20 and 50% in 5 years. Stroke increases commensurate with the severity of carotid stenosis. When a patient has carotid stenosis of 70–90%, there is a 26% risk of ipsilateral stroke and a 28% chance of having a cerebral event within 2 years according to the North American Symptomatic Carotid Endarterectomy Trial (NASCET) [29]. Close to 30% of all strokes are associated with extracranial carotid artery stenosis as the result of embolization of thrombotic or atherosclerotic material, thrombosis, and diminished vessel diameter. Most cerebral symptoms are the direct result of plaque ulceration or rupture. Similar to what is seen in the coronary arteries, foam cell infiltration, fibrous cap thinning, and plaque rupture occur in symptomatic patients.

1.5–2.2% of patients with an asymptomatic carotid bruit have a stroke within 3 years according to the European Carotid Surgery Trial [30]. It is crucial for physicians to appreciate that the presence of a carotid bruit does not necessarily correlate or predict the degree of carotid stenosis. The specificity of a focal bruit to predict high grade ipsilateral stenosis (>70%) was 61%, while the sensitivity was 63% in a substudy of the NASCET. The absence of a bruit lowered the probability of a stenosis >70% to be present from 52 to 40%.

Importantly, however, the incidence of coronary artery disease and subsequent mortality is higher in those with a carotid bruit than those without one, 35% in a study of 506 patients demonstrating severe coronary artery disease requiring revascularization in the *Archives of Internal Medicine* [31].

Not to be overlooked is the role of carotid intimal thickening (CIMT) and its association with the metabolic syndrome and stroke risk. Adolphe and others published a review in the Mayo Clinic Proceedings in 2009, of 2,268 patients and the relationship of carotid intimal thickness to event risk and found that CIMT increased with each component of the metabolic syndrome. Intima media thickness has been shown to be a significant surrogate marker for cardiovascular disease and the addition of this important parameter to the diagnostic criteria for metabolic syndrome enhanced cardiovascular risk prediction.

Patients with diabetes are twice more likely to have a stroke and develop carotid artery disease than non diabetics, with development and progression of carotid disease related to systolic blood pressure, postprandial glucose, and elevated LDL cholesterol levels, while smokers have a relative risk for stroke of 2.58 compared to non-smokers. As much as 60% of all strokes are due to uncontrolled hypertension, but the risk of carotid atherosclerosis increases as the number of risk factors (dyslipidemia, smoking, diabetes, and hypertension) increases.

The American Diabetes Association recommends tight diabetic control to reduce not only the microvascular complications, but lessen the likelihood of vasculopathy in association with type-2 diabetes. Benefits of statin therapy in stroke reduction have clearly been demonstrated and should be used for primary prevention against macrovascular complications in men and women with this disease.

Meta-analysis of results from various diabetes subgroups of six primary and eight secondary prevention trials reported by Vijan and Hayward can be used to substantiate these benefits [32].

In primary prevention, pooled relative risk for cardiovascular events with lipid lowering therapy was 0.78 and the pooled absolute risk reduction was 0.03. The number needed to treat in this high risk group was 34.5 for 4.3 years.

In secondary prevention, pooled relative risk was similar, but the absolute risk reduction is more than twice as high. The number needed to treat in this group to prevent one event was 13.8 for 4.9 years.

Lipoprotein (a) has been shown to be a significant risk factor particularly in the diabetic patients increasing the likelihood of a cerebral vascular event threefold. Aspirin therapy has been shown to be of benefit after carotid endarterectomy in asymptomatic carotid disease and with lacunar infarctions.

The European Stroke Prevention Study (ESPS)-2 showed statistically significant benefits from extended release dipyridamole and aspirin in secondary stroke prevention. Hence according to the latest guidelines, every patient who has experienced a stroke or transient ischemic attack that is non-cardioembolic in origin and has no contraindication should receive an anti-platelet agent [33].

This can be:

1. Aspirin in doses of 50–325 mg/day
2. Aspirin 25 mg and extended release dipyridamole 200 mg twice daily
3. Clopidogrel 75 mg daily,are all exceptional options for initial therapy.

In 2009, prasugrel (Effient), a novel thienopyridine ADP receptor inhibitor received FDA approval to reduce thrombotic cardiovascular events (including stent thrombosis) in patients with acute coronary syndrome. A clinical trial of 13,608 patients with acute coronary syndrome compared clopidogrel and aspirin with prasugrel and aspirin and found that prasugrel reduced the risk of nonfatal stroke (12.1% for clopidogrel vs. 9.9% for prasugrel); however, this newer and more potent drug although being particularly effective in patients with diabetes, also increased the risk of fatal bleeding. Prasugrel is not currently indicated for patients who have had a transient ischemic episode or stroke.

The combination of aspirin 25 mg and extended release dipyridamole, 200 mg twice daily, has been shown to be more effective than aspirin alone, while the combination of dipyridamole and aspirin b.i.d. may be more effective than clopidogrel alone with a favorable adverse effect profile.

In the UKPDS trial, tight blood pressure control in diabetics resulted in over a 40% reduction in the risk of stroke. Statistically significant reduction in the risk of stroke was seen in the Heart Outcomes Prevention Evaluation (HOPE) trial with the ACE inhibitor ramipril and in the Telmisartan, Ramipril or Both in Patients at High Risk for Vascular

Table 9.2
Strategies to reduce risk of macrovascular disease in diabetics

Stop smoking

Reduce blood pressure <130/80 mmHg

Reduce LDL<100 mg/dl with statin therapy

Raise HDL>50 mg/dl in women

>45 mg/dl in men

Reduce triglycerides<150 mg/dl

Take aspirin (81–325 mg daily)

Lose weight with diet and exercise

Add Ramipril (Altace) for overall risk reduction or Telmisartan (Micardis) if ACE inhibitor intolerant

Vinik et al. [*35*]

Events (ON TARGET) trial with telmisartan. ACE inhibitor and angiotensin receptor blocking therapy has been shown to inhibit the progression of arteriosclerotic vascular disease. In some studies this inhibition has been dose dependant.

Thiazolidinediones have also shown to inhibit the progression of early carotid arteriosclerotic vascular disease while the Losartan Intervention for Endpoint Reduction (LIFE) trial has demonstrated that losartan (Cozaar) can be effective in reducing stroke in hypertensive diabetic patients [*34*].

Surgical revascularization has shown some benefit in diabetic patients with carotid artery arteriosclerotic vascular disease, particularly with stenoses greater than 70%. Further data needs to be collected on carotid artery stenting, although this may be prove to be a promising alternative in the future, particularly in those patients who are at high risk for serious complications during carotid endarterectomy.

SUMMARY

From the foregoing discussion, it is clear that although the diabetic patients will suffer from their microvascular disease they will die from their macrovascular disease. Multifactorial risk reduction strategies must be developed early and maintained consistently to have any dramatic impact on arteriosclerotic vascular disease. Table 9.2 summarizes the strategies for macrovascular risk reduction in the type-2 diabetic patient.

REFERENCES

1. Deckert T, et al. Implications for micro-and macrovascular disease. Diabetes Care 1992;15:1181–1191.
2. Greenfield S, Billimek J, Pellegrini F, Franciosi M, DeBerardis G. Comorbidity affects the relationship between glycemic control and cardiovascular outcomes in diabetes. Ann Intern Med 2009;151:854–860.
3. Haffner SM, Lehto S, et al. Mortality from coronary artery disease in subjects with type 2 diabetes and in nondiabetic subjects with and without prior myocardial infarction. N Engl J Med 1998;339:229–234.
4. Kelly TN, Bazzano LA, Fonseca VA, Thethi TK, Reynolds K, He J. Systematic review: glucose control and cardiovascular disease in type-2 diabetes. Ann Intern Med 2009;151:394–403.

5. Stamler J, Caccaro O, Neaton JD, Wentrworth D. Diavetes, other risk factors, and 12 year cardiovascular mortality for men screened in the Multiple Risk Factor Intervention Trial (MRFIT). Diabetes Care 1993;16:434–444.

6. Gilpin E, Ricou F, et al. Factors associated with recurrent myocardial infarction within one year after acute myocardial infarction. Am Heart J 1991;121:457–463.

7. Herlitz J, Malmberg K, et al. Mortality and morbidity during a five year follow up of diabetics with myocardial infarction. Acta Med Scand 1988;224:31–38.

8. Eschwege E, Richard JL, Thibult N. Coronary heart disease mortality in relation with diabetes, blood glucose and plasma insulin levels. The Paris Prospective Study. Horn Metab Res Suppl 1985;15:41–46.

9. Hansson L, Zanchetti A, Carruthers SG. Effects of intensive blood pressure lowering and low dose aspirin in patients with hypertension: principal results of the Hypertension Optimal Treatment (HOT) randomized trial. Lancet 1998;351:1755–1762.

10. Lehto, S, Pyorala K, Miettinen H, et al. Myocardial infarct size and mortality in patients with non-insulin dependent diabetes mellitus. J Intern Med 1994;236:291–297.

11. Uusitupa M, et al. The relationship of cardiovascular risk factors to the prevalence of coronary heart disease in newly diagnosed type 2 diabetes. Diabetolologia 1985;28:653–659.

12. Fuller JH, et al. Coronary heart disease risk and impaired glucose tolerance. The Whitehall Study. Lancet 1980;1:1373–1376.

13. Jarrett RJ, et al. Diabetes mellitus and cardiovascular disease – putative association via common antecedents. Diabetologia 1988;31:737–740.

14. Levine GN, Jacobs AK, et al. Impact of diabetes mellitus on percutaneous revascularization CAVEAT-I Investigators. Coronary Angioplasty versus Excisional Atherectomy Trial. Am J Cardiol 1997;79:748–755.

15. Creager MA. Results of the CAPRIE trial: efficacy and safety of clopidogrel. Vasc Med 1998;3(3):257–260.

16. Van Belle E, Bauters C, et al. Restenosis rates in diabetic patients: a comparison of coronary stenting and balloon angioplasty in native coronary vessels. Circulation 1997;96:1454–1460.

17. Taylor GJ, Moses HW, et al. Six year survival after coronary thrombolysis and early revascularization for acute myocardial infarction. Am J Cardiol 1992;70:26–30.

18. Elliot WJ, Meyer PM. Incident diabetesin clinical trials of antihypertensive drugs: a network meta-analysis. Lancet 2007;369(9557):201–207.

19. Zuanctti G, Latini R, Maggioni AP, Franzosi M, Santoro L, Tognoni G. Effect of the ACE inhibitor lisinopril on mortality in diabetic patients with acute myocardial infarction. Circulation 1997;96:4239–4245.

20. Patti G, Nusca A, DiSciascio G. Meta-analysis comparison (Nine Trilas) of outcomes with drug eluting stents versus bare metal stents in patients with diabetes mellitus. Am J Cardiol 2008;102:1328–1334.

21. FRISC II Investigators. Long term low molecular mass heparin in unstable angina: FRISC-II multicenter study. Lancet 1999;354:701–707.

22. Ridker P, Cushman M, Stampfer M, Tracy R. Inflammation, aspirin and risk of cardiovascular disease in healthy men. N Engl J Med 1997;337(5):356.

23. Hiatt WR. New treatment options in intermittent claudication. In J Clin Pract Suppl 2001;119:20–27.

24. Criqui MH, Langer RD, Fronek A. Mortality over a period of 10 years in patients with peripheral vascular disease. N Engl J Med 1992;326:381–386.

25. Jensen-Urstad KJ, Reichard PG, et al. Early atherosclerosis is retarded by improved long term blood glucose control in patients with IDDM. Diabetes 1996;45:1253–1258.

26. Donnelly R. Assessment and management of intermittent claudication: importance of secondary prevention. Int J Clin Pract Suppl 2001;119:2–9.

27. McDermott MM, Guralnik JM, Greenland P. Statin use and leg functioning in patients with and without lower extremity peripheral arterial disease. Circulation 2003;107:757–761.

28. Hiatt WR. New treatment options in intermittent claudication: the US experience. Int J Clin Pract Suppl 2001:119:20–37.

29. North American Symptomatic Carotid Endarterecdtomy Trial Collaborators. Beneficial effect of carotid endarterectomy in symptomatic patients with high grade carotid stenosis. N Engl J Med 1991;325:445–453.

30. Rothwell PM, Gutnikoff SA, Warlow CP. Reanalysis of the European Carotid Surgery Trial. Stroke 2003;34:514.

31. Sauve JS, Thorpe KE, Sackett DL. The North American Symptomatic Carotid Endarterectomy Trial. Can bruits distinguish high grade from moderate symptomatic carotid Stenosis? Ann Intern Med 1994;120:633–637.

32. Vijan S, Hayward RA. Pharmacologic lipid lowering therapy in type-2 diabetes mellitus. Ann Intern Med 2004;140:650–658.
33. Libby P, Plutzky J. Diabetic macrovascular disease: the glucose paradox. Circulation 2002;106:2760–2763.
34. Dahlof B, Kjeldsen RB, Julius SE, Beevers S, de Faire U. Cardiovascular mortality and morbidity in the losartan intervention for endpoint reduction in hypertension study (LIFE). Lancet 2002;359(9311):995–1003.
35. Vinik A, Vinik E. Prevention of the complications of diabetes. Am J Manag Care 2003;9(3):S63–S77.

SUPPLEMENTARY READINGS

Agewall S, Fagerberg B, et al. Carotid artery wall intima media thickness is associated with insulin mediated glucose disposal in men at high and low coronary risk. Stroke 1995;26:956–960.

American Diabetes Association. Consensus development conference on the diagnosis of coronary heart disease in people with diabetes. Diabetes Care 1998;21:1551–1559.

Aronson D, Bloomgarden Z, et al. Potential mechanisms promoting restenosis in diabetic patients. J Am Coll Cardiol 1996;27:528–535.

Brownlee M, et al. Advanced glycosylation end products in tissue and the biochemical basis of diabetic complications. N Engl J Med 1988;318:1315–1321.

Carrozza J, Kuntz R, et al. Restenosis after arterial injury caused by coronary stenting in patients with diabetes mellitus. Ann Intern Med 1993;118:344–349.

Clark RS, English M, et al. Effect of intravenous infusion of insulin in diabetics with acute myocardial infarction. BMJ 1985;291:303–305.

Fava S, Azzopardi J, et al. Factors that influence outcome in diabetic subjects with myocardial infarction. Diabetes Care 1993;16:1615–1618.

Gum P, O'Keefe JJ, et al. Bypass surgery versus coronary angioplasty for revascularization of treated diabetic patients. Circulation 1997;96(9 Suppl):II7–II10.

Kornowski R, Mintz GS, et al. Increased restenosis in diabetes mellitus after coronary interventions is due to exaggerated intimal hyperplasia. Circulation 1997;95:1366–1369.

Krolewski AS, et al. Magnitude and determinants of coronary artery disease in juvenile onset, insulin dependent diabetes mellitus. Am J Cardiol 1987;59:750–755.

Lyons TJ. Glycation and oxidation: a role in the pathogenesis of atherosclerosis. Am J Cardiol 1993;71:26B–31B.

Sobel BE. Acceleration of restenosis by diabetes. Circulation 2001;103:1185–1187.

Soler NG, Bennett MA, et al. Myocardial infarction in diabetics. Q J Med 1975;44:125–132.

The Diabetes Control and Complications Trial Research Group. The effect of intensive treatment of diabetes on the development and progression of long term complications in insulin dependent diabetes mellitus. N Engl J Med 1993;329:977–996.

UK Prospective Diabetes Study (UKPDS) Group. Intensive blood glucose control with sulfonylureas or insulin compared with conventional treatment and risk of complications in patients with type 2 diabetes. Lancet 1998;352:837–853.

10 Microvascular Disease

CONTENTS

Key Words: Diabetic retinopathy, Diabetic neuropathy, Diabetic nephropathy, Diabetes Control and Complication Trial (DCCT), United Kingdom Prospective Diabetes Study (UKPDS), A1C levels

INTRODUCTION

The microvascular complications of diabetes include:

1. Retinopathy
2. Nephropathy
3. Neuropathy, which includes mononeuropathy, diabetic amyotrophy, symmetric distal neuropathy, diabetic gastroparesis, diabetic diarrhea, neurogenic bladder, impaired cardiovascular reflexes, and sexual dysfunction [1]

Both the Diabetes Control and Complication Trial (DCCT) and the United Kingdom Prospective Diabetes Study (UKPDS) have shown the importance of tight glycemic control in preventing microvascular disease and that the benefits of treatment were not a threshold at 6.5%, but a continuum, where further reductions in A1C levels below 6.5 continue to demonstrate benefit [1].

Diabetes is the leading cause of new cases of blindness in individuals between the ages of 20–74 due to macular edema and retinopathy. By the time diabetes is diagnosed, up to 40% of patients may already have some form of retinopathy, while another 22% will develop it over 6 years and 90% of patients will have retinopathy following 15 years of

From: *Current Clinical Practice: Type 2 Diabetes, Pre-Diabetes, and the Metabolic Syndrome*,
Edited by: R.A. Codario, DOI 10.1007/978-1-60327-441-8_10
© Springer Science+Business Media, LLC 2011

known duration of disease. Retinopathy is responsible for 12,000–24,000 cases of blindness each year [2].

It is critical for the primary care physician to realize that waiting until the diabetic patient complains of blurred vision may be too late, since permanent retinal injury with visual loss may have already occurred. With the use of more sensitive methods of evaluation and early screening, it has become apparent that the relationship between blood glucose and retinopathy tends to vary across a continuum with the 10-year prevalence of retinopathy in individuals with impaired glucose tolerance being similar to those with overt diabetes in the Data from an Epidemiological Study on the Insulin Resistance Syndrome (DESIR) study from France. This study comprised 5,212 men and women 30–65 years of age. Of the 700 participants for eye examinations, 235 had diabetes with 36 already receiving treatment, 238 had normal fasting glucose (<100 mg/dl) and 227 had (IFG) impaired fasting glucose (110–125 mg/dl). Forty-four individuals had diabetic retinopathy (19 with diabetes, 19 with IFG, and 6 with normal glucose). In this study, two factors that were most associated with retinopathy during the 9-year follow-up period were fasting plasma glucose and hemoglobin A1C. The characteristics at baseline that most predicted retinopathy included systolic blood pressure of 142 mmHg (137 for no retinopathy), A1C of 6.4% (5.7% with no retinopathy), and fasting plasma glucose of 130 mg/dl (106 mg/dl with no retinopathy) [3].

There are several interesting theories as to how hyperglycemia wreaks its havoc on the retina [4]. These include:

1. Neovascularization – Vascular endothelial growth factor (VEGF) in response to local tissue ischemia, stimulates the growth of new blood vessels in non perfused areas. This neovascularization causes blood vessels to grow between the internal surface of the retina and the vitreous gel, posteriorly with 45° of the optic disk. Early on in the process only vessels are seen, while white fibrous tissue begins to grow as the condition progresses.
2. Capillary occlusion – In the hyperglycemic state the white blood cells may express more molecules on their surfaces, called integrins. These can interact with the capillary endothelial cells which express intercellular adhesion molecules (ICAMs), which make the white cells adhere to the capillary walls. This causes the capillaries to become plugged and interferes with white cell passage progressively depriving larger areas of the retina of perfusion. Initially surrounding capillaries can compensate by accepting increased flow, but this autoregulation eventually fails with wider retinal areas becoming compromised.
3. Exudative edema and leakage – White cells that have adhered to the endothelial surface release products that increase permeability. With increased permeability of the endothelium, production of VEGF is increased, which acts locally by diffusing into the optic disk, through the vitreous involving the retina and into the anterior chamber of the eye, allowing fluid to leak into the retina, resulting in tissue edema. This edematous fluid and cholesterol begins to accumulate in the retina which impairs visual acuity.
4. Fibrosis – With neovascularization there is a proliferation of fibrous tissue, which causes local and widespread gel retraction, which tears new vessels and results in hemorrhage between the gel and the retina. This can result in floaters or diffuse visual loss. Hemorrhaging can produce more fibrosis, which can cause further retinal distortion detachment with more visual loss.

Diabetic retinopathy can be divided into background and proliferative retinopathy. Background retinopathy involves microaneurysms, intraretinal hemorrhages, clinically significant macular edema, venous beading, cotton wool spots, intraretinal microvascular abnormalities, and circinate retinal abnormalities.

Proliferative diabetic neuropathy can include surface neovascularization, and subsequent complications of proliferation including vitreous hemorrhaging and fraction retinal detachments.

Although the retina may appear to be normal on clinical examination, several biological and physiological changes are occurring at the cellular level accompanied by alterations in retinal blood flow and leukocyte adhesion.

Diabetic retinopathy tends to progress from the mild non-proliferative form simply manifesting increased vascular permeability to the moderate and severe non-proliferative form that involves vascular closer to the finer proliferative form characterized by neovascularizations on the retina and the posterior portion of the vitreous.

Visual loss from diabetic retinopathy can occur as a result of preretinal or vitreous hemorrhaging from neovascularization, distortion of the retina due to new blood vessel formation and contraction of fibrous tissue resulting in retinal detachment and subsequent irreversible vision loss and capillary non-perfusion or macular edema [5].

It is important for the primary physician to understand the importance of preventing or delaying the onset of progression of diabetic retinopathy particularly when the individual is asymptomatic. Referral to an ophthalmologist is important when the diagnosis is established. Timely intervention with laser photocoagulation can decrease the production of vasoproliferative factors and prevent visual loss in a large percentage of patients with severe non-proliferative or early proliferative diabetic retinopathy.

Clinical presentations of the disorder can be varied with the most common presentation being asymptomatic individuals. However, other presentations can include sudden visual loss, marked retinal lipid exudation in association with increased hyperlipidemia, marked vascular narrowing in small vessels usually associated with hypertension, and transient worsening of retinopathy that can occur despite tight control.

Sudden visual loss is usually the result of:

1. Retinal vascular occlusion
2. Vitreous hemorrhaging which usually presents as strings or spots in the vision
3. Central nervous system stroke
4. Sudden onset of bilateral macular edema, usually associated with cardiac or renal decompensation or severe anemia
5. Lens changes due to blood sugar alterations

Clinical trials have shown the relationship of glycemia to the progression of diabetic retinopathy with progression to proliferative retinopathy more likely with the highest A1C quartiles. The DCCT trial in type-1 diabetics demonstrated that intensive glycemic control can significantly reduce the risk of retinopathy compared with conventional therapy and that this benefit also extends to existing retinopathy [5].

The UKDPS trial showed a similar decrease with a relative onset of 21% with a 12-year follow-up. The Diabetic Retinopathy Candesartan Trials Program (DIRECT Prevent 1 and DIRECT Protect-1) involved 309 countries in randomized, double blinded, placebo controlled trials in type-1 diabetics with 1,421 in Prevent-1 and 1,905 in Protect-1. These two trials showed that the use of candesartan, an angiotensin receptor blocker (16–32 mg) reduced the incidence of retinopathy, but had no beneficial effect on the progression of retinopathy [6].

Previous findings from the Eurodiab Controlled Trial of Lisinopril in Insulin-Dependent Diabetes (EUCLID) suggested that the incidence and progression of retinopathy in type-1 diabetes can be reduced with renin-angiotensin system blockade with the use of the angiotensin converting enzyme inhibitor, lisinopril [7].

However, the DIRECT-Protect 2 trial used the same drug, candesartan (16–32 mg) in 1,905 type-2 diabetics in a double blinded, randomized, placebo controlled study over a 4-year period of time and found that progression of retinopathy was non significantly reduced by 13% compared to placebo, but regression was significantly increased ($p=0.009$) by 34%! Candesartan had no effect on macular edema or the incidence of proliferative diabetic retinopathy [8].

Recent research has shown that vasoactive endothelial derived growth factor and protein kinase C play an important role in the progression of diabetic retinopathy with clinical trials currently in progress with the use of inhibitor of protein kinase C both for prevention and treatment.

Laser photocoagulation therapy performed by an ophthalmologic surgeon plays an important role in those patients with non-proliferative diabetic retinopathy, which is why it is essential for diabetic patients to undergo regular ophthalmologic examination even if their vision appears to be normal. Ophthalmologic examination should be performed at diagnosis and yearly.

Non-proliferative or background retinopathy is usually characterized by the microaneurysms and intraretinal hemorrhaging that appear similar to dots and blots. Macular edema can occur in these individuals if significant amount of fluid leaks into the macular area where central vision originates. The presence of macular edema is suggested by the presence of hard exudates in the macular area.

Advanced background retinopathy is sometimes referred to as preproliferative retinopathy. These individuals have an increased risk of progression to fine proliferative retinopathy. This stage is characterized by soft cotton-wool exudates, irregularly dilated and tortuous retinal capillaries, intraretinal neovascularization, and beading of the retinal veins [4].

Proliferative retinopathy imparts most serious threats to vision. The neovascularization in this abnormality usually involves more than 1/3 of the optic disk with these fragile vessels prone to bleeding and disruption of retinal function. This bleeding can cause cobwebs, or floaters, or retinal detachments that result from contraction of fibrous tissue.

In the symptomatic patients with hard exudates near the macula, any proliferative or preproliferative characteristics in the first trimester of pregnancy should have a careful ophthalmologic evaluation. Alarm symptoms include blurry vision persisting for greater than 1–2 days when not associated with a change in blood glucose, cobwebs, flashing lights, or black spots in the field of vision or sudden loss of vision in one or both eyes.

Retinal hemorrhaging or neovascularization covering more than one-third of the optic disk or macular edema places patients at extremely high risk. The Early Treatment Diabetic Retinopathy Study (ETDRS) revealed that argon laser photocoagulation applied locally can be extremely effective in stabilizing vision and treating macular edema [9].

Photocoagulation has been shown to slow visual loss progression in cases of macular edema and improve vision by as much as 50% when used as a preventative measure. Patients with proliferative retinopathy and high risk characteristics are usually given pan-retinal laser treatments with a scattered pattern of 1,200–1,600 burns applied uniformly throughout the periphery of the retina avoiding the macular area [5].

Significant retinal detachments and large vitreous hemorrhages may require vitrectomy. This is usually reserved for patients with poor vision. Hypertension can be an independent significant risk factor in causing and aggravating retinopathy in type-2 diabetics as well as increasing the risk for macular edema.

Clinical trials have shown that elevated systolic blood pressure may significantly increase the risk of retinopathy in type-2 diabetics with most studies confirming an association not only with systolic, but also diastolic hypertension. In the UKPDS trial, 10 mm systolic blood pressure decreases and 5 mm. diastolic decreases reduced diabetic microvascular complications after approximately 8 years by 37%.

There are several mechanisms postulated for the aggravation and promotion of diabetic retinopathy by hypertension. These include:

1. Increased retinal endothelial damage
2. Loss of retinal vascular auto-regulation
3. Increased expression of VEGF resulting in proliferation of small vessels and worsening of retinopathy

Several clinical trials have confirmed that microalbuminuria, macroalbuminuria, and or proteinuria is related to progression of retinopathy with close to 70% of type-2 diabetic patients on dialysis, possessing some form of retinopathy. This is important to keep in mind particularly in those patients with impaired renal function since retinopathy may be progressing as well [10].

An interesting association has been found between anemia and retinopathy, particularly since anemia is more common in patients with renal failure. Next to hyperglycemia, anemia has now been found to be the second highest risk factor for subsequent development of diabetic retinopathy with patients being twice as likely to develop diabetic retinopathy with hemoglobins less than 12 in a recently completed Finnish trial.

The ETDRS showed that severe visual loss and iris peripheral retinopathy were associated with a low hematocrit and increases in hematocrit from 29.6 to 39.5% in treatment with erythropoietin (Procrit and Epogen) resolved macular edema in three of five patients evaluated.

Although there is some literature to support the association between smoking and diabetic retinopathy, the association is much stronger with macrovascular disease and nephropathy. Lipid disturbances can also aggravate prognosis in diabetic retinopathy with elevated triglyceride levels associated with vision loss and proliferative diabetic retinopathy in the ETDRS trial.

Clearly, strict glycemic and blood pressure control can have a dramatic effect on reducing the progression of diabetic eye disease. All intensive glucose therapeutic maneuvers except for chlorpropamide were associated with a clear reduction in the risk of diabetic retinopathy progression in the UKPDS trial, while captopril and the beta blocker atenolol have shown benefit in type-2 patients in the UKPDS.

The anti-angiogenic effects at the cellular level of the thiazolidinediones have been shown to be a benefit in neovascularization. Rosiglitazone (Avandia) has been shown to inhibit VEGF induced proliferation and migration of retinal pigment epithelial cells and has had a direct result in inhibiting neovascularization, hence the thiazolidinediones might play an important role in preventing retinopathy [10].

The Wisconsin Epidemiologic Study of Diabetic Retinopathy (WESDR) showed no association between aspirin use and the severity of retinopathy. This study further provided evidence that aspirin therapy did not increase the risk of vitreous hemorrhaging in diabetics with proliferative retinopathy [11].

Hence there is no contraindication for the use of aspirin in patients with diabetic retinopathy although more evidence needs to be established to determine if aspirin can actually alter the course of the disease.

Although there is insufficient data regarding the effects of clopidogrel on retinopathy, both the Ticlopidine Microangiopathy of Diabetes Study and the Aspirin Microangiopathy of Diabetes Study confirmed that these agents can be used safely in the presence of retinopathy with fewer microaneurysms found in the aspirin group. The use of anti-platelet agents has not been associated with an excess number of hemorrhagic complications in diabetic patients, and hence there is no contraindication for this approach for diabetic patients with acute myocardial infarctions [12].

Further investigation shows that the emerging agents may be effective in treating retinopathy. These include aldose reductase inhibitors, somatostatin analog, and VEGF inhibitors. Whether vitamin E therapy can delay the onset of progression of diabetic retinopathy is currently unclear.

Indications for surgery in diabetic retinopathy include [5]:

1. Visually debilitating persistent vitreous blood
2. Eyes with advancing neovascularization despite maximum photocoagulation
3. Eyes with significant and severe vascular proliferation
4. Severe fibrous proliferation
5. Eyes with severe proliferation in which vitreous hemorrhage precludes photocoagulation
6. Bridging pre-macular fibrosis
7. Progressive macular distortion due to fibrosis
8. Severe posterior pole hemorrhage without significant vitreous detachment

Since diabetic retinal disease presents a significant morbidity problem to the patient, prompt identification and early ophthalmologic referral plays an important role in not only prevention, but treatment.

The prevention and/or treatment of diabetic retinopathy involves:

1. Controlling blood glucose
2. Controlling blood pressure
3. Retinal laser photocoagulation including panretinal scatter photocoagulation for proliferative retinopathy or neovascular glaucoma or focal photocoagulation for macular edema
4. Vitrectomy for nonclearing vitreous hemorrhage or traction detachment of the retina
5. Controlling dyslipidemia with statins and/or fenofibrates

DIABETIC NEUROPATHY

Diabetic neuropathy afflicts up to 70% of patients with type-2 diabetes and it does not represent one distinct disease but rather an adverse group of conditions that affect the peripheral nervous system, attacking the peripheral, proximal, and autonomic nerves causing both focal and systemic disease, and also increasing mortality risk compared to diabetics without the condition. Patients with diabetic neuropathy may have pain, which occurs in up to 20% of patients, or impaired sensation in the feet and hands, slow digestion, carpal tunnel syndrome, and impaired cardiovascular responses [13].

Severe nerve damage has been shown to be a major contributor to lower extremity amputation. Impaired alteration and sensation can lead the diabetic patient to develop asymptomatic severe foot ulcerations, which could lead to subsequent severe infection and loss of limbs. In addition, neuropathic arthropathy can become a major problem in diabetics with impaired sensation. Multifocal neuropathic damage involving abnormalities in the autonomic nervous system and all classes of peripheral sensory axons can occur with this disease.

The specific pathogenic disturbances underlying the etiology of neuropathy have not been completely elucidated even though a recognized link exists between persistent hyperglycemia or neurological dysfunction. As with retinopathy, the incidence of diabetic peripheral neuropathy correlates with the duration of diabetes and glycemic control.

Some theories concern the accumulation of sorbitol in hyperglycemic states or even its increased oxidation to fructose. Whether the culprit is fructose, sorbitol, or a combination of both, the end result is nerve damage and an imbalance of nicotinamide adenosine diphosphate (NADP) and its reduced form NADPH.

Depletion of the cell's NADPH occurs during the conversion of glucose into sorbitol and subsequent conversion of sorbitol into fructose. This decreased NADPH disrupts the oxidation reduction potential intracellularly causing the accumulation of various oxidative free radicals that can cause nerve damage in fibers of the autonomic nervous system and all types of peripheral sensory neurons and the myelin sheaths that surround the motor axons [14]. The hyperglycemic state also results in the glycation of proteins often leading to the formation of advanced glycosylation end products, which subsequently impair blood flow to the nerves and cause ischemia by enhancing the production of these free radicals. This plethora of neurological deterioration results in a wide variety of signs and symptoms that complicates and adds some confusion to the classification process.

Even pre-diabetes and the metabolic syndrome increase the risk for painful, sensory neuropathy. Costa and others reported on 548 patients on the aggregation of metabolic syndrome features and noted that small fiber neuropathy risk was doubled in those with this syndrome complex [15]. In fact impaired glucose tolerance neuropathy could represent the earliest stage of diabetic neuropathic disease. Sumner and others in the journal, *Neurology*, reported a dose response relationship for the severity of hyperglycemia with small fiber neuropathy being found in pre-diabetics and polyneuropathy involving both small and large fibers being more common in the overt diabetic [16].

Vinik et al. classify diabetic neuropathy into the following categories [17]:

1. Large fiber neuropathy characterized by impairments to vibration and touch, loss of tendon reflexes, and occasionally motor deficit loss involving the hands and both legs up to the mid thigh.
2. Small fiber neuropathy characterized by slight sensory loss mostly thermal and allodynia. This can be just as painful as large fiber neuropathy, but is usually not associated with motor deficits and normal to slightly decreased tendon reflexes. This involves the lower extremities from the mid calf to the feet.
3. Proximal motor neuropathy involving the shoulders and popliteal to mid thigh areas bilaterally, involves minimal sensory loss, can be significantly painful with loss of deep tendon reflexes and significant proximal motor deficit.
4. Mononeuritis multiplex, which can involve the third or the sixth cranial nerves and is usually associated with truncal neuropathy with mild sensory loss, significant pain, normal deep tendon reflexes, and motor deficits of varying degrees.

5. Entrapment syndromes which can be either the ulnar or median nerves in the upper extremities and the lateral popliteal nerves in the lower extremities which can be painful, characterized by significant sensory loss in the nerves involved. Deep tendon reflexes are usually normal and motor deficits can be present to a varying degree.
6. Diabetic autoneuropathy, which includes cardiovascular abnormalities with fluctuating heart rates, orthostatic hypotension, gastrointestinal disturbances including diabetic diarrhea and gastroparesis, and genitourinary problems including bladder dysfunction and sexual disturbances [18].
7. Distal symmetric polyneuropathy with damage to small and large nerve fibers resulting in various signs and symptoms that can be evaluated and quantified by sensory testing.

According to the San Antonio Conference on Diabetic Neuropathy there are three main groups of neurologic disturbance in diabetics [19]. These include:

1. Subclinical neuropathy characterized by abnormalities in somatosensory testing and electrodiagnostic evaluations
2. Focal neuropathic syndromes
3. Distal symmetric sensory motor
4. Diabetic amyotrophy
5. Autonomic syndromes with diffuse clinical neuropathy [20]

The diagnosis of subclinical neuropathy is based upon:

1. Decreased amplitudes and conduction velocities in selective electrodiagnostic testing
2. Abnormal quantitative sensory tests for thermal, sensory, and vibration thresholds
3. Abnormalities in quantitative autonomic function testing demonstrating decreased heart rate variation with postural testing with Valsalva maneuver and deep breathing [20]

These patients do not have significant clinical symptoms despite all these demonstrable abnormalities.

Focal mononeuropathies occur primarily in the elderly patient population and usually tend to be self limited resolving in 6–8 weeks and can involve both upper and lower extremities. These occur as the result of vascular occlusions causing infarction of the affected neurons and include mononeuritis multiplex, polyradiculopathies, and plexopathies.

These can be distinguished from other entrapment syndromes that tend to evolve more slowly and persist without intervention. The classic example of this is the 3rd or 6th nerve palsies that can occur in diabetic patients without warning. Nerve entrapment sites in diabetic patients can involve radial, ulnar or median nerves, lateral femoral cutaneous nerve of the thigh, peroneal, medial, and lateral plantar nerves as well as the femoral nerve.

Patients with diabetes are twice as likely to develop carpal tunnel syndrome as a result of edema or accumulation of fluid within the carpal tunnel area.

Distal symmetric sensorimotor neuropathy usually presents following acute stressful phenomenon, but can be insidious in their onset. This type of neuropathy can involve either motor or sensory nerves, small or large fibers or both.

Small nerve fiber dysfunction may usually manifest with symptoms of pain and hypersensitivities in the lower extremities followed by reduced light touch, pin prick, and loss of thermal sensitivities [13]. These patients usually complain of burning discomfort, allodynia (excessive discomfort to light touch), decreased sweating, pain, cold feet, dry skin, and impaired blood flow, and vasomotor function.

Patient symptoms can be varied including burning dysesthesias and allodynia (pain in response to a nonpainful sensation), decreased sweating, impaired vasodilatation, dry skin, cold extremities, impaired blood flow and vasomotor function, defective thermal sensation with normal reflexes, and motor strength with significantly reduced sensitivity to the 1 g monofilament and vibratory sensation with the 128c tuning fork.

Acute painful neuropathy is usually of a duration of less than 6 months characterized by pain and paresthesia early in the course of the disease. These spontaneous episodes of pain can occasionally be severely disabling with the pain varying in character and intensity. Patients may characterize these sensations as stabbing, lancinating, sharp, burning with concomitant altered sensations of pins and needles, coldness, and numbness and tingling [18].

This pain can be so annoying that even basic daily activities can be disrupted and the extremities can be exquisitely sensitive to touch.

Chronic painful polyneuropathy is far more common.

This usually occurs many years later in the course of the disease, lasts for greater than 6 months and can be significantly disabling associated with analgesia and narcotic tolerance. Although the exact mechanism for the severe pain in small fiber neuropathy is not well understood, clearly damage, injury, and subsequent disruption of neurofiber registration of pain occurs in the cerebral cortex rendering the painful stimulus more chronic. On occasion, disappearance of the pain may come with nerve death, but more likely it remains persistent and severely annoying.

Large fiber neuropathy is usually associated with Charcot's neuroarthropathy. This can involve either the motor or sensory nerves or both. These large fibers are responsible for cold, thermal perception, position sense, vibratory and motor function.

These larger fibers are myelinated and synapse in the medulla oblongata with rapid conduction beginning in the lower extremities. Subclinical abnormalities can be detected on electromyography and are characteristic of "dying back" neuropathy. This could also be sometimes seen with toxic chemical exposures to polychlorinated biphenyls and to tetrachlorodibenzoparadioxin (TCDD).

Patients usually have minimal symptoms characterized by a sensation of walking on cotton or an inability to discriminate among coins. These patients classically may have depressed tendon reflexes, impaired vibratory perception and position sense, sensory ataxia, shorting of the Achilles tendon with pes equinus and wasting of the small muscles of the feet with weakness in the muscles of the extremities [18].

This neuropathy can progress to the point where the patients have a great deal of difficulty standing on their toes or their heels with stocking-glove distribution of sensory loss, a consistent finding along with a deep, throbbing, aching, and often crampy pain with increased blood flow and hot feet.

Nerve conduction studies, somatosensory evoked potentials and electromyography remain the mainstay of establishing the diagnosis of peripheral neuropathy helping to distinguish the diabetic from the neoplastic, inflammatory, traumatic, vascular, toxic, autoimmune, and some of the other metabolic and endocrine abnormalities that can cause peripheral neuropathy including acute intermittent porphyria, hypothyroidism, B-12 deficiencies, and uremia.

Physical examination can give important clues, but proper equipment needs to be used. A tuning fork with a vibrating frequency of 128 Hz is preferable for diagnosing the duration of vibratory sensation, which can help quantify, to some extent, the severity of the neuro-pathic process. A 1 g monofilament increases sensitivity to 90% in detecting neuropathy.

To evaluate a patient for entrapment neuropathies, Tinel's sign can not only be used for carpal tunnel syndrome but can also be used for median, plantar, ulnar, peroneal, fibular, and ulnar notch neuropathies. On occasion, in particularly difficult cases, nerve biopsy may be helpful in excluding other causes of neuropathy and special arginine staining can be used to diagnose dying back neuropathy [20].

Diabetic amyotrophy, largely a disorder of the larger fibers, is heralded by painful mus-cle weakness and atrophy, affecting the lower limbs in an asymmetric pattern. This is more common in older men with poor glycemic control and can be associated with elevated cerebrospinal fluid protein and absent knee reflexes.

Diabetic autonomic neuropathy may present with varying signs and symptoms encom-passing damage to the motor and sensory axons of the parasympathetic and sympathetic nervous system including [20]:

1. Pupillary disturbances of the Argyll-Robertson type that are bilaterally small and con-strict when the patient focuses on a close object (accommodates), but do not react to light. This type of papillary reaction is also found in tertiary syphilis
2. Metabolic disturbances including hyperglycemic unresponsive and unawareness
3. Cardiovascular disturbances characterized by orthostatic hypotension, syncope, heat intolerance, cardiac autonomic disturbances and denervation, and inappropriate tachy-cardia with exercise
4. Neurovascular abnormalities including hyperhidrosis, alterations in the skin blood flow, gustatorial sweating in areas of symmetrical distribution and hyperhidrosis
5. Gastrointestinal disturbances including esophageal dysfunction, gastroparesis, diabetic enteropathy, diarrhea, and fecal incontinence including bacterial overgrowth and constipation
6. Genitourinary abnormalities including cystopathy, neurogenic bladder, defective vagi-nal lubrication, retrograde ejaculation, and erectile dysfunction

Cardiac autonomic neuropathy occurs in approximately 22% of patients with type-2 diabetes and can progress from initial manifestation of increased heart rate as a result of vagal denervation to fixed heart rates. In diabetic patients with heart rate variability, 5 year mortality rate is five times greater than those with normal variability with increased risk for sudden death and silent myocardial infarctions.

Cardiovascular autonomic neuropathy can manifest with [20]:

1. Resting tachycardia
2. Beat to beat variations
3. Accelerated heart rate response to standing
4. Postural hypotension with systolic blood pressure drops greater than 15 mmHg
5. Increased diastolic blood pressure greater than 16 mmHg in response to hand grip for 5 min
6. Prolongation of the Q-T interval greater than 444 ms
7. Nocturnal hypertension with early morning decreases in blood pressure
8. Neurocardiogenic syncope

These patients, because of these disturbances, may be more prone to developing a myocardial infarction in the evening as compared to the morning as we see in those individuals with normal autonomic function.

Impaired blood flow to the extremities can cause worsening neuropathy and impaired exercise tolerance. Excessive facial and trunk sweating can be manifested to compensate for impaired lower body sweating. Particularly common is the facial sweating immediately after eating (gustatory sweating). Gastrointestinal symptoms in diabetic patients may be close to 80% as a result of in impairments of both sympathetic and parasympathetic intervations [21].

Patients may experience delayed gastric secretion and emptying presenting with episodes of nausea and vomiting. Other symptoms can include anorexia, bloating, epigastric discomfort, and alternating episodes of constipation and diarrhea with diarrhea being more prominent in patients with autonomic neuropathy. Diarrhea can result due to pancreatic insufficiency, bacterial overgrowth, malabsorption, or intestinal hypermotility.

Diabetic diarrhea tends to present nocturnally, which can distinguish it from other causes of malabsorption including inflammatory bowel disease, tropical and non-tropical sprue (celiac disease), and infectious states.

Neurogenic abnormalities in the detrusor muscles or damaged afferent fibers impairing bladder sensation can cause impaired sensory and motor function in the urinary bladder. Dribbling, overflow incontinence and urinary retention may occur.

Quite often, erectile dysfunction may be the first manifestation of a developing autonomic neuropathy followed by episodes of diminished ejaculation, loss of ejaculatory effort or retrograde ejaculation. Poor glycemic control has shown to be the chief risk factor for autonomic neuropathy, although in the Pittsburgh Epidemiology Study, increased LDL, and hypertension were also contributing factors [22]. Other data has implied associations between systolic and diastolic blood pressure and lipid disturbances with neuropathies [20].

Clearly, exposures to other neurotoxins including pesticides, herbicides, cigarette smoking, alcohol, and adverse medication side effects as well as genetic predispositions can also increase the risk of neuropathy.

The cornerstone of treatment begins with tight glycemic control. Clinical studies have that the highest prevalence of diabetic peripheral neuropathy occurs in those patients with poorest diabetic control. The DCCT trial also confirmed significant benefits with intensive insulin therapy on preventing and inhibiting progression of neuropathy. In the UKPDS trial, tight glycemic control was associated with an improvement in vibratory sensation.

Various clinical trials have shown that ACE inhibitors can improve some of the symptoms of peripheral neuropathy increasing parasympathetic activity and improving heart rate variability. Trandolapril therapy showed improvement in amplitude, latency, and conduction velocities and lisinopril usage showed improvement in electrophysiologic and quantitative sensory tests after 12 weeks of therapy [23].

Other agents that have been tried with mixed success include gamma-linolenic acid, alpha-lipoic acid and other combinations utilizing these two chemical compounds. Daily infusion therapy of 600 or 1,200 mg of alpha-lipoic acid showed significant symptoms improvement compared to placebo in type-2 diabetic patients, with a two year trial in patients with diabetic polyneuropathy showing statistically significant improvement in nerve conduction velocity.

Studies with immunosuppressant agents like azathioprine, intravenous gamma globulin, and plasmaphoresis have been tried in the past with mixed success. Although phase II trials showed some promise with recombinant nerve growth factor therapy, this was not fulfilled or demonstrated in phase III studies. Not only has this diminished the interest in neuro-trophic factors, but these substances can cause pressure discomforts at the injection sites with hyperalgesia [18].

Diabetic neuropathic pain can be severely debilitating and is generally resistant to aceta-minophen, selective COX-2 inhibitors, and other NSAIDs. Treatment of these conditions has centered around the use of tricyclic antidepressants, antiepileptic drugs, selective sero-tonin reuptake inhibitors (SSRIs), sodium channel blockers, capsaicin, dextromethorphan, antiarrythmics, antiepileptics, and opioids.

Tricyclic antidepressants including desipramine, nortriptyline, and amitriptyline have been considered first line drugs in the treatment of neuropathic pain for many years. These agents work well in neuropathic pain by increasing serotonin, blocking sodium channels, and increasing post synaptic concentration of norepinephrine.

Unfortunately as many as 50% of patients will not get significant relief from the severe pain experienced with this condition.

Amitriptyline may cause some unwanted side effects including seizures, hypotension, increased sedation, hyperthermia, and other effects including constipation and pseudode-mentia. This can be significantly problematic in the elderly patient population, which may be prone to develop cardiac and other side effects.

Both first generation agents including carbamazepine, valproic acid, phenytoin and clon-azepam and second generation drugs including gabapentin, topiramate, lamotrigine and oxcarbazepine have been shown to have variable effectiveness in treating this condition.

Carbamazepine has been the drug of choice for treating trigeminal neuralgia for many years. Unfortunately, the multiple side effects of this drug including hepatic enzyme induc-tion, hyponatremia, thrombocytopenia, and multiple drug interactions have limited its use. Alpha-2 delta antagonists like pregabalin (Lyrica) and gabapentin (Neurontin) have shown some significant promise in relieving neuropathic pain. Pregabalin has FDA approval for diabetic neuropathy as well as postherpetic neuralgia. This Schedule V controlled sub-stance has been show to be efficacious in three randomized clinical trials with doses of 50–100 mg three times daily. Dose related dizziness, peripheral edema, and somnolence can occur at the higher doses (300–600 mg daily) with this type of treatment [18].

Topiramate has shown some inconsistent results although some tests have been promising. One placebo controlled double blinded study of 323 patients with diabetic peripheral neuropathy found that 36% of patients treated with topiramate at doses up to 400 mg a day for 12 weeks had greater than 50% reduction in symptoms. The dose of this drug can be quite variable although it is usually given on a twice daily basis.

Lamotrigine has been used with some effectiveness in trigeminal neuralgia and in HIV neuropathy, but is limited because of its significant effects including rash and rare occur-rence of Steven–Johnson syndrome.

The SSRIs have not been particularly effective and somewhat disappointing treat-ments for pain with a lack of consistency of performance in clinical trials. Venlafaxine (Effexor) has been shown to reduce pain by 75–100% in patients with diabetic periph-eral neuropathy, especially when used in higher doses (150–225 mg/day). The serotonin and norepinephrine reuptake inhibitor, duloxetine (Cymbalta), has also received approval for painful diabetic neuropathy at doses of (60–120 mg) daily as the result of two randomized placebo controlled trials. Side effects of decreased appetite, anorexia, weakness, dry mouth, somnolence, and dizziness were more commonly associated with the 120 mg dose.

Sodium channel blockers like the topical agent lidocaine (lidoderm), and mexiletine have been shown to be of benefit. In doses as high as 675 mg, mexiletine demonstrated its efficacy in diabetic peripheral neuropathy. The FDA approved the use of the 5% lidocaine patch in 2001 for the treatment of post herpetic neuralgia and this product has had some effectiveness in relieving the symptoms of peripheral neuropathy particularly when it is confined to smaller rather than diffuse areas of the extremities [13].

Capsaicin has also been shown to be effective in post-herpetic neuralgia and has been shown to have some benefit in diabetic peripheral neuropathy. However, the burning sensation and subsequent increased sensation of warmth can be very annoying to some patients who are already are experiencing a burning sensation from diabetic neuropathy.

Some clinical trials have shown varying benefit with dextromethorphan, but the drug is not available in formulations appropriate to deliver up to 600 mg a day, which appears to be the desired dose for achieving a benefit. In addition, this drug has been recently been a target for abuse and overdosing by adolescents.

Tramadol has been proven to be effective when given at doses of 200–400 mg a day for greater than 4 weeks. This product shares properties with opioid analgesics, but has a low affinity for the mu-opioid receptor. In controlled studies, its efficacy is comparable to the tricyclics and levorphanol. The commonest side effect is central nausea, similar to sea sickness, which can be somewhat attenuated by being well hydrated.

Controlled release oxycodone was shown to be an effective treatment for diabetic peripheral neuropathy with doses of 30 mg BID needed to achieve the desired effect. Dose dependence and drug abuse have raised some concern in primary circles about its ultimate use particularly on a chronic basis. For those patients who require narcotics, fentanyl patches have been shown to have opioid potency with significantly less central nervous system effects and constipation than the opioids. The patch also ensures compliance with the smooth drug delivery causing less fluctuation of analgesic blood levels [18].

Peripheral nerve stimulation has also been shown to be of occasional benefit. This would include percutaneous electrical nerve stimulation (TENS) and vibratory stimulation. These have been effective only for short term. Other alternative therapies include acupuncture and relaxation techniques.

Diabetic enteropathy can impair gastric acid secretion and motility, resulting in gastroparesis which is found in about 25% of diabetics. Typically, these patients present with early satiety, nausea, vomiting, epigastric pain, bloating, and anorexia. These episodes may last for several months on a cyclical basis with vomiting of undigested food particles.

Other conditions like gastric or duodenal ulcer, gastritis, and gastric cancers should be excluded. This problem can interfere with nutrient delivery to the small bowel and impair glucose absorption and even absorption of medication. Wide swings of glycemia occur commonly.

Although the severity of symptoms does not always correlate with scintigraphic imaging, consumption of radionucleotide labeled food can be of value in making the diagnosis, demonstrating impaired gastric emptying.

Diabetic gastroenteropathy remains a difficult condition to treat particularly with the withdrawal of cisapride from the market. Initial treatment should focus on tight glycemic control with patients advised to eat multiple small meals of 4–6 oz daily with reduced fat intake (less than 40 g daily). Fiber intake should be reduced to prevent bezoar formation [21].

Metoclopramide (Reglan) is perhaps the best studied drug and is usually given in a dose of 10–40 mg in divided doses before meals and at bedtime. Although in general this drug is well tolerated, side effects can result in galactorrhea, irregular menses, erectile dysfunction, and may exacerbate Parkinson's disease or cause symptoms of Parkinsonism in other individuals. Other common side effects include gynecomastia, tardive dyskinesia and fatigue.

Macrolide antibiotics, including erythromycin, can be somewhat effective in improving gastric emptying. Very low doses of erythromycin (125 mg in divided doses daily) are often sufficient in relieving symptoms. This dose can easily be administered with a liquid suspension. This lower dose tends to minimize the typical side effects from this antibiotic, including abdominal pain, nausea, and vomiting. Another dopamine antagonist, domperidone, has a central antiemetic effect, but is currently not available in the USA and has had side effects including diarrhea, galactorrhea, and headache. Levosulpiride, a prokinetic selective antagonist for D2 dopamine receptors, at 25 mg three times daily can also be tried to improve gastric emptying.

The topical clonidine patch appears to be a particularly useful agent in treatment of gastroparesis and diarrhea whether as initial therapy or in individuals concomitantly needing the medication for hypertension control.

Diabetic diarrhea affects 20% of diabetics and is characterized by intermittent patterns of episodes lasting from several hours to several days. Here, nocturnal diarrhea and fecal incontinence are common. The patient may have up to 20–30 bowel movements in a 24 h period.

Causes of diarrhea in a diabetic patient include [21]:

1. Diminished sympathetic inhibition
2. Hypomotility with bacterial overgrowth
3. Pancreatic insufficiency
4. Steatorrhea
5. Bile salt malabsorption

Octreotide, 50 mg three times daily, or loperamide 2 mg four times daily, may be helpful for diarrhea.

Diabetic sexual dysfunction and impotence is a very common complaint in the male patient population and is usually caused by circulatory and/or nervous system abnormalities. Females may experience a lack of lubrication, painful intercourse, and difficulty achieving orgasm. Usually most patients can be treated non-invasively with some success.

The three agents currently available for use in the USA for males are:

1. Sildenafil (Viagra)
2. Tadalafil (Cialis)
3. Vardenafil (Levitra)

Sildenafil can be taken in doses of 25, 50, or 100 mg 1 h before sexual activity, but works best on an empty stomach with at least 4–5 h after eating a meal before the pill can be taken. Food can be ingested, however, 1 h after taking sildenafil on an essentially empty stomach [20].

This substance results in increases in nitric oxide levels and has been extremely successful in restoring normal sexual dysfunction to many. The drug should not be used in patients taking nitroglycerin preparations or in individuals with active coronary ischemia. The drug needs to be used with caution in patients who are on medications that are metabolized through the cytochrome P450-3A4 system. Similar caveats exist with the other two sexual dysfunction medications.

Tadalafil (Cialis) has an onset of action similar to sildenafil with a prolonged duration of action of up to 36 h compared to the 4–6 h with sildenafil and vardenafil. Tadalafil is also available in a daily low dose pill (2.5–5 mg). The utility of these drugs have made other options like penile prosthesis, vacuum constriction devices, and intracavernosal injection of vasoactive agents and intraurethral insertions less attractive.

These phosphodiesterase type-5 inhibitors have several cardiovascular effects including:

1. Decrease in blood pressure at rest
2. Increased exercise time and oxygen consumption in congestive heart failure
3. Decreased peak exercise heart rate in congestive heart failure
4. Increased coronary flow reserve
5. Increased coronary blood flow
6. Improved endothelial function
7. Decreased pulmonary artery blood pressure and vascular resistance in pulmonary hypertension
8. Decreased aortic stiffness

The ease of use of these products makes normal sexual activity and performance a realistic possibility for many diabetic males who have been frustrated with this problem. Hopefully, some assistance will be provided for female diabetics in the future.

DIABETIC NEPHROPATHY

Diabetic nephropathy is the most frequent cause of end-stage renal disease in the USA, Japan, and Europe, affecting 20–30% of patients with diabetes. In Europe and the USA, the incidence of diabetic nephropathy has increased substantially arising by 150% in the past 10 years in this country alone. Among those patients who require dialysis, 40% of patients had diabetic nephropathy and a 15% higher mortality at 5 years and a 22% higher mortality at 1 year than their non-diabetic cohorts [24]. Early diagnosis followed by aggressive treatment play important roles in delaying the progression of kidney disease.

Patients with diabetes should be screened annually for nephropathy even with no history of kidney disease since type-1 diabetics will usually develop nephropathy within 5 years of diagnosis, while type-2 diabetics can manifest early nephropathy within 10 years.

Table 1 summarizes strategies to prevent diabetic nephropathy.

Table 1
Recommendations for preventing and treating diabetic nephropathy

Optimize glucose control

Optimize blood pressure control

Reduce LDL <100 mg/dl with statin therapy

Both ACE inhibitors and ARBs can be used to treat albuminuria and hypertension

For hypertensive type-2 diabetics with microalbuminuria, ARBs are the initial agents of choice

With the onset of nephropathy, restrict protein to less than 0.8 g/kg of body weight daily

Combinations of ACE inhibitors and ARBs will decrease albuminuria more than with either agent alone

Direct renin inhibitors may have additive effects when used with ACE inhibitors or ARBs

From American Diabetes Association [42]

PATHOPHYSIOLOGY OF DIABETIC NEPHROPATHY

In 1936, Kimmelstiel and Wilson originally described the nodular intercapillary glomerulosclerosis characteristic of diabetes, although a diffuse pattern of glomerulosclerosis can also be seen. These glomerular changes are usually preceded by thickening of the basement membrane, podocyte loss, mesangial expansion, and glomerular hyperfiltration. These changes are usually associated with retinal capillary microaneurysms. Once macroalbuminuria develops, progressive loss of intrinsic ultrafiltration capacity follows and the glomerular filtration rate (GFR) drops rapidly.

The earliest manifestation of diabetic nephropathy is microalbuminuria usually preceded by nocturnal systolic hypertension. The American Diabetes Association position statement on diabetic nephropathy states that microalbuminuria is present if the microalbumin/creatinine ratio exceeds 30 µg/mg creatinine in a spot urine, greater than 30 mg of albumin in a 24-h collection, or greater than 20 µg of albumin per minute in a 4-h timed specimen. The threshold for macroalbuminuria is reached at greater than 300 µg/mg creatinine. The classification of a patient should be based on at least 2 or 3 abnormal results on specimens collected within a 3–6 month period of time.

This can be measured in different ways [25]:

1. Non-timed or spot urinary albumin collections measured in micrograms of albumin/mg of creatinine
   (a) Normal – less than 30 µg albumin/mg creatinine
   (b) Microalbuminuria – 30–299 µg albumin/mg creatinine
   (c) Clinical or macroalbuminuria equal or >300 µg albumin/mg creatinine
2. Timed specimens with a 4-h collection
   (a) Normal – less than 20 µg of albumin/minute
   (b) Microalbuminuria – 20–199 µg of albumin/minute
   (c) Clinical or macroalbuminuria – equal or >200 µg of albumin/minute

3. Timed specimens with a 24-h collection
   (a) Normal – less than 30 mg/24 h
   (b)   Microalbuminuria – 30–299 mg/24 h
   (c) Clinical or macroalbuminuria – >300 mg/24 h

The preferred method is the spot urine collection with a first morning void specimen, since the time urine collection can present challenges and difficulties with compliance.

It should be kept in mind that the urine dipstick is too insensitive for this purpose, since it will only turn positive when albumin excretion exceeds 300 mg/day. Remember as well that proteinuria without albuminuria may indicate the presence of a paraproteinemia warranting serum protein electrophoresis. False positive results can occur with congestive heart failure, fever, urinary tract infection, and exercise. Commonly, two elevated levels out of three measurements covering a 3–6 month period of time are required to define nephropathy.

Looking deeper into the interplay of factors underlying the mechanisms of diabetic nephropathy, one must appreciate the critical role of glomerular hypertension and its progression from hyperfiltration to overt nephropathy. Adler in 2004 pinpointed mesangial expansion as the defining abnormality in diabetic nephropathy, encroaching on the capillary lumen initiating the progression to renal failure [26]. He also pointed out that other important factors contribute to progressive proteinuria including alterations and injury to the podocyte pore membrane, glomerular basement membrane detachment, and signal transduction changes that result in apoptosis. Proteinuria itself enhances tubulointerstitial atrophy and fibrosis, accelerating nephropathy and compounded by arteriolar sclerotic lesions which foster ischemia. The prime mover in all this physiologic disaster is angiotensin II, which interacts with various cytokines and growth factors that are activated by and travel along the same signaling pathways ultimate leading to fibrosis, inflammation, and nephrological deterioration.

Individuals who have had type-2 diabetes for 10–15 years will develop microalbuminuria in 20–40% of cases. This tends to progress to macroalbuminuria with albumin levels greater than 200 µg/ml or greater than 300 mg/g of creatinine or greater than 200 µg/min or greater than 300 mg in a 24-h period.

Patients with macroalbuminuria are termed as having overt nephropathy. Creatinine clearance begins to decline at a steady rate once macroalbuminuria is present. The rates vary from patient to patient, but the average reduction is 10–12 ml/min per year of creatinine clearance in untreated patient [25].

Uncontrolled hyperglycemia, hypertension, and dyslipidemia can accelerate the progression to end-stage renal disease. Microalbuminuria is indicative of abnormal vascular responses and increased permeability of the endothelium at the glomerular level. Renal cells in Bowman's capsule are particularly vulnerable to the vascular permeability of increased blood pressure that is characteristic of diabetes. Once glomerular pressure begins to increase insipiently, the GFR begins to drop causing glomerulosclerosis and subsequent progression from microalbuminuria to severe proteinuria.

Protein that is normally secreted is 60% non-albumin and 40% albumin. The changes in type-2 diabetes are slightly different than those observed in the type-1 diabetic. Initially in type-1 diabetes, increases in GFR result from an increase in renal size that is generally reversible with glycemic control. Glomerular thickening and widening of the basement membrane occur without proteinuria. These early microscopic cellular changes are then followed by microalbuminuria which tends to progress. After 10–15 years of type-1 diabetes, approximately 80% of patients will have some degree of proteinuria, progressing to overt nephropathy, and end stage renal disease without proper intervention – 50% within 10 years and 75% within 20 years [27].

This differs slightly from the type-2 diabetic in which more of the latter tend to have proteinuria at the time of presentation. Without treatment, 20–40% of proteinuric type-2 diabetics will progress to overt nephropathy and subsequent end-stage renal disease. This probably is related to the fact that type-2 diabetes is often present for many years before being identified. Although the rate of progression to end-stage renal disease is somewhat slower in type-2 diabetes, prolonged periods of increased albuminuria and hypertension are associated with an enhancement in cardiovascular mortality and morbidity risk. In diabetic patients who also have hypertension, glomerular thickening accompanies capillary basement membrane changes. This initiates a decline in renal function by compromising capillary filtration surface.

Subsequently, this continued glomerular thickening can lead to intercapillary glomerulosclerosis, shrinkage, and scarring and if not treated can progress to end-stage renal disease. In recent years treatment guidelines to prevent or slow the progression of diabetic renal disease has included not only tight glycemic and lipid control, but a more aggressive stance on blood pressure [28]. The fact that not all type-1 or type-2 diabetics progress to nephropathy may also suggest a genetic susceptibility triggered by hypertension and inadequate metabolic regulation.

The National Kidney Foundation has defined five stages of renal disease [29]. These are listed in Table 2.

Patients with stages 3–5 renal disease should be referred to a nephrologist.

The Joint National Committee on The Prevention, Detection, Evaluation and Treatment of Hypertension (JNC-6) established a blood pressure of less than 130/85 mmHg in patients with diabetes. This limit has been lowered even lower since then. Several expert panels including the American Diabetes Association and The Canadian Hypertension Society have subsequently adopted a blood pressure goal of less than 130/80 mmHg.

Table 2
Stages of renal disease

Stage 1 – Some degree of kidney damage due to abnormal imaging, urine, blood, or pathology results with a normal or increased glomerular filtration rate (GFR) equal to or greater than 90 ml/min per 1.73 m^2 body surface area

Stage 2 – Kidney damage with a mildly decreased GFR (60–89 ml/min)

Stage 3 – Moderately decreased GFR (30–59 ml/min)

Stage 4 – Severely decreased GFR (15–29 ml/min)

Stage 5 – Kidney failure GFR <15 ml/min or on dialysis

From National Kidney Foundation [29]

As a result of the increased risk of progression to end-stage renal disease in individuals with blood pressures greater than 125/75 mmHg and greater than 1 g a day of proteinuria, the National Kidney Foundation set a blood pressure goal of less than 125/75 mmHg for diabetic patients with proteinuria greater than a gram a day and renal insufficiency. Along with the changes in blood pressure requirements, there have been recommendations for changes of agents to use in patients with diabetic nephropathy.

The first choice agents by JNC-6 were the ACE inhibitors, delaying the onset of microalbuminuria in diabetic patients without nephropathy and reducing all cause mortality in nephropathic diabetic patients. The American Diabetes Association Guidelines released in 2006 recommended ACE inhibitors or angiotensin receptor blockers (ARBs) as the first choice in patients with type-1 diabetes and micro or macroalbuminuria or overt nephropathy except during pregnancy. The National Kidney Foundation has also recommended ARBs as the treatment choice for patients with chronic kidney disease in the absence of proteinuria [30]. ACE inhibitors have been shown to delay the progression of nephropathy in type-1 diabetics with hypertension and albuminuria, while both ACEs and ARBs have been shown to delay microalbuminuria progression in type-2 diabetics with the ARBs shown to delay the progression of nephropathy in those patients with macroalbuminuria and renal insufficiency (serum creatinine >1.5 mg/dl).

The basis of our therapeutic approach is to block the release and subsequent activity of angiotensin II which is the end product of the renin-angiotensin pathway. Angiotensin II is not only one of the most potent vasoconstrictors, but also has significant detrimental effects at the cellular level. Angiotensin II increases the intraglomerular pressure by narrowing the renal efferent arterials. This subsequently increases the glomerular capillary pressure putting significant pressure on the walls.

Angiotensin II may also cause disruption of the supporting cells within the renal glomerulus causing small amounts of protein to leak through the capillary walls. Hence blocking the effect of angiotensin II and decreasing its production has been shown to have direct beneficial effect decreasing the production of interstitial and glomerular matrix protein, reducing proteinuria, and lowering both systemic and glomerular hypertension.

ACE inhibitors block the synthesis of angiotensin II and inhibit angiotensin converting enzyme along with inhibiting the degradation of vasodilatory bradykinin and increasing nitric oxide levels. Approximately 50% of the angiotensin II produced in the body goes through this mechanism with 90% of that produced in the tissues. Angiotensin receptor blockers prevent the binding of angiotensin II to its type II receptor site preventing its vasoconstrictor effects [31].

Thirty percent of patients with type-2 diabetes are hypertensive when the diagnosis is made and 70% are hypertensive when nephropathy develops. Renovascular arteriosclerotic disease is present in up to 40% of those patients with overt nephropathy and contributes to 20% of those with hypertension. ACE inhibitors have established themselves as antihypertensive and renal protective agents in patients with diabetes and are particularly effective in decreasing the risk of development or progression of nephropathy.

These agents are particularly effective in decreasing intraglomerular pressure by selectively dilating glomerular efferent arterioles. This renal protective effect can delay or prevent the development of glomerulosclerosis and in some instances can be independent of its antihypertensive effect. Captopril (Capoten) was shown to slow the progression of nephropathy by 50% in patients with type-1 diabetes despite the fact that median blood pressures in the captopril group and the placebo group were comparable throughout the trial. These individuals had urinary protein excretions of greater than 500 mg/day [32].

Over a 7-year period of time, enalapril was evaluated in 94 patients with type-2 diabetes and normal blood pressure with microalbuminuria. Albumin excretion and serum creatinine levels remained stable over the 7-year course of time in those individuals who were on the ACE inhibitor with subsequent reduction of the absolute risk of nephropathy by about 42%. This was in sharp contrast to those patients who did not take the ACE inhibitor in which albumin rates steadily climbed. When these placebo treated patients were switched to enalapril (Vasotec), the albumin excretion stabilized for the final 2 years and interestingly began to rise again in the enalapril patients who declined treatment after the first 5 years. This served as evidence that the ACE inhibitors can stabilize renal function in previously untreated patients and can offer some significant long-term protection.

The diabetic sub-study of the Heart Outcomes Prevention Evaluation (HOPE) study also called the MICRO-HOPE trial showed that, compared to placebo at equivalent blood pressures, ramipril decreased the rate of progression to overt nephropathy by 24% in patients who were either normal albuminuric or with microalbuminuria. Although the significant benefits in the MICRO-HOPE trial were in the cardiovascular area, the combined microvascular outcomes, including the need for dialysis, retinopathy laser therapy or overt nephropathy was reduced by 16% in the ramipril group with reduction in overall proteinuria regardless of the presence of microalbuminuria at entry [24].

This was the first trial to actually demonstrate that ACE inhibitor therapy can prevent the development of proteinuria in patients who had normal protein upon institution of therapy. Six other small trials involving a total of 352 patients with type-2 diabetes and overt nephropathy showed ACE inhibitors to be superior to other antihypertensive drugs in reducing proteinuria. Angiotensin II receptor antagonists were not part of this study. These studies were not sufficiently empowered, however, to detect an effect on the rate of decline of GFR.

ARBs prevent the binding of angiotensin II at the level of angiotensin II type I receptor. This offers a more complete blockade of the effects of angiotensin II since ACE inhibitors do not eliminate all the production of this substance. The angiotensin type I receptor mediates the presser, arteriosclerotic, and hypertrophic effects of angiotensin II. The unbound angiotensin II then attaches to another receptor site, which renders beneficial cardiovascular vasodilator effects [33].

In animal models, the ARBs attenuate proteinuria, glomerulosclerosis, and renal hypertrophy slowing the progression of albuminuria and subsequent development of overt nephropathy. In addition, the ARBs do not cause cough. In those individuals who develop angioedema from ACE inhibitors, ARBs should not be used because of the crossover effect that has been demonstrated.

Short term effects of losartan and enalapril were evaluated in 16 patients with type-2 diabetes with a crossover design. Reductions in blood pressure and overt albuminuria were similar while there was no change in GFR. Reduction of End-points in Non-insulin dependent Diabetes Mellitus with the angiotensin II Antagonist Losartan (RENAAL) trial compared losartan 50–100 mg once daily with placebo [*34*], evaluating composite end points of doubling of the baseline serum creatinine, onset of end-stage renal disease or death.

In this trial, the ARB demonstrated a 16% reduction in the primary end-point with significant renal protection in patients with type-2 diabetes and nephropathy after a period of 3.4 years. Losartan also reduced the risk of doubling the serum creatinine concentration by 25% and significantly reduced the risk of end-stage renal disease by 28%. This converted into a general delay for the need of dialysis by 2 years [*33*].

The Irbesartan Diabetic Nephropathy Trial (IDNT) was designed to determine which of three treatments, amlodipine, placebo, or irbesartan would most effectively slow the progression of nephropathy in patients with type-2 diabetes. Irbesartan significantly attenuated the rate of progression compared to the placebo or amlodipine despite similar blood pressure reductions. There was also a 37% risk reduction in doubling the serum creatinine with irbesartan [*35*]. The Irbesartan Microalbuminuria in Type-2 Diabetes Mellitus and Hypertensive Patients (IRMA-2) study once again confirmed that irbesartan significantly reduced the rate of progression to overt diabetic nephropathy compared to placebo, with urine albumin excretion decreased by 38% of the group with 300 mg of irbesartan, 24% of the group with 150 mg of irbesartan, and only 2% in placebo, this was despite no significant changes in blood pressure [*36*].

In addition, the group assigned 300 mg of irbesartan began to separate significantly from placebo at 3 months. This stresses the importance of early detection, emphasizing that preventing or delaying the development of diabetic nephropathy can be achieved with proper identification of high risk patients and appropriate renal protective therapy [*37*].

Malacco et al. investigated the efficacy and tolerability of valsartan 80 mg/day with that of lisinopril 5 or 10 mg/day in 188 hypertensive patients and renal insufficiency over a 13-week period of time in the PREVAIL (Blood Pressure and Tolerability of valsartan in comparison with lisinopril) trial [*38*]. This study supported the concept that the effects of ACEs and ARBs were similar resulting from blockade of the renin-angiotensin system. Data from this study showed the changes in both groups with regard to IGG fractional clearance, GFR, albumin clearances, blood pressure changes, and 24-h protein to be similar.

Other studies comparing valsartan and captopril over a 52-week period of time showed comparable effects of the ACE inhibitor and the angiotensin receptor blocker. Further trials were conducted evaluating the efficacy of using both an ACE inhibitor and an ARB in reducing proteinuria. Early indications in animal models are that the combination can be synergistic in proteinuria reduction as is seen with combination ACE inhibitor and calcium channel blocker.

It is important to understand that unopposed dihydropyridine calcium channel blockers may worsen proteinuria, which can increase the progression of renal disease in diabetic patients, this effect can be somewhat attenuated with the addition of an ACE inhibitor. Non-dihydropyridine calcium blockers have not shown this effect [*39*].

Meta-analyses have shown that the dihydropyridine calcium channel blockers in general demonstrated more rapid decline in GFR and more severe proteinuria than other antihypertensive agents in the type-2 diabetic. In the Reduction in Endpoints in Non-insulin Dependent Diabetes Mellitus with the Angiotensin II Antagonist Losartan (RENAAL) trial, dihydropyridines were combined with the ARB losartan and this effect was not seen, lending credence to the fact that not only ACE inhibitors, but perhaps ARBs as well can help prevent proteinuria in diabetic individuals [39].

Beta-blockers have also shown to be of some benefit in treatment of diabetic nephropathy. In the UKPDS trial, both ACE inhibitors and beta-blockers worked equally well in lowering the incidence of micro and macroalbuminuria in the type-2 diabetic study with similar renal protective effects in both the beta-blockers and the ACE inhibitors on renal function.

As of the present time there are no recommendations that beta-blockers are equal to angiotensin receptor agents or even ACE inhibitors in terms of renal protective or protein sparing effect in diabetic kidneys.

Hyperglycemia has been known to be a significant risk factor for diabetic nephropathy, with mean levels of hemoglobin A1C correlating with subsequent loss of renal function. The United Kingdom Perspective Diabetes Study (UKPDS) showed that intensive glycemic control reduced the risk of diabetic nephropathy as well as other microvascular complications. The Kumamoto Study in Japan showed that intensive treatment with three or more insulin injections per day reduced the risk of progressive nephropathy by 28%.

Dyslipidemia is known to be a significant problem in type-2 diabetics especially those with nephropathy. Meta-analyses of 13 controlled studies involving 253 diabetic patients indicated that statins were effective in preserving GFR in patients with chronic renal disease and decreased proteinuria independent of reduction in blood cholesterol. Protein restriction has been shown to reduce decline in GFR and proteinuria in type-2 diabetics with restrictions of protein intake to 0.8 mg/kg/day reducing the rate of progression to end-stage renal disease [40].

The presence of microalbuminuria, while increasing the risk of overall cardiovascular disease two to fourfold, is a surrogate marker for double to triple vessel coronary artery disease with a linear increase demonstrated in type-2 diabetic patients with microalbuminuria compared to non-diabetic non-microalbuminuric controls. In addition, diabetics with microalbuminuria tend to have higher fasting glucose and A1C levels than diabetics without microalbuminuria.

Also to be kept in mind are the dramatic increases in cardiovascular risk associated with the various stages of renal disease.

These are as follows [41]:

Stage cardiovascular risk odds ratio

Stage 1	Increases with amount of proteinuria
Stage 2	1.5
Stage 3	2–4
Stage 4	4–10
Stage 5	10–50
End stage renal disease	20–100

Smoking is known to increase the development and the progression of both macrovascular and microvascular disease and has been shown to be an independent risk factor in the development of nephropathy in type-2 diabetics. Smoking cessation alone may reduce the risk of disease progression by 30%.

Various epidemiologic factors can also effect the progression and development of diabetic nephropathy with race being the best known and most established. Hispanics, African Americans, and Native Americans all have a higher incidence of end-stage renal disease than whites. African American women are 2.3 times as likely as White women to develop end-stage renal disease with African men 1.4 times as likely. Mexicans and Native Americans are nearly 3 times as likely as Whites to develop end-stage renal disease and proteinuria [40].

Gender also appears to play a small role in end-stage renal disease. Fifty-nine percent of men with type-2 diabetes vs. 44% of women need long-term dialysis.

SUMMARY

The current clinical practice guidelines issued by the Canadian Diabetes Association and the American Diabetes Association for the management of type-2 diabetes recommend tight blood pressure control with systolic blood pressures less than 125 and diastolic blood pressures less than 75 in individuals with microalbuminuria, tight glycemic control, and protein intake not exceeding 0.8 g/kg/day along with life style modifications that include exercise, weight loss, cessation of smoking, and reduction of salt intake.

Use of ACE inhibitors and ARBs can be invaluable in preventing and retarding the progression of this disease. LDL cholesterols should be maintained at levels below 100 mg/dl. Early detection of nephropathy remains a cornerstone to diagnosis and prevention. Screening should start with a routine urinalysis with quantitative determination of albuminuria in abnormal cases. Further discussion of treatment will be referred to a later chapter on risk reduction.

REFERENCES

1. UK Prospective Diabetes Study Group. Tight blood pressure control and risk of macrovascular and microvascular complications in type 2 diabetes: UKPDS 38. BMJ 1998;317:703–713.
2. Davis MD, Blodi BA. Proliferative diabetic retinopathy. In: Ryan SJ, Schachat AP, eds. Retina. Vol 2, 4th ed. St. Louis: Mosby, 2006:1285–1322.
3. Geslain Biquez C, Vol S, Tichet J, Caradec A, D'Hour A, Balkou B. The metabolic syndrome in smokers (The DESIR study). Diabetes Metab 2003;29(3):226–234.
4. American Diabetes Association. Diabetic retinopathy. Diabetes Care 2002;26 (suppl 1):S99–S102.
5. Boulton AJ. Treatment of symptomatic diabetic retinopathy. Diabetes Metab Res Rev 2003;29 (suppl 1):S16–S21.
6. Chaturvedi N, Porta M, Klein R, Orchard T, Fuller J, Parvin HH, Bilous R. Effect of candesartan on prevention (DIRECT-Prevent 1) and progression (DIRECT-Protect 1) of retinopathy in type-1 diabetes. Lancet 2008;372:1394–1402.
7. Chaturvedi N, Sjolie AK, Stephenson JM. Effect of lisinopril on progression of retinopathy in normotensive people with type-1 diabetes. The EUCLID Study group. EURODIAB controlled trial of lisinopril in insulin dependent diabetes mellitus. Lancet 1998;351:28–31.
8. Sjolie AK, Klein R, Porta M. Effect of candesartan on progression and regression of retinopathy in type-2 diabetes (DIRECT-Protect 2). Lancet 2008;372:1385–1392.

9. Early Treatment Diabetic Retinopathy Study Research Group. Early photocoagulation for diabetic retinopathy. Ophthalmology 1991;98:766–785.

10. Aiello LP, Gardner TW, King GL, et al. Diabetic retinopathy. Diabetes Care 1998;21:143–156.

11. Klein BD, Moss SE, Klein R, Surawicz TS. The Wisconsin Epidemiologic Study of Diabetic Retinopathy XIII. Ophthalmology 1991;98:1261–1265.

12. The Diabetes Control and Complications Trial Research Group. Four risk factors for severe visual loss in diabetic retinopathy: the third report of the Diabetic Retinopathy Study. Arch Ophthalmol 1979;97:654–655.

13. Wolfe GI, Baroh RJ, et al. Painful neuropathy. Curr Treat Options Neurol 2002;4:177–188.

14. Vinik A. Diagnosis and management of diabetic neuropathy. Clin Geriatr Med 1999;15:293–320.

15. Costa LA, Canani LH, Lisboa HR, Tres GS, Gross JL. Aggregation of features of the metabolic syndrome is associated with increased prevalence of chronic complications in type-2 diabetes. Diabet Med 2004;21;252–255.

16. Sumner CJ, Sheth S, Griffin JW, Cornblath DR, Polydefkis M. The spectrum of neuropathy in diabetes and impaired glucose tolerance. Neurology 2003;60:108–111.

17. Vinik AI, Park TS, Stransberry KB, Pittenger GL. Diabetic neuropathies. Diabetologia 2000;43:957–973.

18. Spruce MC, Potter J, et al. The pathogenesis and management of painful diabetic neuropathy: a review. Diabet Med 2003;20:88–98.

19. American Diabetes Association American Academy of Neurology. Consensus statement: report and recommendations of the San Antonio conference on diabetic neuropathy. Diabetes Care 1988;11:592–597.

20. Ewing DJ, Campbell IW, et al. The natural history of diabetic autonomic neuropathy. Q J Med 1980;49:95–108.

21. Verne GN, Snisky CA. Diabetes and the gastrointestinal tract. Gastroenterol Clin North Am 1998;27:861–874.

22. Maser RE, Pfeifer MA, Dorman JS, Kuller LH, Becker DJ, Orchard TJ. Diabetic autonomic neuropathy and cardiovascular risk. Pittsburgh epidemiology of diabetes complications study. Arch Intern Med 1990;150(6):1218–1222.

23. Locatelli F, Del Vecchio L. How long can dialysis be postponed by low protein diet and ACE inhibitors. Nephrol Dial Transplant 1999;14:1360–1364.

24. American Diabetes Association. Diabetic nephropathy. Diabetes Care 2003;26 (suppl 1):S94–S98.

25. Kidney Disease Outcome Quality Initiative. Clinical practice guidelines for chronic kidney disease: evaluation, classification and stratification. Am J Kidney Dis 2002;39 (suppl 2):S1–S246.

26. Adler AI, Stevens RJ, Manley SE, Bilous RW, Cull CA, Holman RR. Development and progression of nephropathy in type-2 diabetes. BMJ 2004;328:1105–1108.

27. Mogensen CE, et al. Microalbuminuria and potential confounders. A review and some observations on variability of urinary albumin excretion. Diabetes Care 1995;18:572.

28. Nambi V, Hoogwerf B, Sprecher D. Clev Clin J Med. 2002;9(12):985–989.

29. National Kidney Foundation. K/DOQI clinical practice guidelines for chronic kidney disease: evaluation, classification, and stratification. Am J Kidney Dis 2002;39 (suppl 1):S1–S266.

30. Mattock MB, Morrish NJ, et al. Prospective study of microalbuminuria as a predictor of mortality in NIDDM. Diabetes 1992;41:736–741.

31. Sharma K, Ziyadeh FN. Hyperglycemia and diabetic kidney disease: the case for TGF-beta as a key mediator. Diabetes 1995;94:1139–1146.

32. Bakris GL. Microalbuminuria: prognostic implications. Curr Opin Nephrol Hypertens 1996;5:219–223.

33. Keane WF, Lyle PA. Recent advances in the management of type 2 diabetes and nephropathy: lessons from the RENAAL study. Am J Kidney Dis 2003;41 (3 suppl 1)S22–S25.

34. Brenner BM, Cooper ME, de Zeeuw D. Effects of losartan on renal and cardiovascular outcomes in patients with type-2 diabetes and nephropathy. The RENAAL Trial. N Engl J Med 2001;345:861–869.

35. Coats AJ. Angiotensin receptor blockers – finally the evidence is coming in: IDNT and RENAAL. Int J Cardiol 2001;79:99–102.

36. Lewis EJ, Hunsicker LG, Clarke WR. Renoprotective effect of the angiotensin receptor antagonist irbesartan in patients with nephropathy due to type-2 diabetes. N Engl J Med 2001;345:851–860.

37. Lewis EJ, Hunsicker LG, et al. Renoprotective effect of the angiotensin-receptor antagonist irbesartan in patients with nephropathy due to type 2 diabetes. N Engl J Med 2001;345:851–860.

38. Malacco E, Santonastaso M, Vari N, Gargiulo A, Spagnuolo V, Bertocci F, Palodini P. Comparison of valsartan with lisinopril for the treatment of hypertension: the PREVAIL study. Clin Ther 2004;26(6):855–865.
39. Brenner BM, Cooper ME, et al. Effects of losartan on renal and cardiovascular outcomes in patients with type 2 diabetes and nephropathy. N Engl J Med 2001;345:861–869.
40. Pedrini MT, et al. The effect of dietary protein restriction on the progression of diabetic and nondiabetic renal disease: a meta-analysis. Ann Intern Med 1996:124:627–632.
41. Anavekar NS, McMurray JJ, Velasquez EJ. Relation between renal dysfunction and cardiovascular outcomes after myocardial infarction. N Engl J Med 2004;351(13):1285–1295.
42. American Diabetes Association. Standards of medical care for patients with diabetes mellitus. Diabetes Care 2002;25 (suppl 1):S33–S49.

SUPPLEMENTARY READINGS

Benjamin L. Glucose, VEGF-A, and diabetic complications. Am J Pathol 2001;158:1181–1184.
Eddy A. Interstitial nephritis induced by protein overload proteinuria. Am J Pathol 1989;135:719–733.
Kendall DM, Harmel AP. The metabolic syndrome, type 2 diabetes, and cardiovascular disease: understanding the role of insulin resistance. Am J Manag Care 2002;8 (20 suppl):S635–S653.
Lovestam-Adrian M, et al. Diabetic retinopathy, visual acuity, and medical risk indicators. J Diabetes Complications 2001;15:287–294.
Morgensen CE. Natural history of cardiovascular and renal disease in patients with type 2 diabetes: Effect of therapeutic interventions and risk modifications. Am J Cardiol 1998;82:4R–8R.
Valmadred CT, et al. The risk of cardiovascular disease mortality associated with microalbuminuria and gross proteinuria with older onset diabetes mellitus. Arch Intern Med 2000;160:1093–1099.
Ziegler D, et al. Effects of treatment with the antioxidant alpha-lipoic acid on cardiac autonomic neuropathy in NIDDM patients. Diabetes Care 1997;20:369–373.
Zucchelli P, Zuccala A, et al. Comparison of the effects of ACE inhibitors and calcium channel blockers on the progression of renal failure. Nephrol Dial Transplant 1995;10 (suppl 9):46–51.

11 Diabetic Dyslipidemia

CONTENTS

Key Words: Diabetic dyslipidemia, Risk determination, NHANES III, Metabolic syndrome, Insulin resistance, Lipoprotein metabolism

INTRODUCTION

Insulin Resistance represents the central unifying principle of the clustering of abnormalities defining the Metabolic Syndrome and the hallmark of type-2 diabetes. A review of data from NHANES III indicated that 85% of individuals older than 50 with the Metabolic Syndrome were insulin resistant [1]. Even in the absence of over hyperglycemia, or abnormal glucose tolerance, insulin resistance is associated with abnormal lipid and lipoprotein metabolism, characterized by elevated triglycerides and low plasma levels of HDL cholesterol with an increase in the production of small, dense LDL (low density lipoprotein) particles as outlined in Table 1. However, total cholesterol and LDL levels are comparable to individuals who are not diabetic, underscoring the importance of quantitative and qualitative lipid measurement, including total particle number and size, to accurately assess cardiovascular risk.

PATHOGENESIS OF DIABETIC DYSLIPIDEMIA

Lipid disorders in individuals with insulin resistance progressively worsen across a spectrum of glucose tolerance from normal to impaired to frank type-2 diabetes. This pattern of atherogenicity in individuals with insulin resistance extends through ethnic lines including Hispanic and African Americans.

From: *Current Clinical Practice: Type 2 Diabetes, Pre-Diabetes, and the Metabolic Syndrome*,
Edited by: R.A. Codario, DOI 10.1007/978-1-60327-441-8_11
© Springer Science+Business Media, LLC 2011

Table 1
Lipoprotein abnormalities in type-2 diabetes

Increased LDL

Increased VLDL

Increased remnants

Decreased HDL

Increased triglycerides

Increased small, dense LDL

Enhanced glycation of LDL

Enhanced oxidation of LDL

Enhanced antibody formation promoting atherogenesis

Increased triglyceride rich lipoproteins due to decreased

Lipoprotein lipase activity

From Mykkanen et al. [50]

Enhanced cardiovascular risk in women may be partially explained by the fact that insulin resistance and type-2 diabetes have a greater impact on surrogate markers like LDL particle size, HDL, and triglyceride levels. Insulin resistant individuals tend to produce larger and greater VLDL particles which contain a greater concentration of triglyceride that results in a decrease in the size and number of HDL particles with an increase in apolipoprotein B levels, which represent all the atherogenic lipoproteins and correlate with non-HDL cholesterol levels. In addition, insulin resistant individuals also have a reduction in plasma levels of apo A-1, the surface protein that facilitates reverse cholesterol transport. Postprandial dyslipidemia also tends to be more severe in insulin resistant individuals, particularly the clearance of postprandial triglycerides, with plasma levels trending higher and lasting longer across the continuum from normal to impaired glucose tolerant to diabetic individuals, while postprandial hypertriglyceridemia tends to correlate higher with cardiovascular events than fasting levels. The triglyceride rich lipoproteins, including VLDL, chlyomicrons, and metabolites of VLDL including IDL (intermediate dense lipoproteins), are significantly pro-atherogenic, especially when associated with decreased levels of HDL, enhancing the development of inflammatory macrophages and endothelial cells. Triglyceride rich lipoproteins contain apolipoprotein C III, which inhibits lipoprotein lipase, not only promoting further hypertriglyceridemia, but also adhesion of monocytes to endothelial cells.

Postprandially, the incorporation of dietary cholesterol esters and triglycerides into chylomicrons within the enterocytes of the small intestine depends upon the presence of a surface protein, apo B-48. This cell surface protein, present uniquely in chylomicrons, is actually a truncated form of apo B-100, and is combined with core lipids, including apo A-I and apo-A IV, by microsomal triglyceride transfer protein. Type-2 diabetics and individuals with insulin resistance have been shown to have an increased production of triglyceride rich lipoprotein particles containing apo B-48, with an increased expression of microsomal triglyceride transfer protein. Chylomicrons acquire apo C-I, apo-C II and apo C-III from the HDL surface upon entering plasma and are subsequently cleared through the action of apo C-II mediated lipoprotein lipase, releasing free fatty acids and resulting in chylomicron remnants. These chylomicron remnants acquire apo E from HDL and are cleared via the LDL receptors in the liver, while the free fatty acids are taken up by the tissues, enhancing lipoprotein retention and altering the composition of the extracellular matrix produced by smooth muscle cells. This overabundance of free fatty acids worsens insulin resistance, disrupts reverse cholesterol transport, impedes efficient myocyte mitochondrial function, and promotes fatty degeneration within the liver and pancreas. Hence, the inappropriate disposal and metabolism of free fatty acids not only represents a fundamental pathophysiological process in diabetes, but also in accelerated atherogenesis. These fatty acids can come from adipose tissue, from hepatic VLDL and chylomicron uptake, and from peripheral tissue. Chylomicron remnants and triglyceride rich lipoproteins like VLDL are avidly engulfed by the macrophages promoting lipid accumulation within the arterial wall and impairing arterial compliance.

While the hallmark of the postprandial state is chylomicron production, the fasting state is characterized by the production and secretion of VLDL within the rough endoplasmic reticulum of the liver. In order to assemble the VLDL particle, triglyceride is required. The more hepatic triglyceride present, the more apo B-100 is lipidated by hepatic microsomal triglyceride transfer protein and sent to the Golgi apparatus, increasing the VLDL molecule size. The increased flow of free fatty acids from the adipocyte to the liver results from insulin resistance combined with de novo lipogenesis of hepatic triglycerides, enhanced postprandial lipemia, and accelerated production of triglyceride rich VLDL in the fasting state. These VLDL molecules are then hydrolyzed by lipoprotein lipase yielding smaller VLDL particles (intermediate dense lipoproteins-IDL).

These remnants are then taken up by the hepatic LDL receptors and further catabolized by hepatic lipase into LDL particles. Insulin resistant individuals have a reduction in the number of LDL receptors, resulting in a decreased clearance of LDL, which is then converted into a smaller, denser LDL molecules through the action of cholesterol ester transfer protein (CETP) mediated exchange of its core cholesterol for chylomicron or VLDL triglyceride. This small LDL molecule is the hallmark of the insulin resistant and type-2 diabetic individual. In addition, the larger VLDL molecules also participate in exchanging their triglycerides for the cholesterol ester of the HDL molecule due to the action of CETP with these particles, generating additional small dense LDL. These small, dense LDL particles are less likely to be picked up by the hepatic LDL receptors than the larger molecules, are easily oxidized and by virtue of their size, can penetrate and be taken up easier by tissue macrophages after penetrating the endothelial surface, induce a greater production of procoagulant factors, and are immobilized greater by proteoglycans than the larger, more buoyant LDL particles.

HDL cholesterol and circulating apolipoprotein A-I levels are reduced in type-2 diabetics.

In addition, abnormalities in size and composition affect the HDL molecule impairing its ability to participate in reverse cholesterol transport and remove cholesterol from atherosclerotic plaque. In addition, glycation of the apolioprotein A-I moiety of the HDL molecules affects its interaction with the ATP-binding cassette transporter impairing cholesterol removal from cells. The altered chemical composition of the HDL molecule in the type-2 diabetic patient has important adverse consequences at the cellular level, since these alterations can result in impairment of the atheroprotective properties of the HDL molecules and can even result in HDL becoming pro-inflammatory!

Various factors acting alone or in combination lower HDL cholesterol and apo A-I levels in the insulin resistant and type-2 diabetic including decrease in lipoprotein lipase mediated lipolysis, increased postprandial lipemia, overproduction of triglyceride rich

VLDL within the hepatocytes, and increased hepatic lipase activity resulting in a smaller and fewer HDL molecules promoting accelerated atherogenesis due to impaired reverse cholesterol transport activity.

The clustering of dyslipidemic abnormalities in type-2 diabetes of hypertriglyceridemia, low HDL, and a preponderance of small dense LDL particles correlates with direct measurements of insulin resistance and an enhanced risk of cardiovascular diseases. Insulin resistance, however, is difficult to directly measure. The Metabolic Syndrome in Active Subjects (MESYAS) registry has demonstrated that the triglyceride/HDL ratio correlates well with insulin resistance, the metabolic syndrome and the presence of small, dense LDL particles [2]. This study collected data from 18,778 active workers in Spain with a mean age of 42.2 ± 10.7 years with 77.6% men. Those with the metabolic syndrome had a triglyceride/HDL ratio twice as high as those without metabolic syndrome. This ratio correlated to 80% sensitivity and 78% specificity for ratios >2.75 in men and >1.65 in women. In addition, this ratio was also associated with the occurrence of a primary coronary event regardless of the patient's weight. As the triglyceride/HDL ratio becomes greater than 2:1 the likelihood of insulin resistance increases and is highly likely when the ratio exceeds 4:1.

RISK ASSESSMENT

Although severely elevated LDL levels are not a defining feature of the type-2 diabetes, the LDL is more atherogenic, so the measurement of total particle number and the LDL particle size may be more revealing that the LDL measurement alone for determining the risk. This occurs especially in the diabetic patient who may have impaired lipoprotein lipase synthesis, which elevates triglycerides, lowers HDL, and decreases the size while enhancing the atherogenicity of the LDL particle. Measuring apolipoprotein B correlates well with non-HDL cholesterol levels, since apolipoprotein B coats chylomciron (B-48), VLDL, IDL, LDL, and lipoprotein(a) particles.

The American College of Cardiology and the American Diabetes Association have both recommended that patients with diabetes and one or more additional risk factors for coronary artery disease (known cardiovascular event, renal failure, smoking, metabolic syndrome, coronary artery calcium score equal to or >75th percentile, high sensitivity CRP >3.0, HDL <40 mg/dl, triglycerides >200 mg/dl, non-HDL cholesterol >160 mg/dl, and family history of premature coronary artery disease) should be treated to an LDL <70 mg/dl. Diabetic patients with no other major cardiovascular risk factors should have an LDL goal of <70 mg/dl. In addition, their consensus statement advises that all pharmacological decisions should be guided by quantification of atherogenic lipoproteins including LDL, apolipoprotein B, and LDL particle number to not only assess risk, but also serve as therapeutic goals.

Elevated LDL cholesterol has been shown to be a major risk factor for cardiovascular events, while aggressively lowering LDL has been shown to decrease events. However, not all individuals have the same risk requiring an adjustment to account for individual risk variation. Major risk factors that must be taken into account when assessing therapeutic goals include:

1. Hypertension (treated or equal to or >140/90 mmHg)
2. Cigarette smoking
3. Family history of premature coronary heart disease – <55 years of age for male first degree relative or <65 years of age for female first degree relative

4. Age – equal to or >45 years of age in men or equal to or >55 years of age in women
5. Low HDL – <40 mg/dl in men and women (a high HDL >60 mg/dl counts as a negative risk factor, reducing the risk factor tally by one)

The National Cholesterol Education Program (NCEP)-Adult Treatment Panel (ATP)-III classifies patients into five risk categories [3]:

1. Very high risk – These patients have an LDL goal of <70 mg/dl. These include individuals with known or established cardiovascular disease and:
   (a) Acute coronary syndrome or another cardiovascular event
   (b) Metabolic syndrome
   (c) Cigarette smoking
   (d) Renal insufficiency
   (e) Diabetes
2. High risk – Patients with coronary heart disease or coronary artery risk equivalents including diabetes, carotid artery disease, abdominal aortic aneurysm, peripheral vascular disease, and a 10-year Framingham risk >20%. The primary goal is an LDL of <100 mg/dl
3. Moderately high risk – Patients with two or more risk factors and a 10-year Framingham risk of 10–20%. The primary goal is an LDL <130 mg/dl. An additional option in this category is <100 mg/dl if any major risk factors are present
4. Moderate risk – Patients with two or more risk factors and a 10-year Framingham risk of <10%. The primary LDL goal is <130 mg/dl.
5. Lowest risk – Patients with zero to one risk factors and a 10-year risk of <10%. The primary LDL goal is <160 mg/dl.

ATP-III recognized a clustering of major risk factors, life style risk factors (obesity, physical inactivity, and atherogenic diet), and emerging risk factors (plasminogen activator inhibitor-1, impaired fasting or glucose tolerance, high sensitivity C-reactive protein, and high coronary artery calcium score) that tends to be prevalent in those with coronary artery disease, associated with a body type with increased visceral fat. This clustering or metabolic syndrome can improve this high risk status with weight loss, physical activity dietary changes, hypertension and lipid management, and aspirin to reduce the prothrombotic state. Assessment of risk becomes even more important in those patients with the metabolic syndrome, since those with diabetes are at high risk by nature of the disease. A simpler way of looking at the risk categories is that those individuals at low risk for coronary disease should be at an LDL of <130 mg/dl, those with coronary artery disease or coronary risk equivalents should be at <100 mg/dl, and those at high risk should be at <70 mg/dl.

The drive for lower LDL levels was brought about by the Pravastatin or Atorvastatin Evaluation and Infection Therapy-Thrombolysis in Myocardial Infarction 22 (PROVE IT-TIMI 22) trial and the Treating to New Targets (TNT) trial, which showed that treatment to lower LDL level reduced risk for events. In TNT intensive therapy with atorvastatin, 80 mg compared to atorvastatin 10 mg significantly reduced cardiovascular events by 22%. In this trial, atorvastatin 10 mg reduced LDL levels to a mean of 98.6 mg/dl, while the 80 mg dose lowered LDL to a mean of 77 mg/dl [4]. In PROVE IT-TIMI 22, patients with acute coronary syndrome who had their mean LDL reduced to 62 mg/dl fared better than those on pravastatin whose mean LDL was 95 mg/dl [5]. Also of note is the fact that in TNT, patients with metabolic syndrome had more events than those without, while also benefitting from aggressive LDL lowering. It is also important to keep in mind that not all type-2 diabetics will have a 10-year risk >20%, so it is always prudent to evaluate the total risk factors for any given patient.

Although LDL is the main target of lipid lowering for primary and secondary prevention of cardiovascular events in patient with diabetes, one must not ignore the importance of HDL, triglycerides, and non-HDL cholesterol. The NCEP ATP III guidelines clearly specify that non-HDL cholesterol should be an additional goal of therapy when triglycerides are modestly or greatly elevated (200–499 mg/dl). Goals for non-HDL cholesterol, a surrogate marker for apolipoprotein B, are 30 mg/dl higher than LDL goals and correlates well with atherogenic potential.

Several epidemiological studies have shown that low HDL levels are an independent predictor of coronary heart disease morbidity and mortality. This was particularly evident in the TNT trial, where patients with LDL levels <70 mg/dl were risk stratified by their HDL levels. Risk clearly increased with progressively lower HDL levels with individuals having HDL's <30 mg/dl at the highest risk. Several prospective and secondary analysis trials have show a benefit in raising HDL levels in reducing coronary artery disease risk independent of other lipid and nonlipid risk factors. In the Bezafibrate Infarction Prevention (BIP) study, individuals with the metabolic syndrome experienced a reduction in myocardial infarction with increased HDL levels and reduction in triglycerides. In the Veterans Affairs HDL Intervention Trial (VA-HIT), the largest reduction in cardiovascular endpoints was achieved in those with insulin resistance with or without type-2 diabetes [6]. In the Copenhagen City Heart Study, a population of 13,956 men and women aged 20–93 were followed from 1976 through July, 2007 [7]. This study, published in the Journal of the American Medical Association (*JAMA*) in 2008, showed that non fasting triglyceride levels were associated with an increased risk of ischemic stroke, while a study by Nordestgaard published in *JAMA* in 2007, reported a strong association between myocardial infarction, ischemic heart disease, total cardiovascular events, and mortality in men and women with elevated postprandial triglycerides [8].

The leading cause of deaths in the USA is coronary artery disease. The diabetic patient has a two to fourfold increase in likelihood of coronary disease, with 2/3 of diabetics succumbing to their macrovascular disease with double the risk of dying of a myocardial infarction. The metabolic syndrome represents clusters of various surrogate markers that now qualify it as an independent risk factor for cardiovascular mortality and disease.

Clinical Impact of Diabetic Dyslipidemia

The first ATP report of the NCEP was filed in January, 1988. The third report was issued in May 2001 and updated in 2008.

The ATP-III has classified diabetes as a coronary artery disease equivalent. Patients with CAD risk equivalents carry a risk of major coronary events of >20% in the next 10 years. In addition to diabetes the other risk equivalents are:

1. Carotid artery disease
2. Peripheral vascular disease
3. Abdominal aortic aneurysm

The presence of multiple risk factors can increase risk to >20% in a 10-year period. Although not officially listed yet as a coronary artery risk equivalent, the cluster of surrogate markers within the syndrome heightens cardiovascular risk significantly and progressively with the number of markers present.

The risk of coronary heart disease over a 10-year period is based on Framingham data using the following risk factors:

1. Total cholesterol
2. HDL
3. Systolic blood pressure
4. Treated hypertension
5. Cigarette smoking

The data base for these calculations does not include those individuals with existing coronary disease or risk equivalents because these individuals already have an increased risk (20%) of developing a coronary event in the ensuing 10 years with individuals experiencing a stroke also at greater risk for a cardiac event.

The hallmarks of dyslipidemia in Type-2 diabetics and increased risk of cardiovascular disease and accelerated atherosclerosis are [9]:

1. Hypertriglyceridemia.
2. Decreased high density lipoprotein levels (HDL).
3. Preponderance of phenotype B pattern with excessive amounts of small dense LDL and an increase in intermediate dense lipoprotein particles which are more atherogenic than the fluffy large LDL particles.
4. Increased VLDL.
5. Elevated non-HDL cholesterol.
6. Elevated apolipoprotein B.
7. Elevated apolipoprotein C-III.
8. Diminished apolipoprotein A-I.

Most diabetics will also have elevations of total cholesterol presenting with a pattern of mixed dyslipidemia. In diabetic patients, proportionately less cholesterol is carried in the LDL particles. Cholesterol is found in the VLDL molecule and especially the VLDL remnants which are just as atherogenic as the LDL molecule. Hence just measuring LDL actually underestimates atherogenic potential in the diabetic patient.

LDL levels normally obtained through laboratory testing are calculated values based on the Friedewald equation [10]:

LDL = (Total cholesterol) − (HDL) − (Triglycerides/5).

This calculation is really not applicable for triglycerides >150.

The vertical analysis profile (VAP) can measure LDL levels directly eliminating confusion over the calculated LDL.

The presence of small, dense LDL can increase CHD risk threefold. In the Quebec Cardiovascular Study, LDL particle size was predictive of cardiovascular events independent of LDL, HDL, triglycerides, total cholesterol/HDL ratio, and body mass index [11].

The increased atherogenicity of the small, dense LDL molecule can be related to the following [12]:

1. Enhanced predisposition to oxidation
2. Impaired binding to the LDL receptor sites
3. Increased binding to the vessel wall

4. Conformation changes in the apolipoprotein B molecule
5. Presence of other concomitant and synergistic risk factors

The first goal of therapy is to decrease the LDL below 100 mg/dl. This can best be achieved by starting statin therapy in conjunction with therapeutic life style changes.

Dosage of the statin can be increased with doubling of the dose resulting in a 6% decrease in LDL, or adding a second agent for synergistic LDL, and other parameter lowering.

The second goal is to increase HDL to >40 mg/dl in males and 50 mg/dl in females. Once these goals are achieved, attention should be directed to the triglycerides and the non-HDL cholesterol, unless the triglycerides are >500 mg/dl at entry. When triglyceride levels exceed 500 the risk for pancreatitis may be increased, and this makes triglyceride lowering more of an immediate priority.

Not to be overlooked is the significant importance of the non HDL cholesterol, particularly in the diabetic patients. This is determined as follows:

Non HDL cholesterol = (LDL) + (VLDL) = (Total Cholesterol) – (HDL).

This non-HDL cholesterol includes all lipoproteins that contain apolipoprotein B and has been rising significantly in importance in recent years. Since VLDL is closely correlated with atherogenic remnant lipoproteins, it can be reasonably be combined with LDL to enhance the prediction of risk when the serum triglycerides are elevated [13].

Some authorities have even proposed the use of non-HDL cholesterol instead of the LDL cholesterol in the clinical evaluation of risk. The Lipid Research Clinic cohort follow-up study actually showed a stronger correlation with coronary mortality for non-HDL cholesterol than for LDL cholesterol [14]. In addition, levels of non-HDL cholesterol are highly correlated with total apolipoprotein B, which has been shown to be a strong predictor of coronary heart disease events and atherosclerosis in several clinical trials.

Due to the high association between non-HDL cholesterol and apolipoprotein B, non-HDL cholesterol can be an acceptable surrogate marker for apolipoprotein B in clinical practice. This non-HDL cholesterol essentially accounts for the cholesterol that is likely to be deposited in plaque independent of whether it is found in VLDL or LDL. However, the cholesterol within the HDL particles is primarily transported back to the liver and can participate in reverse transport.

DYSLIPIDEMIA THERAPY IN THE DIABETIC PATIENT

Therapeutic lifestyle changes should always be a cornerstone for therapy of patients with type-2 diabetes and metabolic syndrome, while glycemic control can pay important dividends in improving lipid control – especially triglycerides. With just 2 h of weekly exercise and 6% weight loss, a 58% reduction was seen in progression of patients from impaired glucose tolerance to type-2 diabetes in the Diabetes Prevention Program. In general, low carbohydrate diets increase HDL cholesterol, while low saturated fat and low trans fat diets decrease LDL cholesterol and atherosclerosis.

Statins-Hmg-CoA Inhibitors (3-Hydroxy-3 Methylglutaryl-Coenzyme A Reductase Inhibitors)

The statins, the most effective pharmacologic agents for reducing LDL, are competitive inhibitors of HMG-CoA resulting in decreased cholesterol synthesis causing less VLDL particles to be released into the blood, resulting in increased hepatic synthesis of LDL receptors and enhanced clearance of LDL from the blood. These drugs are first line therapy for LDL lowering in individuals with and without type-2 diabetes. Available statins include pravastatin, lovastatin, fluvastatin, rosuvastatin, simvastatin, pitavastatin and atorvastatin. The statins achieve LDL reductions of up to 55% and up to 30% reduction in triglycerides with atorvastatin and rosuvastatin, with modest increases in HDL of from 5 to 15%. In patients with insulin resistance or type-2 diabetes, increased clearance of VLDL and LDL from the circulation reduces apolipoprotein B containing lipoproteins.

Statins may also lower apolipoprotein C- III levels, increasing lipolysis of triglyceride rich particles by increasing lipoprotein lipase activity as shown in the Diabetes Atorvastatin Lipid Intervention (DALI) study [15].

Added to the value of statin monotherapy is its potential for combination therapy with other lipid lowering agents in treating diabetic dyslipidemia. The robust LDL reductions usually required (<70 mg/dl) in high risk diabetic patients along with addressing the other parameters of diabetic dyslipidemia (high triglycerides, low HDL, increased small, and dense LDL particles) may be achieved with up-titrating the more potent statins or by combining a statin with plant stanol and sterol ester, selective cholesterol absorbing agents, bile acid sequestrants, fenofibrates, niacin, omega-3 acid ethyl esters, and pioglitazone.

Niacin (Nicotinic Acid)

The oldest of the lipid lowering drug, nicotinic acid has been used for over 40 years and is the most potent HDL raising agent available, while also reducing VLDL, triglycerides, lipoprotein(a) and LDL. Niacin downregulates the expression of the F1 moiety of F1F10 adenosine triphosphate synthetase, a hepatic cell-surface HDL receptor. This results in increased number of larger HDL particles (HDL-2) and a decreased catabolic rate of apolipoprotein A-1. Niacin also inhibits diacylglycerol acyltransferase 2, which also suppresses triglyceride synthesis. This reduction in triglyceride mass results in decreased activity of hepatic lipase on reducing HDL. By increasing the expression of the adenosine triphosphate binding membrane cassette (ABC) transporters A1 and G1, HDL synthesis is increased and reverse cholesterol transport is enhanced. Although it is not recommended as a first line agent for LDL reduction, niacin will reduce LDL by 10–20%, lipoprotein(a) by 15–25%, and an increase in HDL by 15–35% [16].

Although niacin suppresses free fatty acid release from adipose tissue it can increase insulin resistance. However, the efficacy of niacin monotherapy on cardiovascular outcomes was evaluated in the coronary drug project (CDP) [17]. This study demonstrated a reduction in nonfatal recurrent myocardial infarction and total mortality, while a subset analysis of diabetic patients stratified by glycemic status also showed a reduction in recurrent myocardial infarction and coronary heart disease death at all glucose levels.

The extended release niacin preparation (Niaspan) has been not been associated with any significant glucose abnormalities, while the sustained release niacin (niacin-SR) is available without a prescription and is not recommended for use by the National Lipid Association, since it has been associated with irreversible hepatocellular injury.

Bile Acid Sequestrants

These include colesevelam, colestipol, and cholestyramine and act by binding bile acids in the intestine, reducing their return to the liver, enhancing cholesterol diversion to the bile acid synthesis pathway, decreasing hepatic cholesterol content, upregulating hepatic receptors, and lowering serum LDL levels. These agents lower LDL by 15–30% with minimal increases in HDL of 3–5%. These agents may raise triglyceride levels due to increased VLDL production and are not indicated in patients with triglyceride levels >400 mg/dl and should be used with caution in patients with levels >200 mg/dl.

Some gastrointestinal difficulties (constipation and cramping) can be seen in patients with autonomic neuropathy. A small, randomized, double blinded study in 1994 in patients with type-2 diabetes and triglycerides as high as 300 mg/dl demonstrated a statistically significant 28% reduction in LDL, but a 13.5% increase in triglycerides using cholesty-ramine [18]. In four double blinded 12–26-week placebo controlled trials, in type-2 diabet-ics, colesevelam (Welchol) increased triglycerides only 5%, while lowering LDL by 15% and A1C by 0.5% [19].

Fibrates Selective Cholesterol Absorption Inhibitors

Ezetimibe selectively inhibits cholesterol and plant sterol absorption at the brush border of the intestinal enterocyte by binding to the Niemann-Pick C1-Like 1 (NPC1L1) receptor and acting independent of the cholesterol efflux transporters ABC-G5 and ABC-G8. This agent does not cause fat malabsorption and is converted to ezetimibe glucuronide in the intestine following absorption. This glucuronide, more potent than the parent product, under-goes extensive enterohepatic circulation and is excreted in the feces with <11% renally excreted, making system absorption very low. The 10 mg dose of ezetimibe decreases LDL by 18–20% alone, or in combination with statins or fenofibrates. The ezetimibe/fenofibrate combination can be effective in those patients with muscle cramping from statin therapy although some patients may still get muscle aches with ezetemibe. Combining this drug with the entry dose of any statin results in LDL reduction same as the maximum dose of that statin. Hence 10 mg of ezetimibe and 10 mg of simvastatin will achieve the same LDL reduction as 80 mg of simvastatin (46%). Data in diabetic patients demonstrates the same LDL reduction as those without the disease. It has minimal effects on triglycerides and HDL. Lacking at this time is event reduction data with this product in the type-2 diabetic patient.

Fibrates (Fibric Acid Derivatives)

These include:

1. Fenofibrates – (Antara, Lipofen, TriCor, Lofibra, and Triglide)
2. Fenofibric acids – (Fibricor and Trilipix)
3. Gemfibrozil – (Lopid)
4. Bezafibrate
5. Clofibrate – (Atromid S)

These drugs are useful in treating hypertriglyceridemia and raising HDL – particularly in the diabetic patient and those with metabolic syndrome.

Their mechanisms of actions involve [20]:

1. Increased synthesis of lipoprotein lipase, enhancing the catabolism of triglyceride rich lipoproteins (chylomicrons, VLDL, IDL, and LDL)
2. Increased synthesis of apolipoprotein A-1 and apolipoprotein A-II, which increases HDL level
3. Increased synthesis of ABC-A1, promoting cholesterol efflux into apolipoprotein A-1 during the biogenesis of HDL, increasing reverse cholesterol transport

4. Increased SR-B1 – which increases hepatic uptake of HDL
5. Increased synthesis of mdr2 – which increases biliary cholesterol secretion
6. Increased synthesis of Acyl CoA – which enhances hepatic oxidation of free fatty acids
7. Decreased synthesis of apolipoprotein C-III thereby increasing lipoprotein lipase activity
8. Decreased bile acid synthesis, which enhances biliary cholesterol excretion
9. Peroxisome proliferator activated receptor (PPAR) alpha agonists, binding to the liver X receptor (LXR) and decreasing LXR mediated lipogenesis

Fenofibrates stimulate nitric oxide synthase, enhancing vascular endothelial nitric oxide production, reducing matrix metalloproteinase activity, fostering plaque stability, and decreasing levels of surrogate inflammatory markers like C-reactive protein and interleukin-6 levels.

Fibrates typically decrease apolipoprotein B and lower triglycerides by 35–50% and raise HDL by 10–20%, enhancing intravascular metabolism of VLDL by increasing lipoprotein lipase activity. The fenofibrates can reduce LDL levels by approximately 10%, but LDL levels can rise with treatment of severe hypertriglyceridemia due to a shift to a larger LDL molecule. Fibrates may also diminish the insulin mediated rise in plasminogen activator inhibitor-1, improving fibrinolytic activity in hyperinsulinemic individuals. By increasing uric acid excretion, the fenofibrates can reduce serum uric acid and are more effective than gemfibrozil in reducing non-HDL (especially in those with hypertriglyceridemia) and LDL.

The fibric acid derivatives are conjugated in the liver to glucuronides and then excreted renally. Fenofibrate and clofibrate will accumulate to higher levels with renal insufficiency and require a reduction in dose that is not required with gemfibrozil. However, gemfibrozil is glucuronidized in the same portion of the liver as most of the statins (except fluvastatin and pravastatin), resulting in significant increases in area under the curve with concomitant use. Hence gemfibrozil is not indicated for concomitant use with statins. Fenofibrates do not increase the area under the curve for statins and one fenofibrate (Trilipix) has FDA approval for concomitant statin use.

The fibric acid drugs may increase serum homocysteine up to 35% by a PPAR alpha mediated mechanism, although the clinical importance of this remains to be determined.

There was noted a small, but statistically significant higher incidence of pulmonary embolism in the FIELD (Fenofibrate Intervention and Event Lowering in Diabetes) trial with fenofibrate and the CDP with clofibrate.

Renal transplant patients have experienced reversible fibrate associated renal failure; however, fenofibrates slowed the progression of microalbuminuria in type-2 diabetics in both the FIELD and the Diabetes Atherosclerosis Intervention Study (DAIS) [21].

Omega-3 Acid Ethyl Esters (Fish Oils) (Omega-3 Fatty Acids)

Fish oils decrease synthesis of triglycerides, fatty acids and VLDL, while increasing the beta oxidation of fatty acids and the intracellular catabolism of apolipoprotein B. By stimulating lipoprotein lipase activity they aid in the conversion of VLDL to LDL. They also inhibit diacylglycerol acyl transferase, hormone sensitive lipase, and phosphatidic acid phosphohydrolase activity decreasing the secretion of VLDL triglycerides, and increasing the expression of PPAR alpha activity thus increasing fatty acid oxidation. Based on a meta-analysis of 72 placebo controlled trials, triglyceride reductions of 25–35% have been achieved with 3–4 g of EPA (eicosapentanoic acid) and DHA (docosahexanoic acid) showing greater reduction with very high triglycerides. Individuals with triglycerides >500 mg/dl experienced a 45% reduction [22]. Typically, omega-3 fatty acids do not lower LDL and can increase LDL when given to patients with very high triglycerides do to a shift into producing larger less atherogenic LDL particles. Their effects on HDL are minor in normolipemic individuals (3–5%), but in patients with very high triglycerides (500 mg/dl) HDL increases of 9% have been reported.

A review on the use of omega-3 treatment in type-2 diabetics was published by Hartweg and others in 2009 in the journal *Current Opinions in Lipidology* [23]. This reviewed 243 randomized controlled trials in 1,075 type-2 diabetics and noted 7% decrease in triglycerides compared to baseline. No clinical outcomes were reported in this review.

The omega-3 fatty acids are safe and well tolerated and can be used in combination with any of the other lipid lowering drugs without fear of drug to drug interaction. Thus these agents may have particular advantages in the diabetic patients with renal insufficiency and/ or hypertriglyceridemia with no evidence of worsening glycemic control.

Lipid management is critical in the diabetic patient. With all the options available today, physicians should not be asking themselves why they should institute lipid lowering therapy but why shouldn't they institute therapy.

The first choice in LDL lowering is the HMG coenzyme-reductase inhibitors or statins.

To raise the HDL in the type-2 diabetic patient, statins, fibrates, thiazolidinediones, metformin, triglyceride lowering, omega-3 fatty acids, smoking cessation, weight loss, and increased physical activity are important with the first drug of choice being niacin or fibrates However, statins like rosuvastatin, atorvastatin, pitavastatin, and simvastatin will also raise HDL to a modest degree.

The thiazolidinediones and metformin have been shown to be effective in raising the HDL and are particularly efficacious because of their dual efficacy in diabetic patients in trying to achieve glycemic and lipid goals. Thiazolidinediones will also change LDL composition from the more atherogenic, small dense LDL to the fluffy less atherogenic, buoyant, and larger LDL molecule. The TZD's have also been demonstrated to have anti-inflammatory effects [24]. It is important to appreciate that pioglitazone and rosiglitazone have distinctly discrepant ways of handling lipids, with pioglitazone decreasing triglycerides while rosiglitazone can even raise triglycerides. Two important clinical trials (GLAI and COMPLEMENT) gave important insight into these differences, indicating that although both are equally effective in achieving glycemic control in patients with type-2 diabetes, pioglitazone improved HDL cholesterol, lowered triglycerides and decreased LDL particle concentration, while increasing particle size compared to rosiglitazone in head to head competition.

The GLAI study was a multicenter prospective randomized double blinded parallel group evaluation comparing maximally effective doses of rosiglitazone and pioglitazone monotherapy in type-2 diabetic patients with dyslipidemia. Of the 4,410 patients screened, 802 were eventually randomized, 369 in the pioglitazone group and 366 in the rosiglitazone group with 80% in each group completing 24 weeks of therapy [25]. After a washout period, the patients received 4 weeks of placebo and were then randomized. The effects on A1C were similar in both groups, but by week 4 there was a significant reduction in triglyceride levels (-12%) in the pioglitazone group, but a significant increase (+14.9%) in the rosiglitazone group. Although HDL levels increased in both groups, they were significantly higher in the pioglitazone group (+14.9 vs. 7.8%). Non-HDL cholesterol was stable with pioglitazone, but increased with rosiglitazone (+18.6%). LDL particle size increased in both groups, but was greater with pioglitazone (2.4 vs. 1.7%), while the LDL particle concentration was reduced by pioglitazone (−7.8%), it was increased with rosiglitazone (+12%). Apolipoprotein B significantly increased with rosiglitazone and remained the same with pioglitazone.

The Effects of Pioglitazone on lipid and lipoprotein profiles in patients with type-2 diabetes and dyslipidemia after treatment conversion from rosiglitazone, while continuing stable statin therapy (COMPLEMENT) trial demonstrated significant improvements in lipid parameters beyond those resulting from standard cholesterol lowering statin therapy in patients who had been taking rosiglitazone (Avandia) and then switched to pioglitazone (Actos) [26]. These effects were seen regardless of age or gender or even if patients took fenofibrate in addition to statin therapy. In this trial, triglycerides were reduced by 21% and total cholesterol by 10.5 ($P<0.0001$). Mean LDL particle size increased 0.23 nm and mean LDL particle concentration decreased 189 nm/L, indicating a shift to few and larger LDL particles with pioglitazone therapy. Mean VLDL concentration decreased 44.9 nmol/L and mean levels of apolipoprotein B (apo B) decreased by 2.6 mg/dl. In addition, Szapary and others reported on the effects of pioglitazone on lipoproteins and inflammatory markers in nondiabetic patients with the metabolic syndrome in an article published in the journal, *Arteriosclerosis, Thrombosis, and Vascular Biology* in 2006 [27]. In this study, nondiabetic patients with low HDL and Metabolic Syndrome, pioglitazone significantly raised HDL and favorably affected markers of inflammation, lipoprotein particle size, and adipokines. Pioglitazone increased HDL by 15% and 14% at 6 and 12 weeks compared to placebo and reduced the number of small, dense LDL particles by 18%, while reducing C reactive protein (hs-CRP) by 31% and significantly increasing adiponectin levels by 111%! These were independent of an effect on triglycerides, which were unchanged.

Following LDL reduction, the next important priority in the dyslipidemic diabetic is decreasing the triglyceride and the non HDL cholesterol. Here glycemic control with dietary interventions can have dramatic effects. Fibric acid derivatives or fibrates like gemfibrozil and fenofibrate, niacin, and omega-3 fatty acids are extremely effective in lowering triglycerides. The extended release of niacin is less likely to interfere with glycemic control than their intermediate, or crystalline, and sustained release derivatives. Pioglitazone, but not rosiglitazone, can also be effective in triglyceride lowering.

Statins, particularly rosuvastatin, atorvastatin, and simvastatin can be effective for hypertriglyceridemic patients, but do not seem to be as potent in lowering triglycerides as the fibric acid derivatives (fibrates) or niacin.

The most potent of the statins is the newest member of the class, rosuvastatin (Crestor) with data from the STELLAR (Statin Therapies for Elevated Lipid Levels compared Across doses to Rosuvastatin) Trial indicating greater efficacy in reducing non HDL cholesterol than the other statins across the dosing spectrum [28].

This randomized, open label 6-week trial in 2,431 patients with LDL cholesterols at entry of 160–250 mg/dl and triglycerides <400 mg/dl found that rosuvastatin at 10, 20, and 40 mg daily reduced LDL by 46–55% compared to 37–51% with atorvastatin (10–80 mg), 28–46% with simvastatin (10–80 mg), and 20–30% with pravastatin (10–40 mg).

Rosuvastatin (10–40 mg) also increased the HDL cholesterol by 7.7–9.6%, compared to 21–5.7% with atorvastatin (10–80 mg), 5.2–6.8% with simvastatin (10–80 mg), and 3.2–5.6% with pravastatin (10–40 mg) [9].

More impressive was the fact that at the 10 mg dose, rosuvastatin was associated with a 42% decrease in non-HDL cholesterol, compared with reductions of 34, 26, and 19% with 10 mg of atorvastatin, simvastatin, and pravastatin respectively. At the 40 mg dose, rosuvastatin decreased the non-HDL cholesterol by 51% compared with 45 and 48% among patients treated with 40 and 80 mg of atorvastatin, respectively, and 35 and 42% among those receiving 40 and 80 mg of simvastatin, respectively [29].

Thirty-five percent of the study population in the STELLAR trial had hypertriglyceridemia at baseline. Looking at this subset of people, treatment with 10 mg of rosuvastatin was able to get 80–84% of patients to their LDL and non HDL cholesterol goals.

A randomized trial of 156 patients with triglycerides of 300 mg–800 mg/dl found that treatment with rosuvastatin reduced triglycerides by 37% with the 10–20 mg doses and 40% with the 40–80 mg dose. Pooled analyses of five randomized double blinded trials have shown that rosuvastatin at 10 mg daily lowered triglycerides as effectively as atorvastatin 10 mg and more effectively than 20 mg of simvastatin [30].

A double blinded trial of 216 patients reported by Capuzzi in the American Journal of Cardiology in 2003 with type-2 diabetes and triglycerides 310–372 mg/dl found that rosuvastatin 10 mg daily plus fenofibrate 67 mg t.i.d. lowered triglycerides by 47%, compared to 30% with rosuvastatin 40 mg alone and 34% with fenofibrate alone [31]. An open label, 24-week trial in 270 patients with hypertriglyceridemia and low HDL (45 mg/dl) found that rosuvastatin 10 mg plus with extended release niacin (Niaspan) at 2 g, increased HDL by 24% compared to 11% with rosuvastatin 40 mg alone, 12% with niacin 2 g alone, and 17% with rosuvastatin 40 mg and niacin 1 g. Rosuvastatin 10 mg plus niacin 2 g had less effect on LDL than rosuvastatin 40 mg alone [30].

In the Justification for the Use of Statins in Primary Prevention: an Intervention Trial involving Rosuvastatin (JUPITER), the benefits of rosuvastatin in primary prevention of cardiovascular events were demonstrated in patients with the metabolic syndrome and elevated hs-CRP [32].In this trial, 5,577 of the 17,802 participants had the metabolic syndrome.

Due to the significant vasculopathic and thrombotic nature of type-2 diabetes, diet therapy should always be considered a valuable adjunct rather than substitution for medication to achieve goals. This is because many of the medications, particularly the statins, have shown some significantly pleotrophic benefits in addition to their lipid effects which make them ideally suited for risk reduction in the diabetic patient.

For obese patients with low HDL and elevated triglycerides, avoidance of the white four carbohydrates, like rice bread, pasta, potatoes, high fructose corn syrup, sugar sweetened foods and beverages will aid in reducing lipids and improving glycemic control. Diabetic patients can significantly improve glycemic control with low carbohydrate regimens.

The vascular endothelium in the diabetic patient is the site of significant pathologic alteration including suppression of nitric oxide activity, impaired endothelial function, decreased prostacyclin release, increased adhesion molecule expression, increased platelet aggregation and monocyte aggregation, increased procoagulant activity, increased in advanced glycosylation end products, impairment of fibrolytic activity, and impaired degradation of fibrin. Many of these effects can be attenuated or eliminated with appropriate medication therapy.

The results of large landmark clinical trials support the use of medication in this vasculopathic population. The Scandinavian Simvastatin Survival Study (4S) was a secondary prevention trial using simvastatin 20–40 mg/day. This trial demonstrated a 36% reduction in LDL, a 7% increase in HDL and 11% reduction in triglyceride levels with a 55% reduction of coronary heart disease event rate, which was of statistical significance in the diabetic cohort. There is an overall 30% reduction in total mortality and a 34% decrease in coronary events in the entire population of 4,444 patients followed for 5 years [33].

The primary endpoint of this study was mortality from all causes and its secondary endpoint was major coronary events. Simvastatin also was shown to reduce the risk of mortality for all causes by 43% and reduce the risk of any arteriosclerotic event by 37%. This risk reduction was not dependent on baseline level of total cholesterol, LDL, HDL, or triglycerides.

There was a trend toward better effect for those patients who were in the upper half of triglyceride distribution equal to or >150 and the lower half of HDL distribution <42 mg/dl.

The Cholesterol and Recurrent events or CARE Trial was a 5-year study comparing the effects of placebo and pravastatin in 4,159 patients with known coronary disease of whom 586 were diabetic. The mean baseline lipid concentration in the diabetic group were similar to the nondiabetic group and consisted of triglycerides of 164 mg/dl, HDL's of 38 mg/dl, and LDL's of 136 mg/dl. Patients with diabetes who received pravastatin experienced a 25% reduction in risk of coronary events, which included PTCA, CABG, nonfatal MI, and coronary heart disease death compared with placebo. Similar reductions were seen in the nondiabetic group. This was independent of age and sex. Average duration of follow-up for these patients was 5 years. The P-values were statistically significant for the diabetic patients in this population [34].

The Diabetes Arteriosclerosis Intervention Study (DAIS) was a primary and secondary prevention study of diabetic patients only. Four hundred and eighteen people completed in the cohort using micronized fenofibrate (Tricor) 200 mg/day. In this study there was a 7% reduction in LDL, 8% increase in HDL, and 29% reduction in triglycerides with a 24% coronary heart disease of end rate reduction. P values however were not available because the study was not empowered to examine clinical endpoints [35].

The Veterans Administration HDL-C Intervention Trial also known as VA-HIT, was a secondary prevention study of males of whom 309 were diabetic. After 1 year, patients in the gemfibrozil group had a mean 4% lower total cholesterol level, an HDL that was 6% higher than placebo group, and a 31% lower triglyceride level. The LDL levels were not significantly different between the groups. In this study there was 22% reduction in primary endpoint which was coronary heart disease death and nonfatal MI's with P value of 0.006. There was a 24% relative risk reduction for the combined coronary heart disease death, nonfatal stroke and MI's as well with a 24% risk reduction for combined coronary heart disease [22].

For the subset of patients with diabetes, similar results were achieved with a statistically significant 24% risk reduction in combined coronary heart disease, nonfatal MI and stroke. In this trial, 50% of patients had hyperinsulinemia, diabetes, or both. The absolute risk of a major coronary event was significantly higher in patients with these syndromes than in those patients without (27.2% compared to 16%). The benefits of gemfibrozil were confined to the diabetic group and not to the subset without diabetes or hyperinsulinemia [36].

The Long Term Intervention with Pravastatin and Ischemic Disease (Lipid Study) was a secondary prevention trial using pravastatin 40 mg a day in 396 type-2 diabetic patients. In this study, there was a 25% reduction in LDL, a 5% increase in HDL, and 11% reduction in triglycerides with a 19% decrease in coronary heart disease event reduction [34].

Similar reductions of 33% were seen in the AFCAPS/TEXCAPS (Air Force/Texas Coronary Arteriosclerosis Prevention Study) using lovastatin 20–40 mg daily. Here, 155 patients had diagnosed diabetes at study entry. Lovastatin therapy led to a relative risk of 0.56 for any coronary heart disease event and an absolute risk reduction of 0.04, but neither figure was statistically significant [37].

The landmark Heart Protection Study (HPS) using simvastatin had an entry and maintenance dose of 40 mg and involved 20,536 cohorts of which over 5,000 patients were diabetic. This study was carried out over a 5-year period and demonstrated that reductions in LDL cholesterol below 100 mg/dl showed a statistically significant benefit in reduction in overall cardiovascular mortality events of 25% with no distinct threshold. There was also a 27% reduction in overall coronary events including nonfatal MI and coronary heart disease, 25% reduction in stroke, and 24% major vascular event reduction for the entire cohort [38].

These collective studies involving thousands of diabetic cohorts from many countries and spanning several years, all confirm the benefit of statins and fibrates in this patient subset.

A clinical trial compared the effects of 120 patients without coronary disease using the combination of atorvastatin and micronized fenofibrate 200 mg/day for 24 weeks. The results were that the LDL decreased by 46 with 97.5% of patients reaching their LDL goal. Triglycerides decreased by 50 and 100% of patients achieved triglyceride levels <200 mg/dl. In addition, 60% of patients reached optimal HDL goals with the HDL increasing by 22% [39].

A similar study using fenofibrate and fluvastatin in 333 patients with mixed lipidemia and coronary disease showed similar benefits with HDL increasing by 22%, triglycerides falling by 38%, and LDL falling by 24%. There were no clinically relevant liver or muscular abnormalities reported. It is to be kept in mind as of this time that although adding a fibrate to a statin is a common approach for those people with mixed lipidemia, particularly in diabetes, no large scale controlled trials have confirmed the safety of this combination or established clear cut efficacy in reducing cardiovascular events [35].

Currently available data seems to be very promising in pointing the way toward future approaches and perhaps a softening of the warning of the combination use, particularly in the case of fenofibrate, which is metabolized in a different area of the liver than the cytochrome P450 system and involves glucuronidation in the liver. This is important because the risk for potential toxicity increases when statins are combined with other potentially myotoxic drugs. One fenofibrate (Trilipix) has already received FDA approval for concomitant use with statins.

Pravastatin is not metabolized through the cytochrome P450 system, while fluvastatin and rosuvastatin do not have any significant metabolism through cytochrome P450-3A4. Other agents like atorvastatin, lovastatin, and simvastatin are metabolized mainly through cytochrome P450-3A4 with simvastatin significantly metabolized in first pass through the liver through 3A4. Atorvastatin also is metabolized via 2C9 and is the least renally cleared of all the statins making it an ideal drug to use in the renally impaired patient [40].

The major concern with gemfibrozil interaction with the statins and the reason for the increased area under the curve is largely due to the area of the liver where it is metabolized. Gemfibrozil is glucuronidized in a similar area of the liver to all the statins with the exception of pravastatin and fluvastatin. This is why the area under the curve is increased for all the statins with the exception of those two. Hence the risk of myopathy is increased with gemfibrozil compared to fenofibrate [35].

We should be aware however that fibrate therapy can impair liver function independently, and hence patients with impaired liver function should not receive combination statin-fibrate therapy. Adding a bile acid sequestrant to statin therapy has been shown to enhance LDL reduction, however the combination can raise triglycerides particularly in the earlier preparations like cholestyramine.

The newer preparations like colesevelam (Welchol) do not seem to have a significant triglyceride elevation effect and have been shown to be synergistic in LDL reduction. Omega-3 fatty acids can reduce the triglyceride concentration by 20–50% depending on the dose and will not increase the risk of myopathy if used in combination with a statin. Smaller studies have demonstrated that the addition of omega 3 fatty acids to atorvastatin increased the HDL and decreased the concentration of small dense LDL compared with baseline. Of concern, however, is the purity of these products, particularly the toxic chemical load of oily fish. This has been raised recently through a controversial study in Science Magazine which pointed out the high levels of PCB's and dioxins in some preparations of oily fish, surprisingly the farm grown fish [41]. The prescription omega-3 acid ethyl esters (Lovaza) contain 465 mg of EPA and 375 mg of DHA. This product, by virtue of its unique purification process, has no detectable levels of tetrachlorodibenzodioxin (dioxin), polychlorinated biphenyls, or heavy metals. The Combination of Prescription Omega-3 Acid Ethyl Esters with Simvastatin (COMBOS) trial evaluated the effect of 4 g or 4 capsules of this product on 254 hyercholesterolemic patients over a 16 week period. For the first 8 weeks, patients received 40 mg of simvastatin [42]. They were then randomized to receive an additional 4 g of the omega-3 acid ethyl esters or placebo. The results indicated that non-HDL cholesterol had decreased by 9.0% in the omega-3/simvastatin group compared to 2.2% in the simvastatin/placebo group. In addition, the omega-3 group had a 29.5% reduction in triglycerides compared to 6.3% for placebo and 27.5% reduction in VLDL compared to 7.2% with the placebo group. HDL rose 3.4% in the omega-3/simvastatin group compared to 1.2% drop in the placebo group. There was no significant statistical change in the LDL. This study indicated the additional benefits of the addition of omega-3 acid ethyl esters to statin therapy to further enhance reduction of atherogenic lipoproteins. Combination therapy remains extremely attractive in managing the diabetic patient who usually presents to the primary care physician with a multiplicity of lipid abnormalities including high triglycerides, low HDL's, high total cholesterol, preponderance of small dense LDL, and lipoprotein(a) elevations. For these individuals the benefits of combination therapy have to be weighed and may even be greater than the risk for adverse advents [35].

The benefits of combination therapy include:

1. Synergistic activity in reduction in LDL triglyceride and raising HDL.
2. Reduction of lipoprotein(a) – especially with niacin, estrogen, and to some small extent, fenofibrate.

3. Change in LDL particle size to a less atherogenic, larger, and fluffy type molecule.
4. Decreases in fibrinogen.
5. Regression of arteriosclerotic vascular disease.
6. Reduction in non-HDL cholesterol.
7. Reduction in total LDL particle number.
8. Better tolerance with lower doses of medication--particularly with the statins, minimizing drug interaction and side effects.

The disadvantages of combination therapy involve:

1. Added cost and copays of taking two medications
2. Increased risk of adverse side effects, including rhabdomyolysis particularly with the combination of statin and gemfibrozil
3. The paucity of outcome data and less compliance with the added medications.
4. Hepatotoxicity
5. Increased potential for drug–drug interactions

In general, when faced with the dilemma, the physician must keep in mind to treat the LDL first by starting with a statin. If the LDL is still above goal, while on statin therapy, consider either a higher dose of the statin or adding a second agent. One should also keep in mind that increasing the dose of the statin increases the risk for statin drug interaction and side effects [35].

The HATS trial showed the safety of the combination of simvastatin and niacin in improving arteriosclerotic progression, outcomes, and lipid profiles in composite clinical events [43]. This trial compared treatment regimens with lipid modifying therapy and antioxidant vitamin therapy. This 3-year double blind trial included 160 patients with coronary disease, low levels of HDL, and near normal levels of LDL. Patients were evaluated with (1) simvastatin and niacin (2) antioxidants (3) placebo and (4) niacin, simvastatin, and antioxidants. In all groups, crystalline or immediate release niacin was used. These patients were at a mean age of 53 with HDL's of 31 mg/dl, LDL's of 125 mg/dl and triglycerides of 213 mg/dl [44].

Treatment with a combination of niacin and simvastatin, decreased LDL by 43%, triglycerides, by 38%, and Lipoprotein(a) by 15% with an increase of 29% of HDL from baseline. For the primary angiographic end point, stenosis progressed with placebo, antioxidants, and regressed with the combination of simvastatin and niacin [45].

The composite clinical end point included CHD death, nonfatal MI, stroke, or revascularization for worsening ischemia. Combination of niacin and simvastatin reduced risk by 90% compared with placebo. Curiously, antioxidants tended to diminish the benefits. These risk reductions are comparable to the epidemiological projections of a 1% reduction in risk for each 1% decrease in LDL and for each 1% increase in HDL. In this trial, LDL was reduced by 42% and HDL was increased by 26% for a calculated risk reduction of 68%.

An interesting sidelight of this study was the presence of metabolic syndrome in 69 of 160 patients. Of these, 69, 32 received simvastatin and niacin. In these metabolic syndrome patients, combination therapy reduced LDL by 40%, triglycerides by 30%, while increasing the HDL by 26%. Of greater importance was the fact that patients with metabolic syndrome had a significantly higher rate of atherosclerotic progression and a twofold higher rate of clinical events than patients who did not have the metabolic syndrome. Even in this high risk population, treatment with simvastatin and niacin reduced CHD progression by 90% and clinical events by 40% in patients with this syndrome. The combination did not significantly affect glucose and insulin levels.

Among all the lipid lowering agents, nicotinic acid can favorably modify all of the lipoprotein abnormalities associated with atherogenic dyslipidemia according to the NCEP III report. The problem with niacin has been its side effect profile (flushing, hepatotoxicity, hyperglycemia, and gout), less potency for LDL reduction, and less outcomes data compared to the statins [13].

Niacin is metabolized by two hepatic pathways:

1. Conjugation with glycine to form nicotinuric acid
2. Conversion to nicotinamide by oxidation-reduction metabolic pathways

The first pathway is a low affinity and high capacity route that generates metabolites that are associated with flushing. The second pathway is a high affinity, low capacity route whose metabolites can be hepatotoxic.

It is the absorption rates of different niacin preparations that dictate the degree of metabolism by each pathway and the corresponding side effect profile. Immediate release or crystalline niacin quickly saturates the second pathway, which results in most of the drug being metabolized by pathway-1 which leads to a high incidence of flushing. Niacin SR is metabolized to a greater degree by pathway-2, which causes less flushing, but more hepatotoxicity, which has been reported with this formulation and can be irreversible and severe [24].

The extended release niacin formulations can significantly attenuate the flushing that can be commonly experienced with other niacin preparations. This phenomenon is mediated by nicotinic acid skin receptors, which release prostaglandin D2. Laropiprant (currently in the development stage) can reduce flushing by inhibiting the binding of prostaglandin D2 to its receptor in the Langerhans cells of the epidermis. Both tissue macrophages and the Langerhans cells can elaborate prostaglandin D2 when stimulated by niacin. Aspirin, taken 30–60 min before dosing, can also alleviate flushing.

Niacin was shown to reduce the incidence of coronary events and stroke in the CDP reported in *JAMA* in 1975. This 5–8 year trial showed a reduction of non fatal MI of 27% at 5 years, stroke and TIA of 21% at 5 years, and total mortality of 11% at 15 years [44].

The Stockholm Ischemic Heart Disease Study in 1988 reported similar results when niacin was combined with clofibrate with a 26% reduction in total mortality and 36% reduction in CHD mortality over a 5-year period of time [46].

The CDP was a double blinded, placebo controlled, secondary prevention trial of lipid lowering therapy conducted between 1966 and 1974. Here, over 8,300 hypercholesterolemic men with previous myocardial infarction were randomized to treatment with placebo, crystalline niacin, clofibrate, estrogen, or dextrothyroxine [17].

Patients treated with 3 g daily of niacin experienced significant reductions in coronary events in this study with 14% reduction in nonfatal MI/CHD death, 27% reduction in nonfatal MI, and 26% of stroke/TIA – all statistically significant. Niacin reduced nonfatal MI similarly in patients with normal and impaired FBG, including those with diabetes as defined by current standards. Here, entry cholesterols were 250 mg/dl with triglycerides of 177 mg/dl with niacin resulting in a 9.9% reduction of cholesterol and 26.1% reduction of triglycerides.

In a post trial follow-up, performed 9 years after the study, ended and published in the Journal of the American College of Cardiology in 1986, total and CHD mortality were reduced even among patients with evidence of impaired glucose tolerance.

Niacin in combination with a bile acid sequestrant has also been shown to promote regression of coronary atherosclerotic lesions in several studies confirmed by coronary angiography including the Cholesterol Lowering Atherosclerosis Study (CLAS) I (1987), CLAS II (1990), Familial Atherosclerosis Treatment Study (FATS) (1990), and the University of California at San Francisco Specialized Center of Research (UCSF-SCOR) (1990) [44].

In the FATS, niacin+colestipol resulted in a 39% regression rate compared to 32% for lovastatin+colestipol, and 11% while the UCSF resulted in a 33% regression with niacin, colestipol, and lovastatin compared to usual care [47].

Crystalline niacin, particularly in higher doses, has been associated with increases in glucose levels and insulin resistance. In 1990, Garg and Grundy evaluated the effects of niacin in 13 patients with type-2 diabetes in an 8-week crossover study using 1,500 mg of niacin t.i.d. for 8 weeks. Niacin reduced triglycerides by 45% and LDL by 15%, and raised HDL by 34%. Niacin also increased fasting blood glucose by 16% and A1C by 21%.

Recently, two large studies (ADVENT and arterial disease multiple intervention trial [ADMIT]) reevaluated niacin monotherapy in the type-2 diabetic. The ADMIT evaluated the effects of immediate release niacin in diabetic patients with peripheral vascular disease. This 48-week trial looked at 125 diabetic patients with an average dose of 2,500 mg daily. Niacin produced progressive decreases in triglycerides, total cholesterol, and LDL and progressive increases in HDL as the dose was titrated upward. Although fasting glucose rose in the 12–18 week period, it returned to baseline and below baseline after 24 weeks [44].

The Assessment of Diabetes Control and Evaluation (ADVENT) trial enrolled 146 patients with diabetes controlled with diet, oral agents (except TZD's), or insulin. This study used extended release Niacin (Niaspan) in doses of 1,000 and 1,500 mg, and placebo with 325 mg of aspirin given 30 min prior to dosing to attenuate flushing.

Niaspan increased HDL by 24.3% at the 1,500 mg dose and 19% with the 1,000 mg dose compared to 4.2% for placebo. This was more pronounced for the larger, more cardio-protective HDL-2 particles compared to the smaller HDL-3 particles. Triglycerides were lowered by 27.8% in the 1,500 mg group, 12.8 in the 1,000 mg group, and 54% in placebo. A1C increased by 0.29% with the 1,500 mg Niaspan dose ($P=0.048$), while the changes with the 1,000 mg dose were comparable to placebo. Fasting glucoses rose between 4 and 8 weeks and returned to baseline by 16 weeks. ADVENT also demonstrated a dose related reduction in hs-CRP of 12% with the 100 mg dose and 20% with the 1,500 mg dose, compared to 2% with placebo. Niaspan reduced the concentration of the smaller, dense LDL particles by 50–60%, while increasing the concentration of the larger, less atherogenic LDL particles [45].

Niacin, in the extended release form, is currently available as a combination pill with simvastatin (SIMCOR) and lovastatin (ADVICOR).

Humans obtain cholesterol from the diet in two sources, de novo synthesis in the extra-hepatic tissues and in the liver and ingested saturated fats and cholesterol. In addition, cholesterol that is excreted in the bile is reabsorbed in the terminal ileum, in a process referred to as enterohepatic recycling. The total amount of cholesterol that is synthesized or in the diet must be excreted

Upwards of 300 mg of cholesterol is derived from the diet each day, while 800 mg is synthesized on a daily basis. This combined amount of 1,100 mg must be excreted as fecal sterols.

Cholesterol in the extrahepatic tissues is delivered to the liver in HDL, the majority of which is derived from in vivo synthesis. HDL is taken up by the liver through the scavenger receptor. Cholesterol produced in the liver has two major fates, most is returned to the liver after being taken up by the extrahepatic tissue and the rest is reintroduced in the systemic circulation as VLDL particles, which are subsequently metabolized to LDL, because the intestinal reabsorption of bile salts and the intestinal absorption of cholesterol from diet and bile play an important role in cholesterol metabolism. These represent key targets for cholesterol lowering therapy.

The bile acid sequestrants like cholestyramine, colestipol, and colesevelam inhibit intestinal reabsorption of these bile acids. The plant stanols and sterols along with the selective cholesterol absorptive inhibitors (ezetimibe) prevent intestinal absorption of cholesterol.

Ezetimibe is currently the only agent in the class of the selective cholesterol intestinal absorptive inhibitors and it does not affect the absorption of other lipid soluble nutrients. This newer class of medication affects cholesterol by several distinct mechanisms. Bile acid sequestrants reduce bile acid reabsorption in the ileum causing hepatic bile acid deficiency. This subsequent deficiency results in an increase in the synthesis of bile acid from hepatic cholesterol, which is subsequently replenished through an increased hepatic uptake of LDL and chylomicrons along with an increased hepatic cholesterol synthesis.

Through this increased clearance of LDL particles by the liver, bile acid sequestrants reduce the LDL concentration. The plant stanols and sterols displace cholesterol from micelles preventing their reuptake at the brush border and subsequently reducing cholesterol that is transported to the liver, hence increasing the clearance of LDL from plasma.

Ezetimibe acts by decreasing the absorption of cholesterol in the bile and from the diet inhibiting its uptake into the cholesterol of the micelles and the intestinal epithelial cells. This enhances LDL clearance by the liver and reduces LDL levels. This action is achieved by a selective inhibition of the intestinal epithelial sterol transporter [48].

After 8 weeks, the addition of ezetimibe to ongoing statin therapy improved LDL levels by 21.4% (−25.1 vs. 3.7% with statin therapy alone, P values <0.001). HDL increased by 1.7% (2.7 vs. 1.0% with statin therapy alone, P<0.05) and triglycerides by 11.1% (−14 vs. −2.9% with statin therapy alone, P<0.01). Twenty-one percent of patients who received ezetimibe in addition to ongoing statin therapy achieved their target LDL goal after 8 weeks of therapy [48].

Ezetimibe continues to demonstrate an excellent overall safety in tolerability profile, except for hypersensitivity reactions including rash, and on rare occasions, angioedema. There was no excess myopathy or rhabdomyolysis associated with ezetimibe compared with placebo or statin alone with only a slight increase in liver function tests if coadministered with statins, although patients who experience myalgias with statins may also experience them with ezetimibe.

Stanol esters will lower LDL by up to 14%, triglyceride up to 10%, with no significant effect on HDL and triglyceride. They can be taken 2 or 3 times/day as a spread and can be used very effectively as adjunctive therapy. These agents are well tolerated and palatable

Table 2
Treatment priorities for diabetic dyslipidemia in adults

Decrease LDL

    Statin

    Statin/resin (colesevelam)

    Statin/ezetimibe

    Statin/fenofibrate

    Resin/fibrate

    Ezetimibe/fenofibrate

    Statin/niacin

Increase HDL

    Behavioral modifications

    Fibrates, statins, niacin (extended release)

Decrease triglyceride

    Glycemic control

    Behavioral and dietary modifications

    Fibrates

    Niacin (extended release)

    Omega-3 acid ethyl esters

    Statins (rosuvastatin, atorvastatin, simvastatin, pitavastatin)

Decrease non-HDL cholesterol

    Statins

    Combination therapy (statin/niacin; statin/fenofibrate

        Statin/ezetimibe; statin/omega-3 acid ethyl esters)

Treatment of mixed dyslipidemia

    Improved glycemic control + statin (rosuvastatin, atorvastain, simvas-
      tatin)

    Improved glycemic control + statin + niacin or statin + ezetimibe

    Improved glycemic control + statin + fenofibrate

    Improved glycemic control + statin + ezetimibe + niacin

    Improved glycemic control + statin + omega-3

From American Diabetes Association

with no significant laboratory abnormalities and certainly safe to use in combination with statins and safe to use in diabeticsy.

The major side effects of the bile acid sequestrants include decreased absorption of the fat soluble vitamins A, D, and K, gastrointestinal distress and constipation and triglyceride elevations with cholestyramine, but not with colesevelam. Despite the known ability to reduce LDL and act synergistically with statins, their clinical use has been limited by several factors. Compliance issues in GI toxicity have been a major problem as well as the total amount of pills that one needs to take, or powders with this type of medication.

Plant sterols and stanols also suffer from a lack of selectivity for cholesterol and may add an added expense to patient cost

Hence managing diabetic dyslipidemia centers around three therapeutic endeavors:

1. Lipid lowering therapy with medication –LDL, HDL, Triglycerides, and non-HDL cholesterol and then novel risk factors: Lipoprotein(a), hs-CRP.
2. Strict glucose control, helping to lower the triglyceride.
3. Adjuvant nutritional therapy, smoking cessation, therapeutic life style changes including weight loss and exercise.

Since reduction in the LDL is the first chore, statins become the treatment of choice with elevation of the HDL and decrease in the non HDL cholesterol, important targets once the LDL has been brought to goal. Triglyceride values greater 500 mg/dl can increase the risk of pancreatitis. In those cases that cannot be managed with diet alone, additions of niacin, fibrates, and omega-3 acid ethyl esters or using these agents first line should be considered [49]. Physicians should also be aware that metformin and pioglitazone will also have triglyceride lowering effects.

SUMMARY

Diabetic dyslipidemia causes substantial alterations in major plasma proteins and substantially increases the risk of coronary heart disease and arteriosclerotic disease in general. These abnormalities are far more common in patients with type-2 diabetes than in type-1. In addition, patients with type-2 diabetes who have existing coronary heart disease have a worse prognosis and their outlook for survival is substantially decreased.

Type-2 diabetes warrants an aggressive primary and secondary approach to coronary heart disease prevention by the primary care physician. This is underscored by the elevation of type-2 diabetes as a coronary heart disease risk equivalent with recommendations to treat these patients as if they had established coronary disease.

Treatment priorities for diabetic dyslipidemia are summarized in Table 2.

REFERENCES

1. Miranda PJ, DeFronzo RA, Califf RM, Guyton J. Metabolic syndrome: definition, pathophysiology, and mechanism. Am Heart J. 2005;149:33–45.
2. Cordero A, LaClaustra M, Leon M, Grima A, Casanovas J, Luengo E, del Rio A. Prehypertension is associated with insulin resistance; the MESYAS registry. Am J Hypertens. 2006;19(2):189–196.
3. NCEP Expert Panel. Executive summary of the third report of the National Cholesterol Education Program. JAMA. 2001;285:2486–2497.
4. Shepherd J, Barter P, Carmena R. Effect of lowering LDL cholesterol substantially below currently recommended levels in patients with coronary heart disease and diabetes: the treating to new targets (TNT) study. Diabetes Care. 2006;29:1220–1226.
5. Tung P, Wiviott S, Cannon C, Murphy S, McCabe C, Gibson M. Seasonla variation in lipids following acute coronary syndrome on fixed doses of Pravastatin or Atorvastatin from the PROVE IT-TIMI study. Am J Cardiol. 2009;103:1056–1060.
6. Robins S, Collins D, Wittes J, Papademetriou V. VA-HIT, a randomized trial. JAMA. 2001;285:1585–1591.

7. Lange P, Parner J, Schnohr P, Jensen G. The copenhagen city heart study. Eur Respir J. 2002;20: 1406–1412.
8. Nordestgaard B, Benn M, Schnohr P, Hansen A. Nonfasting triglycerides and risk for myocardial infarction, ischemic heart disease and death. JAMA. 2007;298:299–308.
9. Best JD, et al. Diabetic dyslipidemia, current treatment and recommendations. Drugs. 2000;59:1101–1111.
10. Johnson R, McNutt P, MacMahon S, Robson R. The use of the Friedewald formula to estimate LDL. Clin Chem. 1997;43:2183–2184.
11. St. Pierre A, Cantin B, Dagenais G, Mauriege B. Low density lipoprotein subfractions and the long term risk of ischemic heart disease in men. The Quebec Cardiovascular Study. Arterioscler Thromb Vasc Biol. 2005;25:553.
12. American Diabetes Association. Management of dyslipidemia in adults with diabetes. Diabetes Care. 2000;23(suppl 1):S57–S60.
13. Steiner G. Treating lipid abnormalities in patients with type 2 diabetes mellitus. Am J Cardiol. 2001;88(suppl):37N–40N.
14. Bush T, Barrett-Connor E, Cowan L, Criqui M. The lipid research clinics follow up study. Circulation. 1987;75:1102–1109.
15. The Diabetes Atorvastatin Lipid Intervention group. The DALI study. Diabetes Care. 2001;24(8): 1335–1341.
16. Canner PL, Furberg CD, McGovewrn ME. Benefits of niacin in patients with and without the metabolic syndrome. Am J Cardiol. 2006;97:477–479.
17. The Coronary Drug Project Research Group. Clofibrate and niacin in coronary heart disease. JAMA. 1975;231:360–381.
18. Armani AM, Toth PP. Colesevelam hydrochloride in the management of dyslipidemia. Expert Rev Cardiovasc Ther. 2006;4(3):283–291.
19. Manghat P, Wierzbicki AS. Colesevelam hydrochloride: a specifically engineered bile acid sequestrant. Future Lipidol. 2008;3:237–253.
20. Toth PP, Dayspring TD, Pokrywka GS. Drug therapy for hypertriglyceridemia: fibrates and omega-3 fatty acids. Curr Atheroscler Rep. 2009;11(1):71–79.
21. Vakkillainen J, Steiner G, Ansquer J. Fenofibrate lowers triglycerides and increases LDL particle number in subjects with type-2 diabetes. Diabetes Care. 2002;25(3):627–628.
22. Rubins HB, Robins SJ, Collins D. Gemfibrozil for the secondary prevention of coronary heart disease in men with low levels of high density lipoprotein cholesterol. Veterans Affairs High Density Lipoprotein Cholesterol Intervention Trial Study Group. N Engl J Med. 1999;341:410–418.
23. Hartweg J, Perera R, Montori VM, Dineen SF, Neil A, Farmer AJ. Omega-3 Polyunsaturated fatty acids for diabetes. Cochrane Database Syst Rev. 2010;(4):CD003205.
24. Pan J, et al. Niacin treatment of the atherogenic profile and Lp(a) in diabetes. Diabetes Obes Metab. 2002;4:255–261.
25. Goldberg RB, Kendall DM, Deeg MA, Buse JB, Zagar AJ, Pinier JA, Tan MH, The GLAI Investigators. A comparison of the lipid and glycemic effects of pioglitazone and rosiglitazone in type-2 diabetics and dyslipidemia. Diabetes Care. 2005;28:1547–1554.
26. Khan M, Berhanu P, Perex A, Demisse S, Fleck P, Kupfer S. Effects of pioglitazone in combination with stable statin therapy on lipid levels in subjects with type-2 diabetes and dyslipidemia when switched from rosiglitazone (The COMPLEMENT trial). Diabetes. 2005;54(suppl 1):A137.
27. Szapary P, Bloedon LT, Samaha FF, Duffy D, Reilly M, Chittams J, Rader D. Effects of pioglitazone on lipoproteins, inflammatory markers and adipokines in non diabetic patients with metabolic syndrome. Arterioscler Throm Vasc Biol. 2006;26:182.
28. Jones PH, Davidson MH, Stein EA. Comparison of the efficacy and safety of rosuvastatin versus atorvastatin, simvastatin, and pravastatin across doses (STELLAR Trial). Am J Cardiol. 2003;92:152–160.
29. Tricor Package Insert. North Chicago: Abbott Laboratories; 2001.
30. Jones PH, Davidson MH, et al. Comparison of the efficacy and safety of rosuvastatin vs. atorvastatin, simvastatin, and pravastatin across doses (STELLAR trial). Am J Cardiol. 2003;92:152–160.
31. Capuzzi DM, Morgan JM, Carey CM. Rosuvastatin alone or with extended release niacin; a new therapeutic option for patients with combined hyperlipidemia. Prev Cardiol. 2004;7:176–181.
32. Ridker PM, The JUPITER Study Group. Rosuvastatin in the primary prevention of cardiovascular disease among patients with low levels of low density lipoprotein cholesterol and elevated high sensitivity C-reactive protein. Circulation. 2003;108:2292–2297.

33. Scandinavian Simvastatin Survival Study Investigators. Randomized trial of cholesterol lowering in 4444 patients with coronary heart disease: The 4S Study. Lancet. 1994;344:1383–1389.

34. The Long Term Intervention with Pravastatin in Ischemic Disease (LIPID) Study group. Prevention of cardiovascular events and death with pravastatin in patients with coronary heart disease and a broad range of initial cholesterol levels. N Engl J Med. 1998;339:1349–1357.

35. Shek A, Ferrill MJ. Statin-fibrate combination therapy. Ann Pharmacother. 2001;35:908–917.

36. Prucksaritanont T, Zhao JJ, et al. Mechanistic studies on metabolic interactions between gemfibrozil and statins. JPET. 2002;301:1042–1051.

37. Downs JR, Clearfield M, Weis S. Primary prevention of acute coronary events with lovastatin in men and women with average cholesterol levels: results of AFCAPS/TexCAPS. Air Force/Texas Coronary Atherosclerosis Prevention Study. JAMA. 1998;279:1615–6122.

38. Heart Protection Study Collaborative Group. MRC/BHF Heart Protection Study of cholesterol lowering with simvastatin in 20,536 high-risk individuals: a randomised placebo-controlled trial. Lancet. 2002;360:7–22.

39. Grundy SM, Vega LG, Yuan Z. Effectiveness and tolerability of simvastatin plus fenofibrate for combined hyperlipidemia (the SAFARI trial). Am J Cardiol. 2005;95:462–468.

40. Vrecer M, Turk S, et al. Use of statins in primary and secondary prevention of coronary heart disease and ischemic stroke. Int J Clin Parmacol Ther. 2003;41:567–577.

41. Hites RA, Foran JA, Carpenter DO, Hamilton MC, Knuth BA, Schwager SJ. Risk global assessment of organic contaminants in farmed salmon. Science. 2004;303:226–229.

42. Davidson M. Omega-3 fatty acids enhance statin lipid lowering effects. The COMBOS trial. Clin Ther. 2007;29:1354–1357.

43. Brown BG, Zhao X-Q, Chait A. Simvastatin and niacin, antioxidant vitamins, or the combination for the prevention of coronary disease. N Engl J Med. 2001;345:1583–1592.

44. Elam MB, et al. Effect of niacin on lipid and lipoprotein levels and glycemic control in patients with diabetes and peripheral arterial disease. The ADMIT study: a randomized trial. JAMA. 2000;284: 1263–1270.

45. Zhao XQ. Simvastatin plus niacin protect against atherosclerosis progression and clinical events in coronary artery disease patients with metabolic syndrome. Am Coll Cardiol. 2002;39(suppl A):242A.

46. Carlson LA, Rosenhamer G. Reduction of mortality in the Stockholm Ischemic. Heart Disease Secondary Prevention Study by combined treatment with clofibrate and nicotinic acid. Acta Med Scand. 1988;223:405–418.

47. Brown G, Albers JJ, Fisher LD. Regression of coronary artery disease as a result of intensive lipid lowering therapy in men with high levels of apolipoprotein B. N Engl J Med. 1990;323:1289–1298.

48. Morris MC, Sacks F, et al. Does fish oil lower blood pressure? A meta-analysis of controlled trials. Circulation. 1993;88:523.

49. The NCEP Expert Panel on Detection, Evaluation and Treatment of High Blood Cholesterol in Adults. JAMA. 2001;285:2486–2497.

50. Mykkanen L, Laakso M, Pentilla I, Pyorala K. Asymptomatic hyperglycemia and cardiovascular risk factors in the elderly. Atherosclerosis. 1991;88:153–161.

SUPPLEMENTARY READINGS

Carswell CL, Plosker GL, et al. Rosuvastatin. Drugs. 2002;62:2075–2085.

Castelli WP. Cholesterol and lipids in the risk of coronary artery disease – the Framingham Heart Study. Can J Cardiol. 1988;4(suppl A):5A–10A.

Castelli WP. Cardiovascular disease and multifactorial risk: challenge of the 1980s. Am Heart J. 1983;106:1191–1200.

Despres JP. Increasing high density lipoprotein cholesterol, an update on fenofibrate. Am J Cardiol. 2001;88(suppl):30N–36N.

Garg A, Grundy SM. Nicotinic acid as therapy for dyslipidemia in non-insulin dependent diabetes mellitus. JAMA. 1990;264:723–726.

Goldberg IJ. Diabetic dyslipidemia, causes and consequences. J Clin Endocrinol Metab. 2001;86: 965–971.

Goldberg RB, et al. Cardiovascular events and their reduction with pravastatin in diabetic and glucose intolerant myocardial infarction survivors with average cholesterol levels: CARE trial. Circulation. 1998;98:2513–2519.

Koskinen P, et al. Coronary heart disease incidence in NIDDM patients in the Helsinki Heart Study. Diabetes Care. 1992;15:820–825.

Langtry HD, Markham A. Fluvastatin, a review of it use in lipid disorders. Drugs. 1999;57:583–606.

McKenney J. Combination therapy for elevated low density lipoprotein cholesterol. The key to coronary artery disease risk reduction. Am J Cardiol. 2002;90(suppl):8K–20K.

Miettinen TA, Taskinen MR, et al. Glucose tolerance and plasma insulin in man during acute and chronic administration of nicotinic acid. Acta Med Scand. 1969;186:247–253.

Rubins HB, et al. Gemfibrozil for the secondary prevention of coronary heart disease in men with low levels of high density lipoprotein cholesterol: VA-HIT Study group. N Engl J Med. 1999;341: 410–418.

Steiner F. Lipid intervention trials in diabetes. Diabetes Care. 2001;23(suppl 2):B49–B53.

Superko HR, Krauss RM. Differential effects of nicotinic acid in subjects with different LDL subclass patterns. Atherosclerosis. 1992;95:69–76.

12 Hypertension in Diabetics

CONTENTS

Key Words: Hypertension, Hypertensive diabetic, Combination Therapy, Cardiovascular disease, Osaka Health Survey

INTRODUCTION

The worldwide prevalence of hypertension is expected to increase from approximately 1 billion individuals in 2000 to over 1.5 billion in 2025 and is currently the most frequent medical diagnosis in the USA [1]. Not only is hypertension a powerful risk factor for cardiovascular disease, doubling the risk of mortality from coronary heart disease and stroke for every 20 mmHg increase in systolic blood pressure and 10 mmHg increase in diastolic pressure, but also is closely linked to the risk of developing type-2 diabetes.

In the Osaka Health Survey, the relative risk of developing type-2 diabetes was 1.76 for hypertensive men compared to 1.39 for normotensive men [2]. In this study, high blood pressure was greater than 140/90 mmHg, and high normal was greater than 130/85 mmHg. In the Framingham Heart Study, blood pressures of 130/85–139/89 mmHg are associated with twice the cardiovascular mortality risk than individuals with blood pressures below 120/80 mmHg.

From: *Current Clinical Practice: Type 2 Diabetes, Pre-Diabetes, and the Metabolic Syndrome*
Edited by: R.A. Codario, DOI 10.1007/978-1-60327-441-8_12
© Springer Science+Business Media, LLC 2011

Table 1
JNC-VII Classification of Hypertension

Classification	Systolic (mmHg)	Diastolic (mmHg)
Normal	<120	<80
Prehypertension	120–139	80–89
Stage 1 Hypertension	140–159	90–99
Stage 2 Hypertension	≥160	≥100

Adapted from Chobanian et al. [45]

CLASSIFICATION OF HYPERTENSION (TABLE 1)

The seventh Joint National Committee (JNC 7) on Detection, Prevention, Evaluation, and Treatment of High Blood Pressure defined optimal pressure of <120/80 mmHg. in an adult. Their classification is as follows:

Elevated blood pressure not only increases the risk of developing diabetes, but represents an important predictor of nephropathy, retinopathy, and cardiovascular disease in type-2 diabetics. The incidence of hypertension is markedly increased among patients with diabetes being 1.5–3.0 times more common in patients with type-2 diabetes than in age matched general population. Although the prevalence of hypertension can vary depending on the patient population studied, 40% of people with diabetes have hypertension at age 45 while more than 60% have hypertension by the age of 65. Interestingly, about 30% of people with type-1 diabetes will eventually develop hypertension following the development of diabetic nephropathy.

Hypertension represents a major macrovascular risk factor for patients with diabetes with stroke, accounting for 65% of deaths in addition to markedly increased microvascular complications. Diabetic hypertensives who achieved a diastolic blood pressure of less than 80 mmHg demonstrated a 50% reduction in major cardiovascular events compared with those whose diastolic blood pressure was less than 90 mg. in the Hypertension Optimal Trial (HOT), while the UKPDS trial demonstrated significant reductions in diabetes mortality, macrovascular complications, and the risk of stroke with tight blood pressure control. Major cardiovascular events occur in approximately 5% of people with diabetes and untreated hypertension yearly and the risk increases significantly in the presence of diabetic nephropathy and other risk factors.

The United States Preventive Services Task Force in 2008 recommended screening individuals with treated or untreated sustained blood pressures >135/80 mmHg for type-2 diabetes [3].

PATHOPHYSIOLOGY OF HYPERTENSION IN OBESITY AND TYPE-2 DIABETES

Metabolic syndrome increases the risk for developing hypertension and overall cardiovascular risk reinforcing the need for identifying the clustering of surrogate markers within this operational concept to appreciate the patient's global risk.

Not to be forgotten is the role of obesity, particularly abdominal, as one of the strongest predictors for hypertension development, increasing progressively with increasing body mass index, with even modest weight loss attenuating that risk. The coexistence of obesity and hypertension enhances the risk of developing type-2 diabetes, while the prevalence of hypertension is up to three times greater than non diabetics of the same sex and age. Almost half of all hypertensive patients are insulin resistant and obese. Hyperinsulinemia is not only directly correlated with hypertension, but induces several mechanisms inherent to and promoting the process, including endogenous angiotensin II production, sympathetic nervous system activation, and endothelial dysfunction. In addition, the vasodilatory properties of insulin tend to be attenuated in primary hypertension due to impaired nitric oxide secretion. It should be appreciated, however, that some ethnic groups (i.e., African American) insulin resistance may not be related to hypertension in those with type-2 diabetes, but may involve enhanced salt sensitivity.

Although the cause of hypertension in type 2 diabetic is multifactorial and complex, the risk of hypertension clearly increases with age, with patients about twice as likely to develop increased blood pressure who had at least one parent with the condition. African Americans have a 7–10% increase in prevalence compared to non-Hispanic white Americans. In addition, for each unit increase in BMI, systolic blood pressure increases by 1.0–1.5%. Conversely weight loss has been associated with reductions in blood pressure in many studies.

Body fat distribution patterns have recently been recognized also as a major risk factor for hypertension in type-2 diabetes, particularly with upper body obesity. Clinical assessments of body fat distribution is derived from measuring waist to hip ratio, the ratio of subscapular to triceps skin folds, and central or upper body adiposity. Although there is no uniformly internationally recognized standard as to what constitutes upper body adiposity, waist hip ratios greater than 0.85 in woman and 0.95 in men have generally been accepted as being abnormal.

Some studies have indicated that the association between blood pressure and body fat distribution are independent of one another with central adiposity being related to blood pressure cross sectionally in Hispanics, African Americans, and whites. Interest recently has focused on the ratio of visceral fat measured by computerized tomography compared to the less metabolically active, central, subcutaneous fat, with higher correlations associated with visceral and retroperitoneal adipose tissue mass and blood pressure in normal glycemic humans. Normal glycemic hypertensive patients are more likely to be insulin resistant than those patients who developed hypertension at an early age with an increased frequency of dyslipidemia and elevated insulin levels.

Although the association between insulin levels, insulin resistance, and hypertension is still being explored, the metabolic consequences and association of insulin resistance, mainly enhanced sodium retention, altered fatty acid transport, proliferation of vascular smooth muscle cells, and enhanced sympathetic nervous system activity with its associated increased peripheral vascular resistance makes the connection highly plausible.

One of the main controversies in associating insulin resistance with hypertension stems around the discrepancy that it can exist in some studies involving various ethnic groups. The associations between insulin resistance and hypertension can be seen in lean African American males but not in Pima Indians. Other studies have indicated that the association of hypertension with insulin resistance is related to differences in adiposity. In normotensive men, short term insulin infusions for 2 h can raise catecholamine levels, but not blood pressure with vasodilatation occurring rather than vasoconstriction. The effects of chronic hyperglycemia remain to be elucidated. Mexican Americans and Pima Indians have high rates of type-2 diabetes, insulin resistance, and hyperglycemia, but yet demonstrate a lower prevalence of hypertension.

The general concept of cardiovascular risk factor cluttering with hypertension has been described in familial dyslipidemia hypertension syndrome where the lipid abnormalities may precede the development of hypertension – particularly reductions in high density lipoprotein cholesterol and increased triglyceride levels. When this association is studied in the obese individuals, the impact of insulin resistance is shown to be greater with hypertension increasing in a step wise fashion along with baseline fasting insulin concentrations in cases with BMI's less than 25 kg/m^2. This, however, was not seen in more obese individuals with little insulin resistance in whom hypertension decreased with increasing BMI's.

Nonetheless, it is important to keep in mind that close to 50% of all hypertensive patients are insulin resistant and obese, with an increase of 30% in insulin resistance increasing the risk of diastolic hypertension, suggesting that the effect of insulin resistance on hypertension is even more significant than the effects of increasing obesity or age. In patients with the metabolic syndrome and obesity, both local and systemic renin-angiotensin systems (RASs) are significantly stimulated with the visceral adipose tissue expressing all the components present in the RAS.

This enhanced RAS activity promotes increased production of reactive oxygen species in skeletal muscle, cardiovascular tissue, and adipocytes in addition to promoting further insulin resistance through the stimulation of the angiotensin-2, type-1 receptors combined with enhanced renal tubular sodium absorption and increased aldosterone secretion associated with this disorder.

Accelerated oxidated stress enhances the effects of inflammatory adipokines and fatty acids promoting atherogenesis and endothelial dysfunction with therapeutic blockade of the RAS system reducing the production of reactive oxidative species. The importance of tight blood pressure control was underscored in the UKPDS trial, which demonstrated 45% reduction in risk of fatal, a non-fatal stroke with systolic blood pressure reductions of 10 mmHg and diastolic blood pressures of 5 mmHg compared to a control group [4].

In the Systolic Hypertension in Europe (Syst-Eur) trial, similar trends were observed with reductions in systolic hypertension reducing stroke rates in diabetics older than 60 years of age with use of nitrendipine. Moderate salt restriction and weight reduction have also been shown to reduce blood pressure in both type-1 and type-2 hypertensive diabetic patients in clinical trials with increased dietary sodium sensitivity being demonstrated in hypertensive patients with renal insufficiency, type 2 diabetes, obesity, African Americans, the elderly, and patients with low renin hypertension [5].

Type-2 diabetic patients also demonstrate a loss of a normal nocturnal drop in blood pressure and heart rate when measured with 24-h ambulatory monitoring. This non-dipping is associated with increased left ventricular mass, microalbuminuria, increased risk of stroke, and myocardial infarction.

Diabetic patients who demonstrate autonomic dysfunction may also have lightheadedness, unsteady gait, fatigue, and orthostatic hypotension. This is why it is important to measure supine and erect blood pressures in all diabetic patients, since doses of anti-hypertensive medications may require careful titration particularly when postural hypotension is found.

Therapeutic lifestyle changes can also play a major role in reducing blood pressure in patients with diabetes. Weight loss, smoke cessation, sodium restriction, 30–45 min of aerobic activity four to five times weekly, reduction in alcohol consumption, and intake of potassium 4,700 mg daily and magnesium 500 mg daily, with liberal servings of vegetables and whole grains have demonstrated significant clinical benefits. The Finnish Diabetes Prevention Program demonstrated the importance of therapeutic lifestyle changes in preventing onset of type-2 diabetes in improving overall cardiovascular health [6]. The combination of low sodium, low fat, high fiber diets are a cornerstone of dietary intervention in diabetic patients. Increased fiber intake accompanied with judicious substitution of complex carbohydrates for saturated fats with smaller feedings are important elements in the ADA diet. The benefits of hypertension control in this patient population result from direct reduction in the metabolic effects of angiotensin II and/or the beneficial effects of renin-angiotensin-aldosterone system inhibition, which reduces atherosclerotic and microvascular complications.

Most diabetic patients achieving optimal blood pressure reductions of less than 130/80 require two or more antihypertensive medications, with the average number of drugs required for a pressure reduction to 130/85 being 3.1 medications [7]. Close to 50% of patients will not reach target blood pressure reduction despite being on three medications.

Several possible explanations between the association of obesity and hypertension include:

1. Adiponectin – Progressive increases in body weight and visceral adipose tissue are associated with decreased expression of adiponectin receptors, messenger RNA, and serum adiponectin levels. Adiponectin may play a key role in maintaining vascular homeostasis as well as possessing anti-atherogenic, anti-inflammatory, and insulin sensitizing capabilities. Decreased adiponectin levels have not only been associated with hypertension, but also an important novel surrogate marker for metabolic syndrome.
2. RAS activation – Obesity and the metabolic syndrome activates both local tissue adipose and systemic renin-angiotensin-aldosterone system (RAAS). Human adipose tissue, especially visceral adipose expresses all the components of the RAAS system including the angiotensin-II type 1 receptor and angiotensinogen. Overactivation of the tissue RAS stimulates the angiotensin II type 1 receptors promoting insulin resistance and enhancing the production of reactive oxygen species in skeletal and cardiac muscle, the vascular endothelium, and within the adipocyte. This accelerated oxidative stress promotes atherogenesis and endothelial dysfunction promoting accumulation of free fatty acids and adiponectin deficiency. The impact of insulin resistance on hypertension is even stronger than the effect of increasing age or obesity with reduced blood pressures being associated with increased insulin sensitivity.
3. Activation of the sympathetic nervous system via leptin mediated mechanisms.

This adipocyte secreted hormone exerts its effects via neuropeptides like corticotropin-releasing hormone and melanocortin to increase arterial pressure and overall sympathetic nervous system activity, while decreasing food intake and stimulating the rate of metabolism. Obese individuals develop resistance to leptin's appetite suppressant and metabolic effects, but not its pressor and sympathetic activation properties, resulting in elevated blood pressure.

From a hemodynamic point of view, obesity related hypertension results from expansion of plasma volume, increasing cardiac output associated with an inadequate response to decreased systemic vascular resistance to compensate for these changes. Systolic blood pressure increases by 4.5 mmHg for every 10 pound weight increase [8]. Similar mechanisms underlie the mechanism of hypertension in the diabetic patient who is also prone to accelerated atherosclerosis. The diabetic hypertensive demonstrates a pattern of arterial aging characterized by enhanced arterial stiffness and vascular remodeling resistant to even effective anti-hypertensive control.

Clearly, the prevalence of hypertension is increased in patients with diabetes and vice versa with at least 50% of patients having at the time of diagnosis or diabetes have or will have hypertension [9]. The oxidative stress and nitric oxide reduction promote thrombosis, inflammation, and vasoconstriction seen in the diabetic hypertensive patients.

Hypertension is more commonly seen in the obese diabetic than the obese non-diabetic and in 40% of those who develop diabetic nephropathy [10].

Since diabetes is diagnosed by blood glucose levels, in the past, much of the attention toward diabetic care focused on the management of hyperglycemia and clearly there has been a well established link between hyperglycemia and microvascular outcomes.

TREATMENT FOR THE HYPERTENSIVE TYPE-2 DIABETIC (TABLE 2)

The UKPDS (United Kingdom Prospective Diabetes Study) group investigated the importance of tight verses less tight blood pressure control and discovered significantly reduced micro and macrovascular complications in the tight control group verses the less tight control group [9].

The Hypertension Optimal Treatment (HOT) study was designed to determine if cardiovascular outcomes could be related to diastolic blood pressure levels. In this study, more than 18,000 patients between the ages of 50 and 80 with hypertension and diastolic blood pressures between 100 and 115 mmHg were randomized to achieve diastolic blood pressure readings equal to or less than 90 mmHg, equal to or less than 85 mmHg, and equal to or less than 80 mmHg. In addition to being started on a dihydropyridine antihypertensive agent, patients were randomized to receive low dose aspirin, 75 mg a day, and followed for an average period of time of 3.8 years [11].

One thousand, five hundred and one of these patients had diabetes at baseline and 8% of the patients in each of the target diastolic blood pressure groups had diabetes. Looking at the diabetic subset, the rate of fatal and nonfatal myocardial infarctions, stroke and other cardiovascular events declined in relation to the target diastolic blood pressure group and all were statistically significant. Risks for these events in the equal to or less than 80 mmHg

Table 2
Choice of agents for hypertension in type-2 diabetes

Treating blood pressure to less than 130/85 mmHg provides dramatic benefits
Thiazide diuretics, ARB's and ace inhibitors are first line treatments
Other agents may often be necessary and goals may not be achieved with
Three or four agents
Aggressive blood pressure control may be the most important factor
In preventing adverse outcomes in type 2 diabetics

Adapted from Vijan et al. [46]

group was reduced by 51% relative to the equal to or less than 90 mmHg group. Risk for stroke and myocardial infarction were also reduced with the lower diastolic blood pressure levels.

In comparison to the 90 mmHg diastolic group, the 80 mmHg group demonstrated reductions of 30% for stroke and 50% for myocardial infarctions; however, these risk reductions did not achieve statistical significance, but cardiovascular mortality in the equal to or less than 80 mmHg group was reduced by 67% compared to the other diastolic blood pressure target groups and the *P*-values were significant at 0.016. Hence the HOT trial supported the concept that diastolic blood pressures equal to or less than 85 mmHg were associated with significant reductions in cardiovascular morbidity and mortality in diabetic patients. In patients with coronary artery disease, a diastolic blood pressure <70 mmHg is associated with an increased risk of CAD events according to Messerli [*12*].

Since the coronary circulation receives its perfusion during diastole, Messerli and others feel that an excessive decrease in diastolic blood pressure can decrease coronary perfusion. This is referred to as the "J-curve", which is the point at which mortality and morbidity increase in response to drops in diastolic blood pressure. Hence antihypertensive drugs that are not coronary protective, can compromise coronary circulation in patients with coronary artery disease.

Adler, in the *British Medical Journal* pointed out the relationship between systolic blood pressure over time and the incidence of both micro and macrovascular complications. In this study, 4,801 patients with type-2 diabetes who had been recruited for the UKPDS trial with baseline systolic blood pressures being measured at 2 and 9 months after the diagnosis of diabetes were evaluated [*13*].

The systolic blood pressure exposure over time for each patient was subsequently calculated and the patients were placed into categories at 10 mmHg increments for systolic blood pressure from 120 up to 160 mmHg. After adjusting for age, ethnicity and sex, the incidence of any diabetes related complication was strongly associated with systolic blood pressure with the incidence of complications increasing two fold over the range of systolic blood pressure from less than 120 to greater than 160 mmHg.

In addition, risk reductions were also significant for microvascular disease, amputations or death from peripheral disease, myocardial infarction, and heart failure. There was no threshold systolic blood pressure identified for any complication. However, the lowest risk was associated with systolic blood pressure less than 120 mmHg.

Therefore, treatment of hypertension in type-2 diabetics provides a dramatic beneficial effect. Targets of 135 mmHg or less are advisable and diastolic blood pressures less than 80 mmHg are optimal in this patient subset. Preferred first line agents for the treatment of hypertension in diabetes are the angiotensin II receptor blocker, the angiotensin converting enzyme (ACE) inhibitors, and the thiazide diuretics.

Although beta-blockers and calcium channel blockers are more effective than placebo, these agents may not be as effective as diuretics, angiotensin II receptor blockers, or ACE inhibitors when used first line and are better considered as adjuvant therapy. A recent data points out that intensive hypertension control is an extremely cost saving and cost effective diabetic intervention strategy [*14*].

ACE inhibitors and angiotensin receptor blockers (ARBs) are even more effective in lowering blood pressure with the addition of a diuretic to maximize the effects. These classes of medications have been shown to reduce disease progression, reduce cardiovascular risk, attenuate albuminuria, and reduce mortality and morbidity associated with systolic heart failure. Patients treated with nondihydropyridine calcium channel blockers demonstrated reduction in morbidity and mortality similar to a beta blocker based regimen. However, non-dihydropyridine and dihydropyridine calcium channel blockers have been shown to be less effective than ARBs or ACE inhibitors in delaying the progression of diabetic kidney disease. Therefore, the calcium channel blockers should be reserved for add-on therapy or used in combination with an ACE inhibitor or ARB in the hypertensive diabetic patient.

Dietary management has also been effective, with weight reduction and exercise being cornerstones of therapy. Sodium restriction in general has not been widely tested in the diabetic patient population. However, controlled studies in essential hypertension have shown a reduction to systolic blood pressure of about 5 mmHg and diastolic blood pressure of 2–3 mmHg with moderate sodium restriction of less than 2,000 mg of sodium a day.

In the Antihypertensive and Lipid Lowering Treatment to Prevent Heart Attack Trial (ALLHAT), blood pressures were decreased by 15.2 mmHg systolic and 9.8 mmHg diastolic with chlorthalidone, and 17.9 mmHg systolic and 10.7 mmHg diastolic with lisinopril. It is an important point to keep in mind that a better response is obtained when the patient has been on concomitant salt restriction with or before antihypertensive therapy.

Different drug classes of medications have been shown to be of benefit in the management of hypertension in diabetics including ACE inhibitors and ARBs. The ALLHAT trial showed benefits of chlorthalidone therapy in the hypertensive and diabetic subset [15].

In the vast majority of hypertensive individuals, more than one medication is needed to achieve control. This is truly important in the diabetic patient where lower systolic and diastolic blood pressures are important. Clearly, there is strong evidence that pharmacologic therapy of hypertensive diabetics can provide substantial decreases in cardiovascular and microvascular outcomes.

The alpha-blocker arm of the ALLHAT trial was terminated after a sub-analysis showed that these agents were substantially less effective than diuretic therapy in reducing congestive heart failure.

Clearly, the data supports that patients with diabetes should be treated to a diastolic blood pressure of less than 80 mmHg. Those with a systolic blood pressure of greater than 130 and less than 139 mmHg can be given a trial of therapeutic life style changes and behavior therapy for a maximum of 3 months, but must be treated pharmacologically if this is not successful after this short trial period.

Those individuals with systolic blood pressures greater than 140 mmHg or diastolic blood pressures greater than 90 mmHg should be started on medication therapy. This therapy should be with ACE inhibitors, ARBs, or diuretics. In those hypertensive individuals who have existing microalbuminuria or clinical evidence of nephropathy, ARBs and ACE inhibitors should be given unless there is some contraindication to their use.

For those individuals 55 years of age or over, either with or without hypertension, ramipril at doses titrated up to 10 mg is the agent of choice in view of the outstanding trial from the HOPE trial with telmisartan indicated for those patients intolerant to ACE's [16].

For those patients who have had a recent myocardial infarction, beta-blockers should be added to the regimen. An important therapeutic decision in managing the hypertensive diabetic is the role of beta-blockers and at what point in therapy they should be used.

In a study of diabetic patients with unstable angina, beta-blockers improved the 3-month mortality from 8.6 to 2.5% and the 6 month mortality from 16.79 to 8.6%. Cardiac mortality was reduced by 42% and cardiac events declined from 14 to 7.8% after 3 years of beta-blocker use in diabetic subjects in the Bezafibrate Infarction Prevention (BIP) Trial [17].

Beta-blockers have several beneficial effects on the myocardial vasculature. When the heart rate decreases, diastolic filling time is prolonged, thus increasing the blood flow to the myocardial tissue. By decreasing heart rate and blood pressure, beta blockers play an important role in reducing cardiac work load. These agents can also increase vagal tone lessening the likelihood of arrhythmia, while having an anti-atherogenic effect by decreasing arterial sheer stress, improving endothelial function, decreasing inflammation within the atheromatous plaques, and inhibiting platelet aggregation.

Beta-blockers are also effective in decreasing the hepatic production and myocardial utilization of free fatty acids subsequently increasing myocardial glucose utilization. The subsequent decrease in myocardial oxygen consumption decreases the frequency of myocardial ischemia and results in few cardiac arrhythmias. Beta-blockers have also been shown to lower levels of C-reactive protein, preventing and reversing myocardial remodeling [18].

The effective management of hypertension in the diabetic patients usually requires multiple medications underscoring the need for the utilization of medications that are additive or even synergistic in their effects. The benefits of tight blood pressure control have been clearly illustrated in the United Kingdom Prospective Diabetes Study (UKPDS) outline in Table 3.

Beta-blockers are recommended following myocardial infarction, heart failure or high risk coronary artery disease due to their proven benefits in risk reduction. Since first and second generation beta-blockers may worsen glycemic control and insulin sensitivity, mask hypoglycemia, and promote dyslipidemia, they are not first line agents for the hypertensive diabetic.

The American Association of Clinical Endocrinologists recommends third generation beta-blockers like nebivolol and carvedilol as second or third line agents [19]. Due to their

Table 3
UKPDS: blood pressure study, tight versus less tight control

Endpoint	Risk reduction (%)	P value
Any diabetes related endpoint	24	0.0046
Diabetes related deaths	32	0.019
Heart failure	56	0.043
Stroke	44	0.013
Myocardial infarction	21	NS
Microvascular disease	37	0.0092
Retinopathy progression	34	0.0038
Deterioration of vision	47	0.0036

1,148 type-2 diabetics
BP lowered to average of 144/82 mmHg (controls = 154/87)
Nine-year follow up
Adapted from UKPDS Group [9]

anti-atherogenic properties, beta-blockers can reduce inflammation, improve endothelial function, reduce plaque rupture, and minimize the effects of shear stress. Due to their sympathetic blockade and renin inhibition, they possess anti-arrhythmic and anti-hypertensive properties.

First generation beta-blockers (propranolol) affect both the beta-1 and beta-2 adrenergic receptors, while second generation beta-blockers like metoprolol or atenolol are more beta-1 selective. Third generation beta blockers like carvedilol are non selective in their beta blocking capabilities, but also block alpha adrenergic receptors resulting in vasodilatation. Nebivolol generates its vasodilatory effects from stimulating nitric oxide release. The first and second generation beta-blockers increase insulin resistance. Fasting plasma glucose and serum insulin as well as apolipoprotein B/apolipoprotein A-1 ratios increased when an atenolol/hydrochlorothiazide (HCTZ) regimen was compared to an ARB (candesartan)/calcium channel blocker (felodipine) regimen in the Antihypertensive Treatment and Lipid Profile in a North of Sweden Efficacy Evaluation (ALPINE) study. In addition, patients in the atenolol group were eight times more likely to develop diabetes and had elevated LDL/HDL ratios when compared to the ARB based group [20].

Carvedilol represents an improvement in beta blockade with its beneficial metabolic effects. By virtue of its alpha blocking properties it increases skeletal muscle blood flow and has shown superiority to metoprolol in non diabetic hypertensives with insulin resistance in the carvedilol-metoprolol study in 1996 [21]. In the Glycemic effects in Diabetes Mellitus: Carvedilol-Metoprolol Comparison in Hypertensives (GEMINI) trial, 1,235 hypertensive diabetics were randomized to either metoprolol or carvedilol [22]. Not only did metoprolol worsen glycemic and cholesterol control, but patients on carvedilol decreased their insulin resistance, stabilized A1C, and lowered cholesterol, while decreasing microalbuminuria with a 16% relative reduction in the albumin/creatinine ratio compared to metoprolol treated patients, while fewer patients with normal albumin secretion progressed to microalbuminuria compared to the metoprolol group. Interestingly, in the GEMINI trial, weight gain was more common in the metoprolol group. Carvedilol CR has been shown to be bioequivalent to short acting carvedilol.

Carvedilol has improved both left ventricular ejection fraction and decreased mortality rates in both diabetic and non-diabetic patients with congestive heart failure. In a double blind randomized trial, the effects of the ACE inhibitor, perindopril (Aceon) was compared to carvedilol on blood pressure and endothelial function in 26 diabetic patients with hypertension. Both perindopril and carvedilol significantly reduced mean blood pressure and increased leg blood flow to the same extent.

Interestingly, carvedilol reduced platelet aggregation significantly, but this effect was not seen with perindopril. In other controlled trial, the metabolic and cardiovascular effects of carvedilol and atenolol in 45 hypertensive patients with type-2 diabetes were evaluated. Mean fasting glucose, insulin, and hemoglobin A1-C concentrations decreased during carvedilol treatment and increased during atenolol with P values being equal to or less than 0.01 between the two groups [23].

The Appropriate Blood Pressure Control in the Diabetes (ABCD) trial was primarily designed to evaluate renal endpoints with intensive hypertension control in patients with type-2 diabetes. In this particular study, 470 patients with hypertension and diabetes were assigned to one of two treatment goals, a target diastolic blood pressure of 80–89 or 75 mmHg [24].

In the intensive group, blood pressure level 132/78 mmHg was achieved and in the moderate group, 138/86 mmHg. After 5 years of follow-up, the groups did not differ in progression of normal albuminuria or microalbuminuria, diabetic retinopathy or neuropathy. However, total mortality was 5.5% in the intensively controlled group and 10.7% in the moderately controlled group.

Various studies have evaluated the effects of specific classes of drugs in the management of hypertension in patients with diabetes. Some compared ACE inhibitors with calcium channel blockers.

In a sub-study of the ABCD trial, 470 hypertensive patients with diabetes were randomly assigned to treatment with either nisoldipine or enalapril with equivalent blood pressures being achieved. However, the nisoldipine group had a substantially higher rate of myocardial infarction.

The FACET (Fosinopril vs. Amlodipine Cardiovascular Events Trial) was an open label study that randomized 380 patient with type-2 diabetes to the above two mentioned antihypertensive agents. At the conclusion of the study, systolic blood pressure control was better in the amlodipine group, while diastolic pressure was similar. Fosinopril was shown to have significantly fewer combined cardiovascular events despite having higher systolic blood pressures, although total mortality and changes in albumin secretions did not differ [25].

In the STOP II Trial (Swedish Trial in Old Patients with Hypertension) three drug groups were evaluated: calcium channel blockers, ACE inhibitors, and beta-blockers plus diuretics. In a post-hoc analysis of patients in the group with type-2 diabetes, blood pressure was equal in the treatment group and cardiovascular events or total mortality were not changed. Interestingly, as we saw in the ABCD trial, however, risk for myocardial infarction was lower in patients treated with the ACE inhibitors than with the calcium channel blockers [26].

The previously mentioned ALLHAT trial showed that in a pre-specified sub group analysis of 12,000 patients with type-2 diabetes, there was no significant difference seen between the ACE inhibitors, calcium channel blockers, and the thiazide diuretics in the primary outcomes of non-fatal myocardial infarction plus coronary heart disease death, all cause in mortality. The risk, however, for heart failure was lowest in the diuretic group.

In comparison to the STOP II and ALLHAT trials, two studies have compared traditional beta-blocker or diuretic base therapy with ACE inhibitors. The CAPP trial (Captopril Prevention Project trial) randomly assigned patients with hypertension to treatment with beta-blockers or diuretics, and captopril to patients with target diastolic blood pressure being less than 90 mmHg. In this group, 572 patients had diabetes. Blood pressure control was similar in both groups. In the captopril group, however, the risk for myocardial infarction, all cause mortality and cardiovascular events was lower. The UKPDS also included a sub-analysis in which patients in the intensive control group with blood pressures less than 150/85 mmHg were randomly assigned to atenolol or captopril. In distinction to the CAPP trial, there were no differences in any of the aggregated or individual macrovascular or microvascular events between the two groups [26].

In addition to ALLHAT and STOP II, two other studies have directly compared traditional treatment with beta-blockers and diuretics to calcium channel blockers. The NORDIL (Nordic Diltiazem) Trial compared treatment with beta-blockers or diuretics to diltiazem. Blood pressure was similarly reduced in both groups but in the sub-group analysis of 727 patients with type-2 diabetes, no differences were seen in total mortality or combined cardiovascular end points [27].

The International Nifedipine Study Intervention as a Goal in Hypertensive Treatment (Insight) Trial compared treatment with thiazide diuretics and a long acting nifedipine. Once again blood pressure reductions were similar in both groups, but in the sub-analysis of 1,302 patients with diabetes there was no difference in the risk for total mortality or cardiovascular end points [28].

ARBs and other drugs in treating hypertension and diabetes have been compared in two trials. The Irbesartan Diabetic Nephropathy Trial (IDNT) randomly assigned 1,715 patients with diabetic nephropathy and hypertension into three groups: placebo, amlodipine, and irbesartan. Irbesartan was more effective than amlodipine or the placebo in preventing the primary end point of doubling serum creatinine, death, or a development of end-stage renal disease. No differences were seen between placebo and amlodipine in any of the outcomes or between any of the groups in the secondary outcomes [29].

The Losartan Intervention for End Point Reduction (LIFE) Trial randomly assigned patients with left ventricular hypertrophy and hypertension to an angiotensin II receptor blocker losartan or a beta-blocker atenolol. In the subset of 1,195 people with diabetes, the losartan group had a substantial lower risk for cardiovascular end points and total mortality as well as a lower risk for microalbuminuria [30].

The effects of many of these agents in controlling some of the risk factors associated with hypertension can be understood when we look at the characteristics of those people with hypertension and diabetes. These include decreased plasma renin activity, increased peripheral vascular resistance, increased salt sensitivity, and decreased baroreceptor sensitivity, with an increased tendency to orthostatic hypotension and blood pressure variability along with increased body weight and abdominal girth.

Along with the dyslipidemia associated with diabetes, the metabolic syndrome and insulin resistance comes vascular hypertrophy, accelerated atherogenesis, excessive angiotensin II production, sodium retention, increased sympathetic outflow, and increased mortality and morbidity. The importance in treating hypertension in the diabetic patient cannot be minimized as shown by the complications of hypertension outlined in Table 4.

Table 4
Complications of hypertension in patients with diabetes

Microvascular

Nephropathy

Autonomic neuropathy

Retinopathy

Macrovascular

Cerebrovascular disease

Cardiac disease

Decreased survival and recovery rates from stroke

Peripheral vascular disease

Adapted from American Diabetes Association [47]

Table 5
Interrelationship between type-2 diabetes and hypertension

Interrelationship between type-2 diabetes and hypertension
75% of type-2 diabetics are hypertensive
Insulin resistance enhances sympathetic nervous system activity increasing blood pressure
Hypertensive patients have 2.5 times greater risk of developing diabetes within 5 years of diagnosis
Cardiovascular disease risk doubles with increase of 20 mmHg systolic and 10 mmHg diastolic blood pressure

Adapted from Chobanian [48]

End-organ damage and medical complications are plentiful when we look at this patient population. Cardiovascular complications include congestive heart failure and its sequelae, cardiomyopathies, peripheral vascular disease, and generalized arteriosclerotic vascular disease. Patients are prone to cerebral vascular infarctions, ischemic events, hemorrhages, carotid and intracerebral arteriosclerotic vascular disease. The interrelationship of hypertension and diabetes is shown in Table 5, underscoring the importance of maintaining surveillance for the concomitant presence of these two disorders in patients.

Neurologic manifestations include peripheral nervous system abnormalities of impotence, autonomic dysfunction, peripheral neuropathy, and postural hypotension, and central nervous system disturbances including behavioral changes, memory loss, hallucinations, nightmares, depressions, and insomnia.

Ophthalmologically, patients have an increased risk of retinopathy and blindness, and nephrologically are prone to albuminuria, proteinuria, and atherosclerosis of the renal arteries with subsequent renal ischemia, renal insufficiency, glomerulonephritis; especially membranous, Kimmelstiel–Wilson glomerulopathy, glomerulosclerosis, intrarenal hypertension, and glomerulohyperfiltration, papillary necrosis, pyelonephritis, and frequent urinary tract infections.

In order to determine the risks and the benefits of the various agents it is important to look at the metabolic variables associated with each type of treatment.

Thiazide diuretics will increase glucose intolerance, hypokalemia, hypomagnesemia, total cholesterol and triglycerides, while being relatively neutral with HDL. These agents act as vasodilators with data confirming their ability to reduce left ventricular hypertrophy.

Calcium channel blockers are relatively neutral in terms of their metabolic variables, but the phenylalkylamines (verapamil) and the benzothiazepines (diltiazem) can cause slowing of the heart rate in individuals prone to bradyarrhythmia.

The phenylalkylamines are negatively inotropic whereas the benzothiazepines are negatively inotropic only if the ejection fraction is decreased before therapy is initiated. The ACE inhibitors are likewise neutral to the parameters suggested except for a slight tendency to developing potassium abnormalities, particularly hyperkalemia. This is most often seen when ACE inhibitors are combined with beta-blockers, ARBs or aldosterone antagonists, or if an individual diabetic patient has renal insufficiency [31].

Although alpha-blockers tend to raise HDL and lower total cholesterol and be relatively neutral with other metabolic variables, these agents should not be used as first line therapy in diabetic patients because of unfavorable outcomes in the ALLHAT trial. These agents are better used as adjuvant therapy particularly in patients who have some prostatic outlet obstruction problems.

A newer class of agents, called the direct renin inhibitors, represented currently by aliskiren (Tekturna), has been recently approved for treatment of hypertension. Blockade of the renin-angiotensin aldosterone system results in the attenuation of a wide variety of potentially harmful angiotensin-2 induced factors including activator inhibitor-1, transforming growth factor B, free oxygen radicals, and proinflammatory cytokines, while resulting in beneficial hemodynamic effects including blood pressure reduction with enhanced vasodilatation.

It has been recognized for years that by blocking the RAAS system limiting the interaction of lumen substrate with renin represents an extremely effective modality in reducing blood pressure. When adequate doses of a renin inhibitor are administered, full renin production and release are blocked, rendering the RAS system inactive.

Aliskiren, despite its low bioavailability, possesses considerable potency. Plasma levels of aliskiren peak at 2–4 h with a half life range of 24–36 h. Since the drug is not substantially cleared by the kidneys, a dosage adjustment is required with renal insufficiency or failure. Drug interactions are possible with this product because it is metabolized via the cytochrome P450-3A4 system with irbesartan decreasing the maximum concentration of aliskiren by 50% and atorvastatin increasing the c-max and area under the curve by 40%, and should not be used with cyclosporine, since significantly elevated levels of aliskiren can occur. Coadministration of 75 mg of aliskiren, and 200 and 60 mg of cyclosporine resulted in a 2.5-fold increase in C-max and a fivefold increase in the area under the curve.

Aliskiren has also been shown to be additive in its effects with an ACE inhibitor or an ARB showing better blood pressure reductions than seen when an ACE inhibitor is combined with an ARB. Recent trials have also indicated a favorable benefit of Aliskiren with a reduction in proteinuria in diabetic patients. In addition, the physician should be aware that complete RAS blockade may have adverse effects on renal function, particularly in patients with bilateral renal arteriosclerotic vascular disease, as well as an increased risk of hyperkalemia in patients with renal insufficiency, heart failure, or diabetics with hyporeninemic hypoaldosteronism. The anti-hypertensive effects of this product have been analyzed in six randomized, double blinded placebo controlled 8-week trials in patients with mild to moderate hypertension, involving 2,730 patients given 75–600 mg of aliskiren and 1,231 patients with placebo. Eighty to ninety percent of the blood pressure lowering occurred within 2 weeks of treatment with both the 150 mg and the 300 mg dose [32]. There is no rebound hypertension with aliskiren with blood pressures taking several weeks to return to pre-treatments levels after therapy is stopped.

Aliskiren was also studied alone (150 and 300 mg) and in combination with valsartan (160 and 320 mg) in an 8-week study involving 1,797 patients. Blood pressure lowering was additive when the two drugs were combined. In elderly patients with hypertension, the Aliskiren for Geriatric Lowering of Systolic Blood Pressure (AGELESS) trial, demonstrated that aliskiren monotherapy was non inferior to ramipril monotherapy at 12, 22, and 36 weeks, but was more successful in lowering systolic blood pressure with a smaller number of patients requiring add on therapy with a thiazide diuretic or amlodipine to achieve the desired blood pressure goal [33]. Cough occurred in 305 of the ramipril group and only 4% of the aliskiren group.

Aliskiren has also been shown to have renoprotective effects in patients with type-2 diabetes, hypertension, and nephropathy independent of its blood pressure lowering effects, even in patients receiving the maximal recommended renoprotective treatment and optimal antihypertensive therapy. 805 patients were enrolled in this clinical trial with treatment initiated with losartan (100 mg daily) plus optimal treatment to achieve an optimal bp of <130/80 mmHg. Patients were then randomized to placebo or escalating doses of aliskiren (150–300 mg). Patients treated with aliskiren demonstrated a 20% reduction in their urinary albumin/creatinine ration compared to placebo, with a reduction in albuminuria equal to or >50% seen in 24.7 % of the aliskiren group compared to 12.5% of the placebo group.

THE ROLE OF COMBINATION THERAPY

Due the inability to achieve hypertensive control with a single agent, it is important for the primary care physician to be aware of the importance of fixed dose combinations in treating hypertension. Data from NHANES III demonstrates that only 11% of people with diabetes and hypertension achieved the blood pressure goal of less than 130/85 mmHg.

Initial therapy with fixed dose combinations can achieve the recommended blood pressure goal in patients with type-2 diabetes faster than conventional monotherapy. It is important for the physician to understand that strategic use of early and intensive antihypertensive therapy with combination agents can be an important adjunct in achieving patient goals as well as aiding in compliance.

In the UKPDS trial, more than one half of the participants required two or more drugs to achieve their blood pressure goals with 29% needing three or more medications to maintain the target blood pressure after 9 years of follow-up. Growing evidence now supports the use of fixed dose combination therapy in mixed patient populations demonstrating that they are more effective than commonly used monotherapy, as well as being better tolerated. These trials include the use of a diuretic with a beta-blocker or an ACE inhibitor, or an ACE inhibitor/calcium channel blocker combination.

The SHIELD trial (The Study of Hypertension and the Efficacy of Lotrel in Diabetes) was a 12-week randomized double blinded parallel group multi-centered study. This followed a maximum 3-week placebo run with 214 participants recruited from 22 centers around the USA. This compared the use of amlodipine/benazepril (Lotrel) 5–10 mg daily to enalapril 10 mg/day. From baseline to week 12, combination therapy produced a 20.5 mmHg decrease in systolic blood pressure and a 13.9 mmHg decrease in diastolic blood pressure compared to 14.5 over 9.6 mmHg with enalapril alone which was statistically significant [15].

This provided the support for the use of these fixed dose combinations including ACE inhibitors and CCB's in the management of the diabetic hypertensive. In this trial, the accumulative percentage of patients achieving treatment success was significantly greater with the combined therapy group than with the enalpril alone, and even patients receiving HCTZ add-on therapy were excluded from the combination group, but not the ACE inhibitor group. The rates of adverse events were similar in each group.

The SHIELD trial provided important evidence that this fixed dose combination can successfully treat diabetic hypertensive patients without influencing the glycemic or lipid control.

A study by Fogari and others, published in the *American Journal of Hypertension* in 2002 demonstrated superior blood pressure lowering as well as significant lowering of urinary albumin excretion with the ACE inhibitor/calcium channel blocker combination compared to monotherapy. This 4-year trial showed that a combination of fosinopril and amlodipine was superior to each agent alone in reducing blood pressure and urinary microalbumin. In addition, the decreases in urinary albuminin excretion were also significantly greater in the combination group compared to either monotherapy as the patients were followed up to 4 years [*15*].

These superior reductions in urinary albumin excretion may be related to the renal protective effects of the ACE inhibitors and a synergistic combined effect of ACE inhibitor and dihydropyridines. In addition, a greater percentage of patients who initially received combination therapy maintain their blood pressure treatment goal compared with conventional treatment group. This was maintained regardless of whether the blood pressure target was 130/85 or 130/80 mmHg [*15*].

This study supports the growing concept that one pill containing two different blood pressure lowering agents achieves blood pressure goal in a larger percentage of patients than one pill with a single agent. This certainly lends a great deal of merit to the use of fixed dose combinations in the diabetic patient who is already looking at the distinct possibility of multipharmacy to control other risk factors.

The controversy continues as to the level of blood pressure reduction that optimizes cardiovascular risk reduction. JNC-6 recommends a target blood pressure of less than 130/85 mmHg for individuals with concomitant hypertension and diabetes, while the National Kidney Foundation 2000 Guidelines and The American Diabetes Association 2002 Guidelines for the treatment of hypertension and diabetes recommend an even lower target blood pressure of 130/80 mmHg.

There is also known to be an increased risk for cardiovascular events and mortality risk in diabetic patients with systolic blood pressures greater than 120 mmHg. It is well known that when both hypertension and diabetes co-exist, the risk of nephropathy and arteriosclerotic cardiovascular disease are markedly increased. Hence an important objective in the treatment of the hypertensive diabetic is to reduce the risk of renal and cardiovascular complications without adversely affecting glycemic and lipid controls.

Fixed dose combinations make sense in diabetic patients not only because of the effects on blood pressure and target organ disease, but also the efficient use of different mechanisms of action in reducing cardiovascular risk that is accomplished with the use of beta-blockers and diuretics, ACE inhibitors, or ARBs with diuretics or ACE inhibitors and calcium channel blockers, or a combination of ACE inhibitor/Renin inhibitor or ARB/renin inhibitor. Fixed dose combinations now include a dihydropyridine/ARB (Azor, Exforge, and Twynsta), a phenylalkylamine/ACE inhibitor combination (Tarka), and a dihydropyridine/ARB/thiazide diuretic as well (Exforge HCT) in addition to the ACE inhibitor/dihydropyridine combination (Lotrel), and finally a rennin inhibitor/ARB combination (Valturna).

In addition by using combination therapy, lower doses of each component drug are often used, thus reducing adverse events. This can be seen in the combination of calcium channel blockers containing dihydropyridine and the ACE inhibitors which tend to attenuate venous dilatation and subsequent edema associated with dihydropyridine use.

. The ALLHAT trial also used component classes of antihypertensive agents that were used in both the SYST-EUR and the HOT trials. In addition, the STOP II trial showed that

CCB's were as effective as diuretics, beta-blockers, and ACE inhibitors in reducing morbidity and mortality in hypertensive patients with diabetes [31].

The cardiovascular benefits of the calcium channel blockers appear to be derived from their blood pressure lowering effect. Calcium channel blockers are more efficacious for lowering blood pressure than ACE inhibitors in some patient populations. Although the short-acting calcium channel blockers increase the risk of cardiovascular events, long-acting calcium channel blockers have shown to be safe and effective in reducing cardiovascular outcomes especially stroke in diabetic patients and non-diabetic patients with hypertension [34].

The dihydropyridine calcium channel blockers, however, should be avoided as solo therapy in patients with macroalbuminuria equal to or greater than 300 mg of albumin per gram of creatinine unless these individuals are being treated with an ACE inhibitor or an ARB.

The American Diabetes Association recommends the uses of dihydropyridine calcium channel blockers only in combination with, but not instead of ACE inhibitors or ARB's for patients with diabetes and elevated blood pressure. The combination therapy approach to hypertensive management in the diabetic is extremely appealing. The increased efficacy of the combination over monotherapy has been well established. The decreased side effects with combination therapy along with increased efficacy and improved patient compliance make it important for the physician to familiarize himself with the available antihypertensive drug combinations [35].

Of all these combinations, initiating therapy with combination calcium channel blocker and ACE inhibitor or ARB remains the most attractive. The results here are additive and synergistic with important outcomes data supporting the benefit of both calcium channel blocker use and ARB or ACE inhibitor use. In addition, by selectively dilating renal afferents with calcium channel blockers and dilating renal efferents with the ACE inhibitors or ARB's, optimum renal protection can be established.

The dual effect of the combination ARB or ACE inhibitor/calcium channel blocker optimally reduces intraglomerular pressure and it is the intraglomerular pressure that is associated with the deterioration in renal function that is seen not only with chronic hypertensive in general, but especially in the diabetic state.

In the Veteran's Affairs Cooperative Study group headed by Materson, 1,292 male hypertensive patients received one of six oral antihypertensive drugs [36]. Patients who did not achieve the diastolic blood pressure goal of less than 90 mmHg during the titration were switched to titration of monotherapy with an alternate drug. Those not aided by the second drug were given a combination of the two drugs that had failed initially. Overall 57.8% patients responded to combinations, four of seven patients or 51% who had failed on diltiazem and captopril therapy achieved goal diastolic blood pressures on the combination.

The ACE inhibitor provides potent arterial and venous dilatation, strong positive outcomes data for the diabetic patient, and is beneficial in patients with co-existing congestive heart failure.

The dihydropyridine calcium channel blocker provides potent antihypertensive blood control and the non-dihydropyridines are not only arterial vasodilators, but can have a vagal effect, slowing heart rate. In addition, these agents are extremely effective in the low renin hypertensives, especially the African Americans and obese patients.

Beta-blockers can also blunt the tachycardia and rise in plasma renin activity associated with thiazide diuretic use, hence their synergistic benefit. Any class of antihypertensives to which thiazide diuretics have been added have shown a synergistic benefit, especially the angiotensive converting enzymes and the ARB's. The natriuretic and vasodilatory effects of calcium channel blockers complement the antihypertensive effects of the ACE inhibitor particularly in the presence of a diuretic [37].

It also is important for the management of diabetes to understand the difference between hypertensive and arteriosclerotic heart disease. In many instances these terms are used interchangeably; however, these are two distinct clinical entities.

Despite the fact that they share some clinical manifestations like angina and sudden death associated with dysrhythmia, the pathophysiology and general clinical course of the two entities are different.

In hypertensive disease, the myocardium and the left ventricle respond to chronically elevated systemic arterial pressure (afterload), while in arteriosclerotic disease, the atheromatous lesions in the coronary arteries produce ischemia in addition to occlusive and plaque disruptive disease. Hypertensive disease most commonly progresses to congestive heart failure whereas occlusive disease most commonly progresses to myocardial infarction. More will be discussed about this in the chapter on risk reduction.

There is distinct difference between dihydropyridines and non-dihydropyridine in terms of their renal effects. The dihydropyridines (amlodipine, felodipine, nisoldipine, nifedipine, and isradipine) have a neutral effect on proteinuria and some of the earlier first generation dihydropyridines like nifedipine can even enhance proteinuria particularly if unopposed with an ACE inhibitor, whereas the non-dihydropyridine calcium channel blockers (verapamil and diltiazem) can decrease proteinuria if blood pressures are reduced.

Hence monotherapy with dihydropyridines should be avoided in the type-2 diabetic.

Glomerular scarring is essentially unchanged in animal model data with dihydropyridine calcium channel blockers, but is decreased in non-dihydropyridines [34].

Renal autoregulation is abolished in both animal and human data with the dihydropyridines and a minimal effect in the non-dihydropyridine class. Combinations of ACE inhibitors and dihydropyridines along with ACE inhibitors and non-dihydropyridines have not been compared in terms of their potency to reduce protein excretion. However, combinations of ACE inhibitors and both classes of calcium channel blockers show synergistic effects in proteinuria reduction.

Bakris et al. has shown data to indicate that at similar blood pressure levels, reduction in proteinuria is enhanced with a trandolapril/verapamil combination to a statistically significant value although the cohort size was small with 11 in the verapamil group, 12 in the trandolapril group, and 14 in the combination group [31].

Curiously, if we look at the clinical hypertensive trials over the past 15 years, almost all have actually been trials using combination therapy of one sort or another. The Losartan Intervention for Endpoint Reduction (LIFE) trial reported that losartan was more effective than atenolol in reducing overall cardiovascular events, especially stroke, but only 10% of these patients actually remained on monotherapy, either the ARB or the beta-blocker. Greater than 90% of these patients required combination therapy. So although losartan had an advantage over atenolol, monotherapy had not proven to be effective in lowering blood pressure compared to any combination therapy.

Even the Captopril Study in type-1 Diabetes in Renal Disease [*38*] was presented as a captopril vs. placebo trial, a large number of patients in the captopril group received other drugs and the so-called placebo group actually received many different medications. In the Irbesartan Diabetic Nephropathy Study in Type II Diabetics Trial (IRMA-2), patients who received irbesartan experienced less progression of renal disease than patients on placebo or on amlodipine.

However, a careful review of this data shows that 31% of the irbesartan patients were actually on thiazide diuretics, 43% were receiving beta-blockers, and 67% were receiving loop diuretics. The placebo group was actually receiving different combinations of medications and the third group in the study was receiving amlodipine plus other medications. So irbesartan, addition to the other medications, proved to be effective over amlodipine and its other medications in slowing the progression of renal disease [*39*].

In the RENAAL trial (Reduction in End points in Non-Insulin Dependent Diabetes with Angiotensin II Antagonist Losartan), the use of losartan significantly slowed the progression of renal disease and reduced the occurrence of end-stage renal impairment. This trial again looked at an ARB plus other medications, in most instances, a diuretic. The placebo group also included other medications, but did not include an ARB [*30*].

So although these trials have shown some specific benefits for the agents tested, clearly the advantages of combination therapy are well established.

In the PROGRESS Trial (Perindopril Protection Against Recurrent Stroke), many investigators believed that antihypertensive control in an individual with previous history of stroke was not beneficial in preventing recurrent stroke. This trial showed that an ACE inhibitor-diuretic combination reduced strokes compared to an ACE inhibitor alone. This trial had an ACE inhibitor arm and an ACE inhibitor-diuretic arm. The combination of the diuretic and perindopril was far superior to either agent alone in the reduction of secondary stroke [*15*].

In the recently completed ALLHAT trial, various combinations were included, including chlorothalidone, a thiazide diuretic, amlodipine, lisinopril, and an alpha blocker. This data showed that thiazide diuretics could be the first step drug of choice in some cases.

Another important message from ALLHAT is that most patients will require more than one drug to reach blood pressure goals and one of these should be a diuretic.

The Australian National Blood Pressure II (ANBP-II trial) reported that an ACE inhibitor was marginally more effective in men than a diuretic in reducing cardiovascular events. This too, was not really a monotherapy comparative trial [*40*]. Multiple drugs in both arms were used with less than 40% of the patients on monotherapy. Blood pressure reductions were similar with the ACE inhibitor based program and the diuretic based program. The Australian trial however, was an unblinded study and changes in medication based on even minor side effects may be more common in such a study particularly when an ACE inhibitor is involved and the individual complains of cough.

In individuals with Stage II hypertension, specific indications are to begin therapy with two drugs and it is important to use drugs that act synergistically. There is no question however that the cornerstone of risk reduction in the diabetic patient with or without hypertension remains the ACE inhibitors and/or the ARBs.

The American Heart Association now recommends the use of ramipril in at-risk people with diabetes to prevent stroke, overall cardiovascular mortality and morbidity, and myocardial infarction as a result of the impressive data from the HOPE study. Ramipril also prevented the onset of diabetes and reduced diabetic complications and the need for revascularization in patients with existing vascular disease as well as delaying or preventing the development of microalbuminuria in diabetic patients. The risk reductions were impressive, 37% for cardiovascular event, 22% for MI, and 32% for stroke, all of which were statistically significant.

The rational for using ACE's and ARB's is based on sound physiologic evidence. Angiotensin II remains a significant culprit both in acute and chronic neurohumoral catastrophic effects at the cellular level. Poor tissue profusion as is seen in diabetics elicits compensatory activation of neurohumoral mechanisms like the RAAS/or sympathetic nervous systems. Once activated, these systems attempt to restore perfusion, for various increases in cardiac output and heart rate, sodium and water retention by the kidney, and increase system vasoconstriction [15].

All these mechanisms may result in increased systemic blood pressure. The presence of normal blood pressure does not indicate that angiotensin II is harmless or not presenting harmful effects at the tissue level. Chronic activation of the neuroendocrine system as a result of decreased perfusion at the tissue level will also activate the renin-angiotensin and sympathetic nervous systems leading to myocardial hypertrophy, vascular hypertrophy, glomerular hypertension, and hypertrophy.

Angiotensin II has significant detrimental effects on the heart by increasing left ventricular pressure and left ventricular volume overload, and angiotensin II production results in increased wall tension, aggravating or producing diastolic dysfunction. This increase in wall tension further induces angiotensin II pathways at the tissue level, which cause a vicious cycle resulting in cardiac hypertrophy and dilatation.

Vascular injury at the blood vessel or endothelial level leads to local angiotensin II production and vascular remodeling increasing fibroblastic growth factor, transforming growth factor, beta-1 insulin like growth factor, and platelet derived growth factor, all of which modulate growth in smooth muscle cells. Renal function is an important parameter in both diabetes and hypertension and any renal injury whether local or systemic can result in glomerular capillary pressure, increased glomerular hypertrophy, and aggravation or production of systemic hypertension, all of which induces further production of the angiotensin II hormone, which aggravates glomerulosclerosis and accelerates the process [35].

Angiotensin II has a direct influence on tubular sodium reabsorptive mechanisms increasing its reabsorption with its primary site of action being on the proximal renal tubule. In addition, angiotensin II exerts indirect effects on the distal tubule mediated through aldosterone.

Long-term exposure to angiotensin I at the kidney level stimulates cell growth along with type I collagen synthesis and protein synthesis. Short-term effects include an increase in prostaglandin synthesis, intracellular calcium concentration, and contraction of glomeruli and mesangial cells. When angiotensin II production is increased, there is an enhancement of platelet aggregation, a stimulation of PAI-1, enhancement of endothelial dysfunction, and smooth muscle cell growth, and migration is subsequently increased.

The net result is an enhancement in leukocytic adhesion, thrombosis, oxidative stress, apoptosis, and impairments in endothelial function and nitric oxide production. By interfering with multiple different substrates, ACE inhibitors will reduce angiotensin II formation and decrease the breakdown of bradykinin. Subsequent elevated bradykinin levels, although they may be responsible for enhancement of the cough, also contribute to beneficial therapeutic effects through release of nitric oxide, which is a potent vasodilator, enhancing endothelial function. Nitric oxide also is a direct antagonist to the harmful effects mediated by angiotensin II.

The Prevention of Events with Angiotensin Converting Enzyme Inhibition (PEACE) trial looked at 8,100 patients over a 5.5-year period of time and showed that the ACE inhibitor trandolapril reduced the risk of heart attacks, deaths, and revascularization procedures in patients with coronary disease. By improving endothelial function and vasodilatation, ACE inhibitors improve endothelial function, maintain many protective properties, and enhance endothelial antithrombotic effects [41].

In mild to moderate hypertension, ACE inhibitors can reduce diastolic blood pressure by 3–7 mmHg and 4–12 mmHg of systolic pressure, with these effects enhanced by the addition of thiazide diuretics. The primary side effect of ACE inhibitors is cough which occurs in at least 15% of the patients, this does not respond to a reduction in dose or change of ACE inhibitors. Patients with renal dysfunction or those receiving potassium sparing drugs, non-steriodal anti-inflammatory drugs, or beta-blockers may get concomitant hyperkalemia during ACE inhibitory therapy. This usually occurs with serum creatinines of greater than 2.5. These agents should be used cautiously in creatinines above this level and only when the benefits exceed the risk. Elderly patients are more likely to have increased risk as a result of arteriosclerotic vascular disease because the glomerular filtration rate may decrease with age [16].

A dreaded rare complication with ACE inhibitors is angioedema, which can present initially as lingual swelling, but can progress over a period of time to life threatening respiratory difficulties. This can occur within a matter of days or several weeks after therapy is initiated. Once an individual develops angioedema, from any cause, an ACE inhibitor or ARB is not indicated. The presence of angioedema is not considered a dose-dependent effect. Concomitant use of non-steriodal anti-inflammatory drugs may decrease the ACEs antihypertensive effects. ACE inhibitors should not be used in pregnancy.

Although the renin-angiotensin system plays a central role in the control of systemic blood pressure and has a distinctive role in the pathogenesis of hypertension, it is important to understand that angiotensin II can be generated via alternative pathways independent of the ACE, with angiotensin II being generated directly from angiotensinogen by cathepsin G and TPA. In fact it is estimated that at least 50% of the angiotensin II that is produced in the body bypasses the renin-angiotensin mechanism.

The ARBs have been a critical advance in risk reduction and hypertensive control. The angiotensin II type I receptor mediates all the known cardiovascular effects of angiotensin II including decreased renal blood flow and renal renin inhibition, vasoconstriction, renal tubular reabsorption, and stimulation of the aldosterone synthesis and release. The angiotensin II type I receptor is not known to mediate vasodilatation. Hence the ARB's provide more complete blockade of the renin-angiotensin system than the ACEs.

Whereas the major benefits of the ACE inhibitors seem to derive largely from their inhibition of bradykinin breakdown and subsequent increase in nitric oxide generation, the major benefit of the ARB's is by inhibiting the binding of the angiotensin II to its receptor site without effecting bradykinin. In doing so, the ARBs prevent target organ damage than it may occur from activation of the ACE system [42].

Whether ARB's are clinically equivalent, superior, inferior, or can be used synergistically with ACE's remains to be determined by several large clinical trials in process. Certainly the limited data as of the present time would point toward a synergistic benefit of ACE's and ARB's in the vast majority of patients except perhaps patients with heart failure who are already on beta-blockers, where mixed results in terms of benefit vs. risk have been demonstrated.

The Valsartan Heart Failure Trial (VALHEFT) showed that adding valsartan to an ACE inhibitor reduced hospitalization from heart failure in patients on the combination group, but the mortality and morbidity tended to be increased when the patients were taking a beta-blocker, ACE inhibitor, and ARB [43].

The Candesartan in Heart Failure Assessment of Reduction in Morbidity and Mortality (CHARM) trial showed that beta-blockade, ACE inhibitor therapy, and ARB therapy (candesartan) did not have a deleterious effect. Results of the Evaluation of Losartan in the Elderly II (Elite II) Study differed from the Elite I trial. Elite I looked at 722 elderly patients demonstrating a decrease in admissions for congestive heart failure among those randomized to losartan particularly for sudden death. Elite II involved 3,152 patients and this failed to show the superiority of losartan over captopril although losartan was better tolerated in the ACE inhibitor. There is also no difference in renal function in either study [44].

The American Diabetes Association recommends the ARB's as first line therapy for Type II diabetics who have microalbuminuria or clinical albuminuria. The agent should not be used in patients who cannot tolerate an ACE inhibitor because of hypotension, angioedema, progressive renal dysfunction, or hyperkalemia. There are some differences among the seven ARBs available on the market. Some have insurmountable binding to the angiotensin II type I receptor (telmisartan, irbesartan, candesartan, olmesartan, and the exp-3174 metabolite of losartan).

Although all agents are approved for once a day dose by virtue of their trough to peak ratios exceeding 0.5, losartan and eprosartan demonstrate the need for twice daily dosage because of slight drifting after 17–18 h. Additionally, telmisartan has trough to peak ratios greater than 100% at the 80 mg dose in systolic and diastolic blood pressure readings and has the longest terminal half life of 24 h.

As of the present time, irbesartan (Avapro) in doses of 300 mg once a day and losartan (Cozaar) 100 mg daily have formal approval for inhibition of progression of microalbuminuria in diabetics at those doses. Of all the available ARB's, only losartan is metabolized to some extent in cytochrome P450-3A4 which can be clinically significant only if a patient is on several other 3A4 metabolized medications.

In placebo controlled trials, the ARBs reduced blood pressure by 5–13 mmHg systolic and by 3–8 mmHg diastolic with the effects enhanced with diuretic therapy. Slight improvement in diastolic blood pressure reduction of 1–3 mmHg has been shown with olmesartan (Benicar) compared to losartan and valsartan (Diovan) in head trials with candesartan (Atacand) showing better antihypertensive therapy in head to head trials with shorter acting ARB's like losartan and valsartan [30].

Despite the fact that these agents do not interfere with bradykinin generation, angioedema has been reported particularly in patients who developed angioedema with ACE's. Hence these agents should not be used in patients who have angioedema from any cause. None of the ARB's have been reported to have any significant drug interactions or effect on pharmacodynamics with the exception of telmisartan, which may raise digoxin levels slightly and a worsening of serum potassium levels when concomitant salt substitutes potassium supplements or potassium sparing diuretics or ACE inhibitors are administered.

These agents should not be used to treat pregnant patients or nursing mothers and have the same contraindications in patients with renal dysfunction and renal artery stenosis as the ACE inhibitors.

Diuretics exert their primary effect by vasodilatation and this effect is retained by using lower doses. The efficacy of the lower dose diuretic reduces the incidence of hyperuricemia, aggravating glycemic control, and hypokalemia making them more attractive for use in the diabetic patient population. By decreasing peripheral vascular resistance, these agents may have additional utility as add-ons or even first choices in the low renin hypertensive patient (African American or obese patient).

Thiazide diuretics, however, increase plasma renin activity and aldosterone secretion, and hence, synergistic benefit with agents that lower plasma renins and aldosterones have been demonstrated (beta-blockers, centrally acting agents, ACE inhibitors, and ARB's). The loop diuretics act on the ascending limb of Henle, and proximal and distal tubule and have less of a vasodilatory effect than the thiazide diuretics exerting their antihypertensive effects mainly from volume depletion. Hence the thiazide diuretics are used more often to control hypertension than the loop diuretics.

In the distal convoluted tubules, spironolactone kinetically binds with receptors at the aldosterone dependant sodium potassium exchange site to inhibit the exchange of sodium for potassium. Hence the efficacy of the potassium sparing drugs in reducing hypertension has been demonstrated. These agents still have to be used with caution, particularly if an ACE inhibitory or angiotensin blocker is also used, because of the risk of hyperkalemia in the diabetic patients. Since diabetic patients may be prone to developing hyporeninemic hypoaldosteronism, the physician should be on guard for the potential for hyperkalemia [18].

Thiazide diuretics have been most often associated with aggravating glycemic control because by induction of hypokalemia, they may inhibit insulin output from the pancreas. Indapamide (Lozol) in low doses reduces blood pressure without worsening glycemic control or lipid profile. Long-term trials with this product did not show an increased incidence of diabetes compared with that associated with other diuretic agents. In addition, low dose thiazide therapy is generally not associated with adverse metabolic effects as previously been mentioned.

High dose diuretics should be avoided because of the risk of hypokalemia, hypomagnesemia, and subsequent ventricular arrhythmias. Judicious use of these agents can be effective in reducing stroke. Smaller doses are extremely effective when used in combination therapy [18].

Patients with sensitivity to sulfonamides may be sensitive to most diuretics. Caution should be exercised in concomitant therapy with lithium due to decreased lithium clearance and subsequent increasing blood levels predisposing to toxicity.

Concomitant use of thiazides and non-steroidal anti-inflammatory drugs (NSAIDS) may increase plasma renin activity or increase the risk of renal failure. Patients on diuretic therapy should be carefully observed for hyponatremia, hypokalemia, and hypomagnesemia.

Thiazides are generally ineffective with serum creatinines greater than 2–3 mg/dl. In these patients, loop diuretics work more efficiently. All diuretic agents can predispose the patient to hyperuricemia precipitating and aggravating gout.

SUMMARY

Since aggressive blood pressure reduction has yielded significant improvement outcomes in many trials regardless of the agent used, it is important for physicians to recognize that hypertension management is a critical aspect of risk reduction in the diabetic patient. Choice of which class agents to use as first line therapy depends on the degree of blood pressure reduction needed, the impact on metabolic parameters, side effect profile, cost, and the presence of other compelling indications.

Since the average number of antihypertensive agents needed to reach target blood pressure control with diabetes is three to four, combination therapeutic approaches may be necessary and even efficient as first line choices. Hence, knowing which combinations will work synergistically by treating hypertension physiologically in each individual patient is critically important.

The ultimate choice of antihypertensive regimens in a type-2 diabetic should be dictated by the patient's degree of hypertension and any other concomitant promorbidities.

The ARBs and ACE inhibitors, with or without diuretics, are considered as first line therapy. In patients with angina, calcium channel blockers and beta-blockers should also be part of the regimen as ACE inhibitors, diuretics, and beta blockers in patients with heart failure. ARBs, ACE inhibitors, diuretics, and calcium channel blockers have all shown beneficial effects in stroke prevention whereas patients with a prior myocardial infarction have a beta-blocker regimen to reduce the risk of second myocardial infarction.

ACE Inhibitor therapy alone, or in conjunction with ARBs have been shown to be beneficial in preserving renal function and reducing proteinuria in patients with diabetic nephropathy. Direct renin inhibitors can also be used with either an ACE or an ARB for additive blood pressure lowering.

REFERENCES

1. Hajjar I, Kotchen TA. Trends in prevalence, awareness, treatment and control of hypertension in the United States 1988–2000. JAMA 2003;290:199–206.
2. Hayashi T, Tsumura K, Suematsu C, Okada K, Fujii S, Endo G. The Osaka Health Survey. Ann Intern Med 1999;131(1):21–26.
3. US Preventive Services Task Force. Screening for coronary heart disease: recommendation statement. Ann Intern Med. 2004;140:569–572.
4. United Kingdom Prospective Diabetes Study Group. Tight blood pressure control and risk of macrovascular and microvascular complications in type-2 diabetes. BMJ 1998;317:703–713.
5. Staessen JA, Fagard R, Thijs L. Randomised double blind comparison of placebo active treatment for older patients with isolated systolic hypertension. The Systolic Hypertension in Europe (Syst-Eur) Trial Investigators. Lancet 1997;350:757–764.
6. Tuomilehto J, Lindstrom J, Eriksson JG. Prevention of type-2 diabetes mellitus by changes in lifestyle among subjects with impaired glucose tolerance. N Engl J Med 2001;344:1343–1350.
7. Gifford RW. A missed opportunity; our failure to control hypertension optimally. J Clin Hypertens 2000;2:21–24.
8. DeSimone G, Roman MJ, Alderman MH. High pulse pressure as a marker for preclinical cardiovascular disease. Hypertension 2005;45:575–579.

9. United Kingdom Prospective Diabetes Study (UKPDS) Group. Tight blood pressure control and risk of macrovascular and microvascular complications in type 2 diabetes. BMJ 1998;317:703–771

10. Van Itllie TB. Health implications of overweight and obesity in the United States. Ann Intern Med 1985;103(6):983–988.

11. Hansson L, Zanchetti A, Carruthers SG. Effects of intensive blood pressure lowering and low dose aspirin in patients with hypertension; principal results of the Hypertension Optimum (HOT) trial. Lancet 1998;351:1755–1762.

12. Hansson L, Zanchetti A, et al. for the HOT Study Group. Effects of intensive blood pressure lowering and low dose aspirin in patients with hypertension. Lancet 1998;351:1755–1762.

13. Adler A, Stratton I, Neill H. Association of systolic blood pressure with macrovascular and microvascular complications of type-2 diabetes (UKPDS-36). BMJ 2000;321:412–419.

14. Curb JD, Pressel SL, et al. Effect of diuretic based antihypertensive treatment on cardiovascular risk in older diabetic patients with isolated systolic hypertension. JAMA 1996;276:1886–1892.

15. Basile J, Lackland D, et al. A statewide primary care approach to cardiovascular risk factor control in high risk diabetic and non diabetic patients with hypertension. J Clin Hypertens (Greenwich) 2004;6(1):18–25.

16. Ravid M, Lang R. et al. Long term renoprotective effect of angiotensin-converting enzyme inhibition on insulin dependent diabetes mellitus. Arch Intern Med 1996;156:286–289.

17. Goldbourt U, Behar S, Reicher-Reiss H, Agmon J, Keplinsky E. The bezafibrate infarction prevention (BIP) trial. Am J Cardiol 1993;71(11):909–915.

18. American Diabetes Association. Treatment of hypertension in adults with diabetes, Diabetes Care 2002;199–201:213–229.

19. American Association of Clinical Endocrinologists Ad Hoc Task Force for Standardized Production of Clinical Practice guidelines. AACE protocol for standardized production of clinical practice guidelines. Endocr Pract. 2004;10;353–361.

20. Lindholm L, Persson M, Alaupovic P,Carlberg V, Svensson A, Samuelsson O. The Antihypertesnive Treatment and Lipid Profile in a North of Sweden Efficacy Evaluation (ALPINE) study. Journal of Hypertension 2003;21(8):1563–1574.

21. Poole-Wilson P, Swedberg K, Cleland J, Lenarda A, Hanrath P, Komajda M. The Carvedilol or Metoprolol European (COMET) Trial. Lancet 2003;362(9377):7–13.

22. Bakris Gl, Fonseca V, Katholi RE. Metabolic effects of carvedilol vs. metoprolol in patients with type-2 diabetes mellitus and hypertension. GEMINI trial. JAMA 2004;292:2227–2236.

23. Giugliano D, Acampora R, et al. Metabolic and cardiovascular effects of carvedilol and atenolol in non-insulin dependent diabetes mellitus and hypertension. Ann Intern Med 1997;126:955–959.

24. Estacio RO, Jeffers BW, Hiatt WR, Biggerstaff SL, Gifford N, Schrier RW. The effect of nisoldipine as compared with enalapril on cardiovascular outcomes in patients with non-insulin dependent diabetes and hypertension. (ABCD Trial). N Engl J Med 1998;338:645–652.

25. Tatti P, Pahor M, et al. Outcome results of the fosinopril versus amlodipine cardiovascular randomized events trial (FACET) in patients with hypertension and non-insulin dependent diabetes mellitus. Diabetes Care 1998;21:597–603.

26. Joint National Committee on Detection, Evaluation and Treatment of High Blood Pressure: The sixth report of the Joint National Committee on Detection, Evaluation and Treatment of High Blood Pressure (JNC VI). Arch Intern Med 1997;154:2413–2446.

27. Hansson L, Lund-Johansen P, Hedner T. Randomized trial of effects of calcium antagonists compared with diuretics and beta blockers on cardiovascular morbidity and mortality in hypertension: the Nordic Diltiazem (NORDIL) study. Lancet 2000;356:366–372.

28. Brown MJ, Palmer CR, Castaigne A. Morbidity and mortality in patients randomized to double blind treatment with a long acting calcium channel blocker or diuretic in the International Nifedipine GITS study: Intervention as a goal in Hypertension treatment (INSIGHT). Lancet 2000;356:366–372.

29. Walker WG, Herman J, et al. Elevated blood pressure and angiotensin II are associated with accelerated loss of renal function in diabetic nephropathy. Trans Am Clin Climatol Assoc 1985;97:94–104.

30. Brenner BM, Cooper ME, et al. Effects of losartan on renal and cardiovascular outcomes in patients with type 2 diabetes and nephropathy. N Engl J Med 2001;345:861–869.

31. Bakris GL, Williams M, et al. Special Report: Preserving renal function in adults with hypertension and diabetes: A consensus approach. Am J kidney Dis. 2000;36:661.

32. Oh B, Mitchell J, Herron J, Chung J. Khan M. Aliskiren, an oral rennin inhibitor, provides dose dependent efficacy and sustained 24 hour blood pressure control in patients with hypertension. J Am Coll Cardiol 2007;49(11):1157–1163.

33. Duprez D. Aliskiren, the next innovation in the rennin-angiotensin-aldosteronesystem blockade. Aging Health 2009;3(5):269–279.

34. Tuomilehto J, et al. Effects of calcium channel blockade in older patients with diabetes and systolic hypertension. Lancet 1997;6:357–364.

35. Estacio, RO, Jeffers BW, et al. Effect of blood pressure control on diabetic microvascular complications in patients with hypertension and type 2 diabetes. Diabetes Care. 2000;23(Suppl 2):B54–B64.

36. Materson BJ, Reda DJ, Cushman WC. Single drug therapy for hypertension in men. A comparison of six antihypertensive agents with placebo. The Department of veterans Affairs Cooperative Study group on Antihypertensive Agents. N Engl J Med 1993;328:914–921.

37. Adler AI, Stratton IM, et al. Association of systolic blood pressure with marovascular and microvascular complications of type 2 diabetes. BMJ 2000; 321(7258):405–412.

38. Laffel LMB, McGill JB, et al. The beneficial effect of angiotensin converting enzyme inhibition with captopril on diabetic nephropathy in normotensive IDDM patients with microalbuminuria. Am J Med 1995;99:497–540.

39. Lewis EJ, Hunsiker LG, et al. Renoprotective effect of the angiotensin receptor blockers irbesartan in patients with nephropathy due to type 2 diabetes. N Engl J Med 2001;345:851–860.

40. Reid CM, Ryan P, Nelson M. General practitioner participation in the second Australian National Blood Pressure Study (ANBP2). Clin Exp Pharmacol Physiol 2001;28:663–667.

41. Solomon S, Rice M, Jablonski K, Jose P, Domanski M. Renal function and effectiveness of angiotensin converting enzyme inhibitor therapy in patients with stable coronary artery disease in the Prevention of Events with ACE inhibition (PEACE) Trial. Circulation 2006;114:26–31.

42. Anderson S, Tarnow L, Rossing P, et al. Renoprotective effects of angiotensin II receptor blockade in type I diabetic patients with diabetic nephropathy. Kidney Int 2000;57:601–606.

43. Cohn JN, Tognoni G. A randomized trial of the angiotensin receptor blocker valsartan in chronic heart failure. The (VALHeFt) Trial. N Engl J Med 2001;345:1667–1675.

44. Pitt B, Poole-Wilson PA, Segal R. Effects of Losartan compared with captopril on mortality in patients with symptomatic heart failure: the Losartan Heart Failure Survival Study (ELITE II). Lancet 2000;355:1582–1587.

45. Chobanian AV, Bakris G, Black HR. Seventh Report of the Joint National Committee on Prevention, Detection, Evaluation and Treatment of Hypertension JAMA 2003;289:2560–2571

46. Vijan S, et al. Treatment of hypertension in type 2 diabetes mellitus: blood pressue goals, choice of agents and setting priorities in diabetes care. Ann Int Med 2003;138:593–602.

47. American Diabetes Association. Hypertension in type-2 diabetes. Diabetes Care 2007;30:S4–S41.

48. Chobanian AV. Interrelationship of hypertension and type-2 diabetes. Hypertension 2003;42:1206–1252.

SUPPLEMENTARY READINGS

Bell DSH. Beta-adrenergic blocking agents in patients with diabetes – friend or foe? Endocr Pract 1999;5:51–53.

Chirstensen PK, Gall MA, et al. Course of glomerular filtration rate in albuminuric type 2 diabetic patients with or without diabetic glomerulopathy. Diabetes Care 2000;23(Suppl 2):B4–B20.

Cooper M, Johnston C. Optimizing treatment of hypertension in patients with diabetes. JAMA 2000;283(24):3177–3179.

Cooper ME, Pathogenesis, prevention and treatment of diabetic nephropathy. Lancet 1998;352:213–219.

DeStefano F, Ford ES, et al. Risk factors for coronary heart disease mortality among persons with diabetes. Ann Epidemiol 1993:3(1):27–34.

Elkeles RS, Diamond JR, et al. Caridovasccular outcomes in type 2 diabetes. Diabetes Care 1992;15:820–825.

Fu Y, Deedwania P. Management of hypertensive patients with diabetes mellitus. Cin Ger 2001;9(7):22–36.

Factor SM, Minase T, et al. Clinical and Morphological features of human hypertensive diabetic cardiomyopathy. Am Heart J 1980;99:446–458.

Giese M, Lackland DT, et al. The hypertension initiative of South Carolina. Promoting cardiovascular health through better blood pressure control. J S C Med Assoc 2001;97:57–62.

Gustaffson I, et al. Effect of the angiotensin converting enzyme inhibitor trandolapril on mortality and morbidity in diabetic patients with left ventricular dysfunction after acute myocardial infarction. J Am Coll Cardiol 1999;34:83–89.

Harris MI. Racial and ethnic differences in health care access and health outcomes for adults with type 2 diabetes. Diabetes Care 2001;24:454–459.

Heart Outcomes Prevention Evaluation Study Investigators. Effects of ramipril on cardiovascular and microvascular outcomes in people with diabetes mellitus: results of the HOPE study and MICRO-HOPE substudy. Lancet 2000;355:253–259.

Larme AC, Pugh JA, et al. Attitudes of primary care providers toward diabetes: barriers to guideline implementation. Diabetes Care 1998;21:1391–1396.

Lazarus JM, Bourgoignie JJ, et al. Achievement and safety of a low BP goal in chronic renal disease. Hypertension 1997;29:641–650.

Parving HH, Lehnert H, et al. The effect of irbesartan on the development of diabetic nephropathy in patients with type 2 diabetes. N Engl J Med 2001;345:870–878.

Pyorala K, Pedersen TR, et al. Cholesterol lowering with simvastatin improves prognosis of diabetic patients with coronary artery disease. Diabetes Care 1997;20:614–620.

Ritz E, Orth SR. Nephropathy in patients with type 2 diabetes mellitus. N Engl J Med 1999;341(19):1127–1133.

Staessen JA, Fagard R, et al. Randomized double blind comparison of placebo and active treatment for older patients with isolated systolic hypertension. Lancet 1997;350:757–764.

Sowers JR, Lester MA. Diabetes and cardiovascular disease. Diabetes Care 1999; 22(Suppl 3):C14–C20.

Sniderman A, Michel C, et al. Heart disease in patients with diabetes mellitus. J Clin Epidemiol 1992;45:1357–1370.

Van Hoeven KH, et al. A comparison of the pathological spectrum of hypertensive, diabetic and hypertensive diabetic heart disease. Circulation 1990;82:848–855.

13 The Pathophysiology and Metabolic Impact of Hyperglycemia

CONTENTS

INTRODUCTION
PATHOPHYSIOLOGY OF HYPERGLYCEMIA
CLINICAL IMPACT OF HYPERGLYCEMIA
SUMMARY
REFERENCES
SUPPLEMENTARY READINGS

Key Words: Hyperglycemia, Vascular injury, Inflammation, Hyperglycemia, Monocyte derived macrophages, Vascular smooth muscle cells

INTRODUCTION

Accelerated vascular injury and inflammation are intimately associated with the devastating complications of type-2 diabetes. This process is initiated and perpetuated by the pathophysiological consequences of the hyperglycemic state. The vascular devastation of hyperglycemia can occur by several mechanisms, impacting the vessel wall, monocyte derived macrophages, and vascular smooth muscle cells.

Nuclear factor kappa B, activated by elevated glucose concentrations, increases the expression of divergent genes in the vascular smooth muscle cells, tissue macrophages, and the cells of the endothelium. In addition, continued exposure of lipids and proteins to these high glucose concentrations generates advanced glycation end products (AGE) including low molecular weight residue, fluorophores, and protein cross links, inducing the formation of reactive oxygen species, binding to cell surface receptors and increasing oxidative stress. Enhanced oxidative stress has several devastating effects at the cellular level within the arterial wall, contributing to macrovascular disease. LDL and glucose oxidation generate the formation of superoxide anions within the mitochondria, generating hydroxyl radicals and NADPH (reduced form of nicotinamide adenine dinucleotide phosphate)

From: *Current Clinical Practice: Type 2 Diabetes, Pre-Diabetes, and the Metabolic Syndrome*
Edited by: R.A. Codario, DOI 10.1007/978-1-60327-441-8_13
© Springer Science+Business Media, LLC 2011

production within tissue macrophages. In the journal, *Circulation*, Davi and others reported in 1999, that prostaglandin F-2, a derivative of arachidonic acid within cell membranes, was elevated in the 24-h urine of diabetic patients [*1*]. The presence of this prostaglandin in increased quantities was a strong indicator of free radical production and was found in the highest quantities in individuals with the highest glucose levels.

PATHOPHYSIOLOGY OF HYPERGLYCEMIA

Hyperglycemia generates the production of nuclear factor kappa-B, which enhances the expression of inflammatory genes within the endothelial cells promoting the attraction, adhesion, and subsequent transmigration of monocytes into the subendothelial space by means of a chemotactic gradient. In addition, nitric oxide production is inhibited by increased glucose states via advanced glycation end products (AGE) mediated mechanisms. The result is significant endothelial dysfunction, impairing vasodilatation, and promoting vascular injury, all due to the deadly triad of hyperglycemia, oxidative stress, and advanced glycation end products.

Poorly controlled diabetics contain monocytes in an inflammatory, activated state which then differentiate into macrophages within the endothelial space, accumulating within the arterial wall. These macrophages then begin to proliferate significantly in the presence of oxidized LDL particles. In addition, exposure to elevated glucose concentrations affects reverse cholesterol transport by inhibiting the uptake of cholesterol esters from HDL and affecting the apo A-1 moiety on the HDL molecules.

Vascular smooth muscle cells proliferate in vitro in a high glucose milieu. Matrix molecules and proteoglycans, produced by the vascular smooth muscle cells, bind atherogenic lipoproteins enhancing their retention within the endothelial space. Increased non-enzymatic glycation of collagen, synthesized by proliferating vascular smooth muscle cells, enhances the deposition and retention of LDL within the vessel wall promoting the growth of unstable plaque formation. This may give some insight into the accelerated atherogenesis experienced by diabetic patients despite lipid values that are not alarmingly increased.

Not to be overlooked is the role of inflammatory mechanisms in the pathogenesis of the arteriosclerotic process particularly in the diabetic patient – both in causing type-2 diabetes and promoting cardiovascular events. In a hyperglycemic and dyslipidemic environment, the endothelium responds by increasing its production of inflammatory cytokines, coagulation promoting proteins, and adhesion enhancing molecules. Tissue macrophages accelerate the inflammatory process by morphing into foam cells, secreting growth factors and matrix metalloproteinases; these also inhibit peroxisome proliferator activated receptors increasing insulin resistance. The central figure in the regulation and promulgation of inflammation is nuclear factor kappa-B, which orchestrates vascular smooth muscle proliferation, cytokine and chemokine expression, apoptosis, macrophage growth and proliferation, and governs LDL oxidation. Many of the bad actors conspicuous in the genesis and promotion of type-2 diabetes (free fatty acids, AGE pathways, and hyperglycemia) play a crucial role in signaling the nuclear factor kappa-B response, recruiting tumor necrosis factor (TNF) alpha in the process.

Cells that have lost their ability to handle increased intracellular glucose concentrations promote activation of protein kinase increasing intracellular injury, inflammation, and oxidative stress with increased flux of free fatty acids due to impaired insulin sensitivity.

The intimate connection between inflammation, insulin resistance, and arteriosclerotic vascular disease is underscored by the role of hypertriglyceridemia, free fatty acids, and hyperglycemia to the endothelial damage brought about by the diabetic state, and also promoting oxidative stress within the endoplasmic reticulum of adipose and liver tissue.

The distressed and embattled adipocyte also plays an important role as an initiator and ultimately an unfortunate victim of the hyperglycemic state. The diseased and abnormally functioning adipocytes, plagued by the harmful effect of oxidative stress and nuclear fact kappa-B activation, release cytokines that act directly on the hepatocyte to increase the production of C-reactive protein and amyloid A, which modifies the structure of the HDL molecules coating the surface of the apo-A1 attachment, impairing reverse cholesterol transport. Inflammatory cytokines also alter the expression of apolipoprotein which affect lipid metabolism within the adipocyte. Adipocyte generated leptin exerts pro-inflammatory effects with the endothelial cells and tissue macrophages, while adiponectin concentrations are decreased, especially within the visceral fat.

The concept of cellular injury and vasculopathy with hyperglycemia has been supported by clinical studies evaluating the vasculature. Compared to normal patients, those with impaired glucose tolerance and those with diabetes, demonstrated a significant increase in lipid rich plaque. Intravascular ultrasound studies in humans have demonstrated a higher percentage of lip volume and area within the coronary artery plaque of those with metabolic syndrome compared to normal individuals with multivariate analyses showing that metabolic syndrome to be an independent predictor of lipid rich plaque. When carotid plaque removed at surgery is analyzed from patients with diabetes compared to normals, the increased presence of dense infiltrations of mononuclear cells associated with inflammation can be seen in the diabetics with cell surface receptors for advanced glycosylated end products (RAGE) present in increased quantities in accordance with the patient's glycemic control. The binding of advanced glycosylated end products (AGE) to their receptor site (RAGE) initiates a chemotactic response accelerating the inflammatory reaction, revealing why patients with diabetes are not only more likely to develop accelerated atherosclerosis, but also more predisposed to developing unstable more dangerous plaque.

Other studies have demonstrated a decrease in coronary blood flow due to impaired endothelial function and vasodilatation with impaired glucose tolerance and control with intramyocardial triglyceride concentration differentially increasing in the normal, obese, impaired glucose tolerant, and frankly diabetic patients. In addition, diastolic dysfunction is progressively more prevalent in the obese, impaired glucose tolerant, and diabetic patients compared to normal, giving insight into the pathophysiology of cardiac lipotoxicity in the evolution of diabetic cardiomyopathy and diastolic and systolic heart failure associated with diabetes.

The association between hyperglycemia and increased mortality and morbidity with multi-organ dysfunction, cardiovascular disease, and adverse neurological outcomes including prolonged ventilator dependence, renal insufficiency, anemia, and increased risk for sepsis and infections is well known. The relationship, however, between control of hyperglycemia and macrovascular disease, particularly cardiovascular disease has, nonetheless, been controversial in light of two clinical trials and an older landmark trial.

The United Kingdom Prospective Diabetes Study (UKPDS), the Action in Diabetes and Vascular Disease: Preterax and Diamicron Modified release Controlled Evaluation

(ADVANCE) trial and the Action to Control Cardiovascular Risk in Diabetes (ACCORD) study included over 25,000 cohorts to evaluate the cardiovascular outcomes with glycemic control in type-2 diabetics. The disparate results of these three trials will be discussed in greater detail in Chap. 14.

CLINICAL IMPACT OF HYPERGLYCEMIA

For many years glycemic control has been a determinate of the micro and macrovascular complications from diabetes. The United Kingdom Perspective Diabetes Study in type-2 diabetics and the DCCT trial (Diabetes Control and Complication Trial) in type-1 diabetics have shown reductions in microvascular and macrovascular complications with tighter glycemic control. From these and many other clinical trials the message is clear; effective diabetic management including glycemic control reduces complications [2].

Insulin was first isolated in 1921 and purified and quickly applied as therapy for type-1 diabetes. The first oral agent drugs were introduced in the 1940s and have had a profound impact on glycemic control and outcomes in type-2 diabetics.

The biggest problem with managing type-2 diabetes is that many patients have already had complications when the disease is finally diagnosed with retinopathy present in 18%, cardiovascular complications in 17%, absent foot pulses in 12%, diminished reflexes in 8%, and microalbuminuria in 4% [3].

Current data indicates that 44% of patients with diabetes have a hemoglobin A1C greater than 7.0 with 40% having an A1C greater than 8.0. To complicate the matter, type-2 diabetes is a known progressive disease that requires increasing levels of intervention with progressive loss of beta-cell function. It is this loss of beta-cell function and first phase insulin response that increased postprandial hyperglycemia and elevated postprandial glucose increases the risk for vascular complications.

Hence, effective management must not only target postprandial glucose, but fasting hyperglycemia and hepatic gluconeogenesis as well. In the DCCT trial, a reduction in hemoglobin A1C from 9 to 7% reduced retinopathy by 63%, nephropathy by 54%, and neuropathy by 60%. There were reductions in cardiovascular disease as well, but they were not statistically significant with the P values of 0.052 [4].

The Kumamoto trial and the UKPDS trial evaluated patients with type-2 diabetes. In the Kumamoto trial, reductions in hemoglobin A1C from 9 to 7% reduced retinopathy by 69% and nephropathy by 70%. In the UKPDS trials, reduction in hemoglobin A1C from 8 to 7% reduced retinopathy by 17–21% and nephropathy by 24–33%. Cardiovascular disease was reduced by 16%, but this was not statistically significant [5].

It is important for physicians to understand that while fasting glucose is an indication of control and is often used as screening for identifying diabetics we can see that postprandial glucose is the initial driver of A1C, and initiates the macrovascular complications. Postprandial glucoses begin to rise in response to progressive deterioration of beta-cell function and subsequent loss of first phase insulin release.

In healthy subjects, large amounts of insulin are released almost immediately in response to nutrient intake whereas patients with type-2 diabetes lack sufficient immediate insulin response, allowing postprandial glucoses to rise and stay elevated when the diabetic condition has manifested itself.

In individuals with impaired glucose tolerance, there is a much slower insulin release although the actual amount of insulin released is greater than in healthy subjects. Nevertheless, postprandial glucose is higher as a result of progressive insulin resistance.

In 1995, greater than 50% of diabetic patients in this country were on monotherapy with 40% taking insulin. By the year 2000, 30% of patients were taking combinations, and in 2009 close to 70% of type-2 diabetics were taking more than one medication – often as a combination pill [6]. Clearly, this is now the era where combination therapy is becoming the trend rather the exception with importance of adding insulin therapy earlier in the regimen to achieve tight glycemic control being emphasized [7].

Although the oral agents are convenient for most patients, they still have their limitations. These include drug interactions, cost of treatment, compliance issues, and effective manipulations of adjustments of polypharmacy. There is absolutely no question as to the positive impact of insulin on management of the disease.

Enough insulin will always overcome insulin resistance. In the USA, primary care physicians and internists are responsible for 65% of initiation of insulin therapy. Further evidence of the increasing mortality in rising glucose concentration has been demonstrated in other studies.

The Diabetes Epidemiology Collaborative Analysis of Diagnostic Criteria in Europe (DECODE) studied the relationship between impaired glucose tolerance, cardiovascular mortality, and overall mortality. In this study, there were 25,000 cohorts, 95% of whom were not known to have diabetes. The patients were followed for up to 10 years. All patients received a 75 g glucose tolerance test and had 2-h postprandial and fasting glucose measuring [8].

Those individuals with the lowest mortality were those with fasting and 2-h postprandial glucose levels below 110 and 140 mg/dl respectively. As the postprandial sugars rose from 150 to 200 mg/dl, there was a progressive increase in mortality and morbidity.

In the UKDPS trials, any improvement in glycemic control was associated with significant reduction in the risk for progression of microvascular complications. A 1% difference in hemoglobin A1C between intensively and conventionally treated patients, reduced microvascular complications by up to 29% [9].

In both the DCCT and Kumamoto studies, a 2% difference in hemoglobin A1C was associated with close to a 60% reduction in microvascular complications. Also demonstrated in UKPS was that for every 1% reduction in hemoglobin A1C, there was a 43% reduction in the risk of amputation or death from peripheral vascular disease, a 30% reduction in the risk of microvascular endpoints, a 21% reduction in the risk of any diabetes related endpoint, 19% reduction in the risk of cataract extraction, 16% reduction in the risk of heart failure, 14% reduction in the risk of myocardial infarction, and 12% reduction in the risk of stroke [9].

Treatment targets for all patients should be individualized attempting to achieve the best glycemic control without increasing the risk for drug interactions, complications of therapy, or hypoglycemia. Table 1 gives an overall therapeutic guide to achieving glycemic control in the type-2 diabetic.

In general, most pharmacologic agents will lower hemoglobin A1C between 1 and 2% with the exception of nateglinide and the alpha-glucoside inhibitors, which will have a 1% reduction in hemoglobin A1C for their effects. The addition of a second drug from a different class will lower the hemoglobin A1C by another 1–2%.

Table 1
Therapeutic guide to achieving glycemic goals in type-2 diabetics

Initial A1C	Therapeutic target	Preferred intervention	Alternative intervention	If A1c is not <6.5%
6–7	PPG assess FPG	Metformin and or TZD AGI glinides DPP-IV inhibitor	Low dose SFU incretin mimetic	Increase doses combination therapy
7–8	PPG assess FPG	Synergistic combinations of all oral agents	Incretin mimetic	Increase doses of oral agents Insulin analogues
8–9	FPG assess PPG	Synergistic combinations of all oral agents	Basal and/or bolus insulin	Intensify therapy combining insulin with oral agents
9–10	FPG and PPG	Synergistic oral agent combinations with basal insulin	Supplement with bolus insulin	Intensify insulin therapy
>10	FPG and PPG	Insulin therapy	May retain sensitizers and SFU's	Intensify insulin therapy

Nathan [22]

Table 2
Contributions of postprandial glucose (PPG)
and fasting plasma glucose (FPG) to A1C

A1C (%)	PPG (%)	FPG (%)
<7.3	~70	~30
7.3–8.4	~52	~48
8.5–9.2	~45	~55
9.3–10.2	~41	~59
>10.2	~30	~70
$P<0.05$		

Monnier [24]

Elevated postprandial glucose is the earliest detectable glycemic abnormality, while the hemoglobin A1C is the sum of the fasting glucose and the postprandial glucoses. Hence in many patients, targeting postprandial glucose can have a major effect on hemoglobin A1C, particularly with A1C levels less than 8.5%, and knowledge of the impact of postprandial hyperglycemia remains critical to diabetic management [10]. Table 2 illustrates the contribution of fasting plasma glucose and postprandial glucose to the A1C.

This is important to know because the diabetic patient spends most of the day in the postprandial state. In the normal weight non-diabetic, glucose returns to premeal values at different rates depending on the caloric content with a large meal taking up to 4.7 h for the glucose to return to normal in non-diabetics, 4.1 h for a medium meal, and 2.4 h for a small meal. A large meal is defined as 50% of the total daily calories, while a medium meal is 25%, and a small meal 12.5%. Exercise during the post meal period can also influence the duration of hyperglycemia with postprandial exercising increasing insulin sensitivity.

Temelkova-Kurktschiev and others in Diabetes Care (2000) showed that post challenge oral glucose tolerance test glucoses are more strongly associated with arteriosclerotic disease than fasting blood sugar or hemoglobin A1C, correlating these values with changes in intimal media thickness. This study involved 582 subjects, aged 40–70, at risk for type-2 diabetes with only the post-challenge glucose levels significantly correlating with intimal medial thickness, not fasting glucose or A1C [11].

The Honolulu Heart Study, a large epidemiologic study of non-diabetic individuals demonstrated as the 1-h post challenge glucose increased, cardiovascular events increased. In this study 6,394 patients were evaluated in terms of their 1-h post challenge serum glucose after receiving a 50 g glucose load [12]. Patients were divided into five quintiles according to their 1-h postprandial sugar as follows: 40–114 mg/dl, 115–135 mg/dl, 134–156 mg/dl, 157–189 mg/dl, and 190–532 mg/dl.

Fatal heart attacks were almost three times higher in the fifth quintile compared to the first quintile with nonfatal MI's doubled between the first quintile and the fifth quintile.

Other studies have compared the evidence of association with meal time glucose spikes and the risk of cardiovascular disease and mortality [13].

The Pacific and Indian Ocean Trial in 1999 published in Diabetes Care showed that 2-h postprandial hyperglycemia doubled the risk of mortality [14].

The Funagata Diabetes Study in 1999 showed that impaired glucose tolerance not impaired fasting glucose was a better risk factor for cardiovascular disease [15].

The Whitehall Study in 1998 found that men in the upper 2.5% of 2-h post meal glucose distribution had significantly higher coronary heart disease mortality [16].

The Diabetic Intervention Study in 1996 published in Diabetologia showed that post meal glucoses, but not fasting glucoses were associated with coronary heart disease [6].

Finally, the Rancho-Bernardo Study in 1998 showed that 2-h post glucose hyperglycemia more than doubled the risk of fatal cardiovascular disease and heart disease in older adults [17].

Data from Bastyr and others published in *The Journal of Clinical Therapeutics* in 1999 compared two regimens of NPH insulin at bedtime and an oral sulfonylurea during the day with lispro, short-acting insulin at meal time and oral sulfonylurea during the day. The lowest fasting glucoses were observed during treatment with the NPH and sulfonylurea, and the highest fastings found with lispro and the sulfonylurea [18].

Bastyr further went on to study 135 patients with type-2 diabetes who failed sulfonylurea therapy and were subsequently randomized to metformin and glyburide/NPH at bedtime and glyburide or pre-meal insulin lispro and glyburide.

The highest fasting glucoses were found with the lispro-glyburide combination and lowest fasting glucoses were observed during treatment with NPH and glyburide. However, it was the patients on lispro and the sulfonylurea who showed the most improvement in glycemic control with lowered hemoglobin A1C's despite the elevated fasting glucoses.

The lispro-sulfonylurea group lowered hemoglobin A1C by 1.6% compared to the NPH-sulfonylurea group, which lowered the hemoglobin A1C by 1.2%. Hence, this data supported the concept that controlling postprandial glucose had a greater impact on lowering hemoglobin A1C than just targeting fasting glucose.

Targeting postprandial glucose in gestational diabetics improved hemoglobin A1C and outcomes over a 6-week period of time compared to preprandial glucose control. This study published in the *New England Journal of Medicine* in 1995, included 66 women with gestational diabetes who were evaluated, comparing preprandial vs. postprandial glucose measurements [19].

The baseline hemoglobin A1C's were 8.6 and 8.9% for the preprandial and postprandial respectively. Although both groups lowered their hemoglobin A1C levels, it was the postprandial group that showed a decrease of twice that of the preprandial group with a change of close to 3% in hemoglobin A1Ccompared to less than 1% in the preprandial group. Sugars were adjusted strictly based on either preprandial or postprandial self monitored data.

This improvement in hemoglobin A1C with postprandial monitoring resulted also in better outcomes for three significant fetal outcome measurements; lower weight for gestational age, lower rate of C-sections, and lower neonatal hypoglycemia. The benefit of controlling postprandial vs. fasting glucose in the gestational diabetic was clearly obvious in this study.

In the DIGAMI trial (Diabetes Mellitus Insulin Glucose Infusion and Acute Myocardial Infarction) prevention of excessive hyperglycemia (blood glucose levels below 215 mg/dl) in the acute phase after a myocardial infarction was associated with significant improvement of survival in these acutely ill diabetics. This study was the only large, placebo controlled, randomized clinical trial of insulin-glucose infusion therapy in patients following an acute myocardial infarction in the era of thrombolytic therapy.

This study enrolled 620 diabetics randomized to receive either standard treatment for MI plus insulin-glucose infusion for at least 24 h followed by multidose insulin treatment or standard treatment alone. In this study, insulin-glucose infusion followed by sub cutaneous insulin treatment improved long-term survival by nearly 1/3 and this effect persisted for at least 3.5 years with an 11% absolute reduction in mortality. The reduction was most apparent in those patients with low cardiovascular risk and no previous insulin treatment [20].

Van Den Berghe looked at the effects of intensive insulin therapy in 1,548 patients to maintain normal glycemia during a critical illness. These patients were receiving mechanical ventilation and admitted to the surgical intensive care unit and randomly assigned to receive insulin therapy to maintain blood glucose between 80 and 110 mg/dl or conventional treatment (infusion of insulin if blood glucose exceeds 215 mg/dl and maintenance of glucose between 180 and 200 mg/dl).

At the time of admission, only 13% of the patients in the intensive treatment arm had a history of diabetes and 5% were receiving insulin. At the 12-month period, 35 patients (4.6%) in the insulin treatment group had died compared with 63 (8% in the standard treatment group). This represented a risk reduction of 42%. About 10.6% of the insulin treated group stayed in the ICU for more than 5 days, compared to 20% of the conventional group. The intensively treated group had reductions in:

1. Sepsis by 46%
2. Acute renal failure requiring dialysis by 41%
3. Critical illness acute polyneuropathy by 44%
4. Hospital mortality by 34%
5. Blood transfusions by 50%
6. Reduction in prolonged requirement for antibiotics by 36% [20]

The risk of mortality and morbidity was high for those conventionally treated individuals who succumbed to excessive inflammation, sepsis, polyneuropathy, and multiple organ failure. All of these values were statistically significant.

Further analysis demonstrated that it was control of blood glucose rather than insulin administration that resulted in the observed clinical benefit. This was an important compelling conclusion because hyperglycemia is common in critically ill patients even with no previous history of diabetes. Patients in this setting are prone to significant stresses on insulin release and insulin resistance.

Treating patients in the intensive care unit of course is always a challenge since insulin requirements in individual patients may vary widely depending on insulin sensitivity before and during the critical illness, caloric intake, severity, and nature of the illness, other concomitant medications that may aggravate insulin sensitivity, the presence or absence of renal or hepatic disease and insulin reserves.

After the sugars are normalized, patients should be monitored closely to determine any subsequent needs for insulin or other medication. Clearly any changes in the patient's clinical condition, especially worsening infection, can increase insulin requirements and aggravate insulin sensitivity.

Current targets for glycemic control include hemoglobin A1C of less than 6.5%, fasting glucoses less than 110 mg/dl (with benefits being shown below 100 mg/dl), postprandial glucoses less than 140 mg/dl with limitations of postprandial glucose excursions to 40 mg/dl from the preprandial values.

Although postprandial glucose is defined as being measured 2 h after the meal, clearly, several studies have indicated the prognostic importance of elevated 1-h postprandial glucose levels as well.

It has been well established that chronic hyperglycemia is very closely related to the subsequent development of microvascular disease and aggravating existing macrovascular disease. It is important to understand that postprandial glycemic spikes do have acute effects on the cellular level causing transient increases in retinal profusion and glomerular filtration rate.

Postprandial hyperglycemia interferes with vascular dilatation enhancing endothelial dysfunction. The Rancho/Bernardo study identified 70% of women and 48% of men with no prior diagnosis of diabetes and no fasting blood glucose elevation who had post challenge hyperglycemia. This was associated in women with a 2–3 fold increase in mortality from cardiovascular disease or ischemic heart disease. This was not seen in the male cohort [11].

The Paris Perspective study, including a cohort of 7,000 men, found a significantly large increase in annual coronary heart disease mortality both in patients who were confirmed as being diabetic and in subjects with 2-h post challenge blood glucoses equal to or greater than 200 mg/dl, subsequently marking them newly diagnosed diabetics. Even more striking in the Paris Perspective data was the difference between normal glycemic men and the men who were classified as having impaired glucose tolerance (between glucoses of 140 and 240 mg/dl) [13].

Similar results were demonstrated in the Honolulu Heart study looking at 8,000 non-diabetic Japanese men followed for 12 years. In this study, coronary heart disease increased in a linear fashion with increases in 1-h post challenge glucoses with men in the fourth quintile (postprandial glucoses 157–189 mg/dl), having twice the adjusted rate of fatal heart disease [21].

The Diabetes Epidemiology Collaborative Analysis of Diagnostic Criteria in Europe Trial (DECODE) compared the performance of the U.S and European diabetics in predicting mortality. DECODE included a very large study population of more than 18,000 men and 7,300 women equal to or greater than 30 years of age from 13 prospective European cohort studies. One thousand five hundred study participants were diagnosed as having diabetes at baseline and the rest had unknown glucose tolerances. Patients were followed for a median of 7 years and a maximum up to 10 years. At any level of fasting glucose, even the lowest quintiles, the risk of deaths were substantially increased in patients with post challenge glucoses equal to or greater than 200 mg/dl [13].

This supported the evidence that postprandial hyperglycemia is independently related to mortality and is actually a better predictor of mortality than fasting hyperglycemia. Hence it is clear that postprandial hyperglycemia is an important emerging and largely overlooked risk factor with important deleterious macrovascular consequences.

Chaisson and others in the STOP-NIDDM (Study to Prevent Non insulin Dependent Diabetes Mellitus), showed that acarbose was the first oral agent to demonstrate reductions in the risk for cardiovascular disease and hypertension in an impaired glucose tolerant population [22]. This was the first evidence for an oral agent that lowers postprandial glucose to also reduce the risk for cardiovascular disease and hypertension. This occurred despite 30% of the participants stopping the drug during the trial.

Acarbose inhibits enzymatic cleavage of dietary carbohydrates into simple sugars and is similar to dietary modifications. The patients receiving the drug showed reductions in blood pressure, waist circumference, weight, triglycerides, and postprandial glucose, improving insulin resistance and carbohydrate metabolism. Many of these are targets of risk reduction in the metabolic syndrome as well.

In January 2002, Baron published a large review of 48,858 patients from the Keiser Permanente Medical Care Program of Northern California showing that the large cohorts of diabetic patients, after a multivariant adjustment, demonstrated an 8% increased risk of heart failure for each 1% increase in hemoglobin A1C, with a hemoglobin A1C of 10% or greater associated with a 1.6% fold greater risk of heart failure compared with normal levels [11].

Data suggested that, independent of clinically recognized coronary disease, poor glycemic control could well be associated with an increased risk of heart failure. Diabetes was known to be a well established independent risk factor for heart failure, supporting the concept of subclinical diabetic cardiomyopathy.

The Permanente study, however, showed a graded association between glycemic control and the incidence of complications due to heart failure among diabetics in an HMO setting. The association appeared to be much stronger in men than women and persisted after adjustment for interim MI, diabetes related factors, ACE inhibitor therapy at baseline and use of beta-blockers. This data also suggested that tight control could lower the risk of heart failure and that this relationship was linear [11].

Poor glycemic control may predispose to heart failure by three possible mechanisms:

1. Contributing to the development of subclinical diabetic cardiomyopathy and systolic dysfunction
2. Promoting atherosclerotic vascular disease with the ensuing occlusive coronary artery involvement
3. Contributing to myocardial fibrosis, impaired ventricular relaxation and diastolic dysfunction

In addition, hyperglycemia is associated with a preponderance of small dense LDL, low HDL, endothelial dysfunction, deranged fibrinolysis, and a predisposition to arteriosclerotic vascular disease. The small vessel vascular disease that is caused by diabetes may play a critical role in the etiology of diabetic cardiomyopathy.

In the DCCT trial, more than 1,400 individuals with type-1 diabetes were stratified on the basis of their microvascular disease at entry. The study had to be stopped prematurely because of a profound difference between both primary and secondary outcomes of tight diabetic control. Intensive therapy reduced the development of diabetic retinopathy by 76%. The albumin excretion rate was reduced by 35% and clinical neuropathy reduced by 70%. In those individuals who had evidence of microvascular disease at trial entry, progression of retinopathy was reduced in 54% with 46% experiencing a reduction in proliferative and severe non-proliferative diabetic retinopathy. Clinical neuropathy in these patients was reduced by 58% where fixed proteinuria greater than 300 mg for 24 h was reduced by 56% [23].

As we saw earlier, data from the Kumamoto trial were very similar to the DCCT trial in a population of thin Japanese type-2 diabetics. Intensive therapy here, reduced hemoglobin A1C level to a mean of 7.1% and it was sustained for up to 6 years. The intensively treated group noted a 12% overall reduction in diabetes related endpoints with a 25% reduction in specific microvascular disease outcomes. In this study, retinopathy was reduced by 21% and albuminuria by 33% at 12 years of follow-up. Once again the difference in myocardial infarction rate was reduced, but not achieving statistical significance.

The obese cohort of the UKPDS was randomized to metformin and this group demonstrated a 32% reduction in diabetes related endpoints, 42% in diabetes related deaths, and a 39% reduction in myocardial infarctions. This was a post-hoc analysis with some crossover, and hence there were some patients who were not exclusively assigned to receive metformin. Nonetheless, the UKPDS trial confirms that microvascular complications in diabetes can be prevented as well as in the type-1 diabetic.

In an office managed setting, intensive control of type-2 diabetes was also demonstrated by Meldrum. Reduction in A1C levels from 8.7 to 7.5% resulted in a 16% increase in outpatient visit costs, a 42% increase in outpatient pharmacy costs, but a 47% reduction in hospital professional costs. Interestingly, evaluating this data also indicates the importance of glycemic control independent of the agent used in reducing the microvascular complications. Although the initial cost of initiating intensive therapy are increased, these are more than offset by subsequent reduction in emergency room visits, long-term complications, and reductions in hospitalizations with this approach, hence justifying the cost effectiveness of tight control [23].

The failure to statistically reduce the incidence of macrovascular disease is undoubtedly a reflection of the multifaceted nature of macrovascular complications with their incipient onset with insulin resistance, emphasizing the need to attack macrovascular disease by controlling multiple parameters as early as possible.

Clinical trials in patients with both type-1 and type-2 diabetes have demonstrated that the risk of development of progression of diabetic retinopathy is not increased in patients treated with the long-acting insulin analog glargine compared to those patients who receive NPH. Clearly, better glycemic control is associated with the reduced progression of retinopathy in diabetic patients regardless of the agent used.

Some data suggest that retinopathy may worsen initially with the onset of improved glycemic control mediated in part by the effects of insulin like growth factor I. In vitro studies have raised a concern about potential growth factor activity of the insulin analogs via this receptor, although in a recent review of 2,207 patients with type-1 or type-2 diabetes no such increased risk was noted [23].

Clearly, early insulin therapy can be extremely invaluable in achieving tighter glycemic controls. Hence by shifting the paradigm for the treatment of type-2 diabetes to more flexible individualized and multi-optioned approaches, the physician should make effective use of all the available options, set the right goals for the patient, and keep in mind the patient's preferences and motivation for cooperation.

It is important to keep in mind that the improvement of the macrovascular risk factors in the type-2 diabetic must emphasize not only tight glycemic control, but also lipid and blood pressure management with the insulin resistant stage. It is only by that comprehensive approach that we can achieve better outcomes.

In the past, the sulfonylureas were labeled under the dark cloud cast by the University Group Diabetes Study in the early 1970s, which were concerned about possible cardiotoxicity of these first generation secretagogues in patients with diabetes. Other studies such as the UKPDS did not find any such association.

Both the first generation and the second generation sulfonylureas had no increase in cardiovascular events associated with their use. The newer sulfonylureas such as glimepiride (Amaryl) do not affect acute ischemic compensatory responses in the myocardial cell because of less binding to the adenosine triphosphate dependent potassium channels.

SUMMARY

Clearly, hyperglycemia contributes to micro and macrovascular disease. An important take home message from the UKPDS trials is that tighter glycemic control will reduce microvascular complications with the effect on cardiovascular events certainly not as impressive as could be achieved with tighter blood pressure control combined with a sound lipid lowering strategy and inhibition of platelet aggregation.

The aggregation of prediabetic impaired glucose tolerance, hypertension, obesity, and dyslipidemia with insulin resistance paves the groundwork for significant cardiovascular complications from the diabetic state when and if it develops.

REFERENCES

1. Davi G, Ciabattoni G, Consoli A, Mazzetti A, Falco A. In vivo formation of prostaglandin F2 and platelet activation in diabetes mellitus. Circulation 1999;99:224–229.
2. UK Prospective Diabetes Study. Overview of six years of therapy of type 2 diabetes. Diabetes 1995;44: 1249–1258.
3. Brownlee M. The pathobiology of diabetic complications: a unifying mechanism. Diabetes 2005;54: 1615–1625.
4. The Diabetes Control and Complications Trial Research group. The effect of intensive treatment of diabetes on the development and progression of long term complications in insulin dependent diabetes mellitus. N Engl J Med 1993;329:977–986.
5. Fonseca V, Rosenstock J, et al. Effect of metformin and rosiglitazone combination therapy in patients with type 2 diabetes. JAMA 2000;283:1695–1702.
6. Hanefeld M, Fischer S, Julius U. Risk factors for myocardial infarction and death in newly detected NIDDM: the diabetes Intervention Study, 11 year follow up. Diabetologia 1996;39:1577–1583.

7. O'Keefe JH, Miles JM, et al. Improving the adverse cardiovascular prognosis of type 2 diabetes. Mayo Clin Proc. 1999;74:171–180.

8. The European diabetes Epidemiology group (DECODE). Glucose tolerance and cardiovascular mortality: comparison of fasting and 2-hour diagnostic criteria. Arch Intern Med 2001;161:397–405.

9. Nathan DM, Meigs J, et al. The epidemiology of cardiovascular disease in type 2 diabetes mellitus. Lancet 1997;350(Suppl 1):S14–S19.

10. Panaram G. Mortaliaty and survival in type 2 diabetes mellitus. Diabetologia 1987;30:123–131.

11. Renders CM, Valk GD, Franse LV, et al. Long term effectiveness of a quality improvement program for patients with type 2 diabetes in general practice. Diabetes Care 2001;24:1365–1370.

12. Donahue RP, Abbott RD, Reed DM, Yano K. Postchallenge glucose concentration and coronary heart disease in men of Japanese ancestry. Honlulu Heart Program. Diabetes 1987;36(2):689–692.

13. Kannel WB, McGee DL. Diabetes and cardiovascular disease: the Framingham Study. JAMA 1979;241:2035–2038.

14. Geiss LS, Herman WH, Smith PJ. The Pacific and Indian Ocean trial. Diabetes Care 1993;16:434–442.

15. Tominaga M, Eguchi H, Manaka H, IgarashiK, Kato T, Sekikawa A. Impaired glucose tolerance is a risk factor for cardiovascular disease, but not impaired fasting glucose. The funagata diabetes Study. Diabetes Care 1999;22:920–924.

16. Balkau B, Shipley M, Jarrett RJ. High blood glucose concentration is a risk factor for mortality in middle aged nondiabetic men. The Whitehall study. Diabetes Care 1998;21:360–367.

17. Barrett-Connor E, Ferrara A. Isolated postchallenge hyperglycemia and the risk of fatal cardiovascular disease in older women and men. The Rancho Bernardo Study. Diabetes Care 1998;21:1236–1239.

18. Turner RC, et al. Glycemic control with diet, sulfonylurea, metformin or insulin in patients with type 2 diabetes. JAMA 1999;281:2005–2012.

19. de Veciana M, Major C, Morgan M, Asrat T, Toohey J, Lien J. Postprandial versus preprandial glucose monitoring in women with gestation diabetes mellitus requiring insulin. N Engl J Med 1995;333(9): 1237–1241.

20. Holmboe ES. Oral antihyperglycemic therapy for type 2 diabetes: clinical applications. JAMA 2002;287:373–376.

21. Donahue RP, Abbott RD, Reed DM, Yano K. Postchallenge glucose concentration and coronary heart disease in men of Japanese ancestry. Honolulu Heart Program. Diabetes 1987;36:689–692.

22. Nathan DM, Buse MB, Davidson JB. Medical management of hyperglycaemia in type-2 diabetes; a consensus algorithm. Diabetologia 2009;52(1):17–30.

23. Ohkubo Y, Kishikawa H. Intensive insulin therapy prevents the progression of diabetic microvascular complications in Japanese patients with noninsulin dependent diabetes mellitus. Diabetes Res Clin Pract 1995;28:103–117.

24. Monnier L. Contributions of postprandial glucose and fasting plasma glucose to A1C. Diabetes Care 2003;26:881–885.

SUPPLEMENTARY READINGS

Bailey CJ. Biguanides and NIDDM. Diabetes Care 1992;15:755–772.

Cefalu WT, et al. Inhaled human insulin treatment in type 2 diabetes. Ann Intern Med 2001;134: 203–207.

Chiasson JL, Josse RG, Hunt JA. The efficacy of acarbose in the treatment of patients with non insulin dependent diabetes mellitus. The STOP_NIDDM trial. Ann Intern Med 1994;121:928–935.

Chiasson JL, Josse RG, et al. Acarbose for prevention of type 2 diabetes mellitus. The STOP-NIDDM randomized trial. Lancet 2002;359:2072–2077.

DeFronzo R, et al. Efficacy of metformin in patients with NIDDM. N Engl J Med 1995;333:541–549.

Effect of intensive blood-glucose control with metformin on complications in overweight patients with type 2 diabetes. Lancet 1998;352:854–862.

Groop L. Sulfonyureas in NIDDM. Diabetes Care 1992;15:737–754.

Harrigan RA, et al. Oral Agents for the treatment of type 2 diabetes mellitus: pharmacology, toxicity and treatment. Ann Emerg Med 2001;38(1):68.

Horton ES, Clinkingbead C, et al. Nateglinide alone and in combination with metformin improves glycemic control by reducing mealtime glucose levels in type 2 diabetes. Diabetes Care 2000;23:1660–1665.

Inzucchi SF, Maggs DG, et al. Efficacy and metabolic effects of metformin and troglitazone in type II diabetes mellitus. N Engl J Med 1998;338:867–872.

Lenhard MJ, Reeves GD. Continuous subcutaneous insulin infusions: a comprehensive review of insulin pump therapy. Arch Intern Med 2001;161(19):2293.

Loh KC, Leow MK. Current therapeutic strategies for type 2 diabetes mellitus. Ann Acad Med Singapore 2003;31:722–729.

Nathan DM. Roussell A, et al. Glyburide or insulin for metabolic control in noninsulin dependent mellitus: a randomized, double blind study. Ann Intern Med 1988;108:334–340.

Saudek CD, et al, Implantable insulin pump vs. multiple dose insulin for noninsulin dependent diabetes mellitus; a randomized clinical trial. JAMA 1996;276:1322–1327.

Sinha R, et al. Prevalence of impaired glucose intolerance among children and adolescents with marked obesity. N Engl J Med 2002;346:802–810.

Stratton IM, Adler AI, et al. Association of glycemia with macrovascular and microvascular complications of type 2 diabetes: prospective observational study. BMJ 2000;321:405–412.

Turner RC. Glycemic control with diet, sulfonylurea, metformin, or insulin in patients with type 2 diabetes: progressive requirement for multiple therapies. JAMA 1999;281:2005–2012.

UKPDS. Effect of intensive blood glucose control with metformin on complications in overweight patients with type 2 diabetes. Lancet 1998;352(9131):854–865.

14 Risk Reduction in the Diabetic Patient

Contents

Key Words: Glycemic control, Lipid control, Blood pressure control, Thrombosis prevention, Multiple factor risk reduction

INTRODUCTION

Diabetic patients are at high risk for cardiovascular mortality, the greatest cause being atherosclerotic vascular disease and its subsequent sequelae. Diabetic patients have greater risk of permanent brain damage with carotid emboli, threefold greater mortality from stroke, poor prognosis for survival, and a two to fourfold greater risk of cardiovascular disease. In the Framingham Heart study, men with type-2 diabetes are twice as likely to develop heart failure compared to non-diabetics and women are five times more likely. The management and control of cardiovascular disease may be the most challenging and elusive task since cardiovascular damage may already be present even before the disease is diagnosed.

The economic impact of this disease has been devastating. In 1997 alone, diabetes was responsible for 88 million disability days, 14 million work loss days, 30.3 million office visits, 13.9 million hospital days, cardiovascular death rate per 10,000 patient years has increased depending upon the number of risk factors with the diabetic fairing far worse than the non-diabetic in each of the risk categories on a linear basis.

Accelerated atherosclerotic vascular disease demonstrated by the diabetic is a result of the metabolic cascade including insulin resistance, hyperinsulinemia, hypertension, endothelial dysfunction, and subsequent increases in triglyceride LDL and VLDL synthesis and decreased clearance for HDL.

From: *Current Clinical Practice: Type 2 Diabetes, Pre-Diabetes, and the Metabolic Syndrome*
Edited by: R.A. Codario, DOI 10.1007/978-1-60327-441-8_14
© Springer Science+Business Media, LLC 2011

Table 1
Cardioprotective effects of ramipril

| Endpoint | *Risk reduction %* | |
	HOPE	*MICRO-HOPE*
Stroke	32	33
Nonfatal myocardial infarction	20	22
Cardiovascular death	26	37
All cause mortality	16	24

From HOPE Study Investigators [97]
Ramipril is indicated to reduce the risk of stroke, myocardial infarction, and death from cardiovascular causes in patients 55 years or older who are at increased risk for these events

Insulin resistance and the metabolic syndrome are at the heart of the deadly quartet of obesity, dyslipidemia, hypertension, and hyperglycemia, which contributes to earlier cardiovascular disease and the microvascular complications of blindness, nephropathy and neuropathy, and the macrovascular complications of stroke, peripheral disease, and coronary artery disease. There may be multiple reasons for the cardiovascular risk associated with type-2 diabetes including impaired vasodilatation, enhance coagulability, excess free fatty acids, insulin resistance, hypertension, and dyslipidemia.

The benefits of ramipril in this high risk patient population were clearly demonstrated in the HOPE and MICRO-HOPE trials as illustrated in Table 1.

Comprehensive risk reduction involves careful attention of the primary care physician to four categories as seen in Table 2 [1]:

1. Glycemic control including control of the hemoglobin A1C <6.5%, fasting glucose less than 100 mg/dl, postprandial sugars less than 140 mg/dl
2. Lipid control including LDL less than 100 mg/dl, HDL greater than 40 mg/dl in men and 50 mg/dl in women, triglycerides less than 150 mg/dl, non-HDL cholesterol <130 mg/dl
3. Blood pressure less than 130/85 mmHg and 125/75 mmHg with any evidence of end-organ disease (retinopathy, neuropathy, and nephropathy)
4. Inhibition of platelet aggregation with aspirin

GLYCEMIC CONTROL

Several studies have evaluated the relationship between blood glucose levels – fasting and postprandial – to cardiovascular risk and have demonstrated that this relationship is graded, continuous, and even reaches below the threshold for diagnosing diabetes. The key principles of glycemic control are outlined in Table 3.

However, what has not been established with crystal clarity is the relationship between glycemic control and reduction of cardiovascular risk. There are five major clinical trials that have looked into this relationship with mixed results. These include the University Group Diabetes Program (UGDP), the Veterans' Affairs Diabetes Trial (VADT), the

Table 2
Cornerstones of therapy for comprehensive risk reduction in type-2 diabetes [1]

Tight glycemic control

    A1C <6.5% (7.0% for patients at high risk for cardiovascular disease with type-2 diabetes greater than 12 years)

        Postprandial glucose <140 mg/dl

        Fasting glucose <100 mg/dl

Tight lipid control

    LDL <100 mg/dl (<70 mg/dl in very high risk patients)

    HDL >45 mg/dl in men

        >50 mg/dl in women

    Triglycerides <150 mg/dl

    Non-HDL cholesterol <130 mg/dl for triglycerides >200 mg/dl

Tight blood pressure control

    Systolic blood pressure <130 mmHg

    Diastolic blood pressure <80 mmHg (BP should be less than 125/75 mmHg with evidence of end organ damage)

Aspirin (75–325 mg/day) for all patients greater than age 30

Ramipril is indicated for overall risk reduction in patients greater than 55 years of age (telmisartan may also be used in ACE intolerant patients)

Irbesartan (Avapro) 300 mg and losartan (Cozaar) 100 mg for existing microalbuminuria

United Kingdom Prospective Diabetes Study (UKPDS), the Action in Diabetes and Vascular Disease (ADVANCE) study, and the Action to Control Cardiovascular Risk in Diabetes (ACCORD) trial. All of these trials studied type-2 diabetics and the impact of glycemic control on atherosclerotic vascular disease, cardiovascular events, and all cause mortality.

The UGDP released its data in 1971 and included approximately 1,000 cohorts that were randomized to one of five treatment arms; phenformin, insulin adjusted to fasting glucose, insulin in a body weight based fixed dose, a sulfonylurea (tolbutamide), and a placebo. In this study, the cardiovascular events and deaths were more than double in the sulfonylurea group compared to placebo (25 vs. 12/1,000 patient years). There was no difference in the insulin groups compared to placebo. The results from this trial prompted many at that time to avoid sulfonylureas altogether and switch to insulin and prompted the FDA to issue a black box warning for all sulfonylureas.

The VADT study included 1,791 type-2 diabetics with a mean entry A1C of 9.4%, a history of coronary heart disease in 40%, and a mean age of 60 years. This study, released in June 2008, showed no difference in cardiovascular outcomes or mortality despite achieving A1C levels of 6.9% in the intensive group and only 8.4% in the standard therapy group. Mean follow-up in this group was 5.6 years. There was also no difference in the microvascular events, while hypoglycemia occurred more commonly in the intensive therapy group (24.1%) compared to the standard therapy group (17.6%) [2].

Table 3
Key concepts in glycemic control

Treat physiologically addressing the dual impairments of

    Impaired beta-cell function (insulin secretion)

    Impaired insulin action (insulin resistance)

Hyperglycemia aggravates both impairments

Keep A1C below 6.5% (7.0% in patients with type-2 diabetes over 12 years at high risk for cardiovascular events)

Keep postprandial glucose below 140 mg/dl

Keep fasting glucose below 100 mg/dl

Add insulin as soon as necessary to achieve and maintain glycemic goals

For fasting and preprandial glucose control

    Decrease hepatic glucose production with metformin

    Increase insulin sensitivity with thiazolidinediones

    Increase insulin availability with long or intermediate insulins and/or DPP-IV inhibitors, sulfonylureas

For postprandial glucose control

    Decrease carbohydrate absorption rate with alpha-glucosidase inhibitors

    Decrease carbohydrate intake

    Increase insulin availability with rapid acting insulins or glinides

    Use DPP-IV inhibitors

    Exenatide/liraglutide

From Nathan [99]

The UKPDS in 1998 included 3,867 patients with a mean age of 54 years who were newly diagnosed with type-2 diabetes. There were two intensive arms in this trial: insulin/sulfonylureas (chlorpropamide, dibenclamide, or glipizide) and metformin in the obese patients. These groups were compared to standard care at that time. Mean A1C levels during the trial were 7.0% in the intensively treated group and 7.9% in the standard treatment group. The metformin group had a statistically significant 30% reduction in macrovascular events including myocardial infarction, stroke, sudden death, angina, and peripheral vascular disease with P values of 0.20, while the insulin/sulfonylurea group experienced a non significant reduction in myocardial infarctions of 16%. Interestingly, in a 10-year follow up study of the UKPDS cohort, this benefit in reduced macrovascular disease (myocardial infarctions and mortality) continued in those who stayed on metformin and was lost in those that stopped the drug. In addition, a post hoc analysis of the original trial revealed that a 10% relative decrease in A1C levels was associated with a statistically significant 14% reduction in myocardial infarction ($P < 0.001$) [3].

The ADVANCE trial included 11,140 cohorts with a target A1C of 6.5% in the intensive arm vs. 7.3% in the standard arm. In this study, there was no difference in the major macrovascular events or all cause mortality between the two groups. However, hypoglycemia was more common in the intensive arm. Participants in this study had an average

age of 66 years, 32% with a history of cardiovascular disease and an average of 8 years with diabetes [4].

The ACCORD trial had a double two by two factorial design of 10,251 patients, 35% of whom had known cardiovascular disease, a mean age of 62 years, mean A1C of 8.3% and were diabetic for an average of 10 years [5]. The standard arm target was 7.0–7.9% while the intensive glucose arm was 5.9%. In addition, half were randomly assigned to receive a lipid lowering regimen of statin/placebo vs. statin/fenofibrate, while the other half were randomly assigned to receive standard hypertensive therapy in one of two groups: <120 mmHg systolic or <140 mmHg systolic. After 1 year, the median A1C values had decreased from 8.1% at baseline to 6.4% in the intensive treatment group and to 7.5% in the standard treatment group and remained stable for over 6 years. After 3.4 years, non fatal myocardial infarction, nonfatal stroke, or cardiovascular deaths occurred in 7.25% of the standard therapy group compared to 6.9% of the intensive therapy group; however, this was not statistically significant ($P=0.16$). There was a statistically significant difference in the rate of nonfatal myocardial infarction in the intensive therapy cohort compared to the standard therapy group (3.6 vs. 4.6%) with a P value of 0.004. However, statistically significant, but small differences in the rates of death from any cause were 14/1,000 in the intensive group vs. 11/1,000 in the standard treatment group with a P value of 0.04.

Rosiglitazone use did not contribute to the mortality (91.2% of the intensive group vs. 57.5%) of the conventional treatment group that received rosiglitazone. Due to the increased mortality, the intensive glucose control arm was terminated. In addition, further analysis of ACCORD and ADVANCE indicated that benefits of lower A1C levels were seen in those individuals with type-2 diabetes less than 10 years with the benefits of tighter control in those having the disease greater than 10 years being less likely.

The BARI 2D (The Bypass Angioplasty Revascularization Investigation 2 Diabetes) Trial evaluated the optimum treatment for patient with both type-2 diabetes and stable ischemic heart disease, evaluating in the process, two treatment strategies for these patients [6]. In this study, 2,368 patients with heart disease and type-2 diabetes were assigned to two treatment arms in a 2×2 factorial design into to two main groups: one group which underwent prompt revascularization with intensive medical therapy and the other with intensive medical therapy using a thiazolidinedione (TZD) sensitizer or insulin therapy.

After 5 years, survival rates did not differ significantly between the revascularization group and the medical therapy group or between the insulin group and the insulin sensitizer group. Similar to the findings in the Clinical Outcomes Using Revascularization and Aggressive Drug Evaluation (COURAGE) trial, patients who were treated with percutaneous cardiac intervention (PCI) had similar mortality and major cardiovascular events compared to those managed medically [7]. So in those diabetic patients who have coronary arteries that can be treated with PCI, medical management can be a reasonable conservative approach to be considered. In addition, the study also indicated that a medical strategy using insulin sensitization or insulin therapy is a reasonable strategy to glycemic control in these patients.

A study by Greenfield and others published in the *Annals of Internal Medicine* in 2009 reviewed the effects of comorbidity on glycemic control and cardiovascular outcomes. In this analysis, 2,613 patients with type-2 diabetes were evaluated for their comorbidities including vision loss, arthritis, genitourinary, lung and heart disease to determine whether achieving A1C levels of 6.5 vs. 7.0% had any cardiovascular benefits [8]. This study concluded that at

A1C levels of 6.5% or lower and 7.0%, cardiovascular events were decreased to a more significant degree in those with low comorbidity suggesting that cardiovascular benefits are highest in those with the lowest comorbidity. For those with substantial comorbidities the overall benefits of trying to achieve a lower A1C to 6.5% might be outweighed by the risk associated with a greater likelihood of hyperglycemia.

It is also important to consider the cardiovascular risks association with the various drugs used to treat type-2 diabetes. Figure 1 summarizes the metabolic effects of the various oral agents used to treat the type-2 diabetic.

The sulfonylureas received a better rating from the UKPDS trial than the earlier UGDP with the United Kingdom study showing that use of these second generation sulfonylureas did not worsen nor improved macrovascular complications of type-2 diabetes. The UKPDS trial, however, did not show any evidence of beta-cell preservation with these oral agents, but rather a slow rise in A1C during the study period. In addition, there have been subsequent studies expressing concern over a worsening prognosis in patients on sulfonylureas if they experience a myocardial infarction, due to the relative non specific affinity for the potassium ATP channel. Inhibition of this channel within the pancreas sets in motion, a sequence of events that ultimately results in insulin release. However, within the cardiac muscle, inhibition of compensatory vasodilatation during an ischemic episode may result. Nateglinide, by virtue of its very short duration of action and increased specificity for the pancreatic potassium ATP channels seems to be less likely to have this effect than the sulfonylureas with the exception of glimepiride which is highly specific for the pancreatic potassium ATP channels despite its longer duration of action. Evans and others in the journal, *Diabetologia*, in 2006 published a retrospective cohort review to evaluate cardiovascular risk of patients on sulfonylureas and metformin [9]. In this analysis, the patients with sulfonylurea monotherapy had a significantly higher risk of cardiovascular mortality than patient's taking metformin, while patients on both drugs were at higher risk than metformin alone, suggesting, as did the UKPDS, a metformin cardioprotective effect. In the ADVANCE study, intensive therapy with sulfonylurea arm did not show an improvement in cardiovascular outcomes – it also did not demonstrate an enhanced mortality with these drugs [4].

METABOLIC EFFECTS OF ORAL AGENTS

DRUG	FPG	PPG	LDL	HDL	TG	hs-CRP
SFU	↓ ↓↓		↔	↔	↔	↔
TZD	↓ ↓	↓	↑	↑	↓↓	↓↓
Metformin	↓ ↓ ↓		↓	↔	↓	↓
AGI		↓ ↓ ↓	↔	↔	↔	
DPP-IV inhib	↓	↓	↔	↑ / ↔	↓ / ↔	
Nateglinide		↓ ↓ ↓	↔	↔	↔	
Repaglinide	↓	↓ ↓ ↓	↔	↔	↔	

Fig. 1. Metabolic effects of oral agents [98]

Metformin was first shown to reduce cardiovascular outcomes in the UKPDS, which demonstrated a 42% reduction for diabetes related deaths and 36% for all cause mortality. Metformin use alone or in combination with a sulfonylurea reduced all cause and cardiovascular mortality compared with sulfonylurea alone in an extensive review of 12,272 new users of these agents published in the journal, *Diabetes Care*, in 2002 [10]. As a result of an increased risk for lactic acidosis, metformin should not be used in patients with heart failure requiring pharmacological therapy and may have pharmacokinetic interactions with cardiovascular medications like furosemide and nifedipine, which can cause an increase in metformin levels, while the drug competes with triamterene, quinidine and digoxin for proximal tubular transport.

Insulin use and its subsequent effects on macrovascular events in patients with type-2 diabetes were evaluated in both the UKPDS and UGDP analyses. The UGDP did not demonstrate an increased risk of cardiovascular events with insulin therapy. In the UKPDS, the intensive therapy insulin arms did not demonstrate any reduction in macrovascular events despite a significant reduction in microvascular outcomes.

However, neither of these two large trials demonstrated a harmful effect of insulin therapy.

The impact of TZDs, rosiglitazone, and pioglitazone, on cardiovascular events were compared in a review by Shaya and others and published in the journal, *Pharmacy and Therapeutics* in September 2009 [11]. This review, using retrospective medical encounter and prescription data analyses in over 14,000 patients with type-2 diabetes, concluded that "rosiglitazone was associated with a significant increase in cardiovascular events among high risk patients with type-2 diabetes, whereas pioglitazone was not." They also recommend further research be done to evaluate this concern. In addition, another large review of 28,361 patients with type-2 diabetes was reported in *The Archives of Internal Medicine* in November 2008 by Winkelmayer et al. [12]. In this large inception cohort of patients 65 years of age or older, 50.3% started treatment with pioglitazone and 49.7% with rosiglitazone with similar baseline characteristics in both groups. Cox regression analysis revealed a 13% increased risk of congestive heart failure and a 15% greater mortality with rosiglitazone compared to pioglitazone, with a 95% confidence interval. There were no differences in stroke or myocardial infarction between the two drugs. The Food and Drug Administration issued a black box warning against use in patients with pre-existing heart failure. In the Prospective Pioglitazone Clinical trial in Macrovascular Events (PROACTIVE) trial, there was no increase in mortality from congestive heart failure in the pioglitazone arm although hospitalization for heart failure was increased by 1.6% [13]. However, a composite reduction in nonfatal myocardial infarction, stroke, and all cause mortality with pioglitazone compared to placebo was also demonstrated as a secondary outcome.

The meta-analysis by Nissen and others in 2007 included 42 trials including 15,560 patients published in *The New England Journal of Medicine* [14]. Although this trial was criticized for combining large trials in which cardiovascular risk was not a primary outcome, its impact has been significant. This meta-analysis indicated that rosiglitazone was associated with a statistically significant increased risk of myocardial infarction. A subsequent follow up meta-analysis by Singh and others in the *Journal of the American Medical Association* (*JAMA*) involving 14,291 patients and including only those trials that were randomized and controlled and used rosiglitazone for 12 months or more were utilized [15]. This large analysis demonstrated that rosiglitazone use was associated with a significantly higher risk of myocardial infarction and heart failure, but not increased cardiovascular mortality. The rosiglitazone evaluated for Cardiovascular Outcomes and Regulation of Glycemia in Diabetes (RECORD) trial enrolled 4,447 patients with type-2 diabetes who were currently taking a sulfonylurea or metformin [16]. These patients could have either rosiglitazone, metformin, or a sulfonylurea randomly assigned as add on therapy (depending on which agent they were taking at the time). There was no increase in myocardial infarctions or death from cardiovascular causes after 3.75 years. In the Veterans Affairs Diabetes Trial (VADT), there was no increased rate of death from any cause after 5.6 years in those patients taking rosiglitazone.

Another meta-analysis, including 19 trials involving pioglitazone that enrolled 16,390 patients by Lincoff et al., published in (JAMA) in 2007, showed a significant 18% decrease in the risk of death, myocardial infarction and stroke, but a higher rate of heart failure than other oral agents [17]. The Pioglitazone Effect on regression of Intravascular Sonographic Coronary Obstructive Prospective Evaluation (PERISCOPE) sought to compare the effects of pioglita-zone to glimepiride to the progression of coronary arteriosclerosis. Five-hundred and forty three patients were enrolled in this 8-month trial [18]. Pioglitazone significantly reduced the progression and the amount of coronary atherosclerosis compared to glimepiride as measured by intravascular ultrasound determinations of atheroma volume. The Carotid Intima Thickness in Atherosclerosis Using Pioglitazone (CHICAGO) trial compared glimepiride to pioglita-zone for progression of carotid intimal thickening (CIMT), a known marker of coronary atherosclerosis and predictor of subsequent cardiovascular events [19]. This trial demonstrated a slowing of the progression of CIMT compared to glimepiride during the study period.

As early as 2003, both the American Diabetes Association (ADA) and the American Heart Association (AHA) issued a consensus statement concerning congestive heart failure and increased fluid retention with the TZDs recommending a multi-step approach prior to initiating therapy including a history and physical examination, electrocardiogram, and providing patient education regarding weight gain, fluid retention, and shortness of breath. An echocardiogram was also added to evaluate for diastolic dysfunction and/or valvular disease along with other risk factors like renal disease, concomitant insulin therapy, age greater than 70 years pre-existing edema. These products should not be used in patients with a New York Heart association Class II or IV, or with an ejection fraction less than 40%. Therapy should always be initiated at the lowest possible dose.

Based on these extensive analyses and in view of the distinct differences in the way the two TZDs handle lipids, it seems prudent to use only pioglitazone for those patients who are candidates for TZD therapy.

The importance of achieving and maintaining glycemic control in type-2 diabetics has been shown to significantly reduce the incidence of microvascular complications like neuropathy, retinopathy and nephropathy, particularly when these levels are maintained less than 7%.

It is important to the clinician to understand that at the time of diagnosis with a fasting glucose greater than 120 mg/dl, at least 50% and as much as 80% of pancreatic beta-cell function has been lost [20]. Hence, even with the best of combination therapies with the oral antidiabetic agents, long term glycemic control is unlikely with persistence in insulin resistance and progressive decline in insulin secretion.

When insulin is added to oral agents, whether it be long acting analogs like detimir and glargine, or twice daily biphasic insulin, or even bedtime administration of neutral pro-tamine hagedorn (NPH) insulin, reductions in hyperglycemia are seen with less weight gain compared to using simply insulin alone.

Microvascular complications were reduced by 12% in the UKPDS with use of either basal/bolus or once daily insulin [21]. In the DIGAMI trial (Diabetes Mellitus Insulin

Glucose Infusion and Acute Myocardial Infarction) study, outpatient subcutaneous insulin therapy preceded by in hospital insulin infusion resulted in 11% reduction in mortality and long-term survival [22]. However, these results were not confirmed by the DIGAMI-II trial, in which glycemic control and all cause mortality were comparable in both the acute insulin glucose infusion group without added insulin, and the acute insulin glucose group.

In addition to maintaining LDL and blood pressure goals, reducing fasting plasma glucose below 110 and 2-h postprandial glucose below 140, reduction in A1C to less than 6.5% meet the goals of therapy for the American Association of Clinical Endocrinologists (AACE) and the American College of Endocrinology (ACE), with the ADA goals being slightly higher (A1C less than 7%; fasting plasma glucose less than 130; and 2-h postprandial glucose less than 180).

Frequent monitoring of blood glucose by the patient can be an important factor to enhance compliance with dietary and exercise requirements in addition to monitoring adherence to the therapeutic regimen. Hypoglycemia can be prevented by avoiding rapid titration in addition to patient education programs instructing patients on acute therapy treatment initiation and symptom recognition. However, hypoglycemic unawareness can occur and sometimes can be associated cryptic symptoms of nightmares, generalized weakness, mental confusion, and unexplained sweating.

In general, oral agent monotherapy is recommended if the hemoglobin A1C is less than 7.0 with combination therapy being necessary for A1Cs greater than 7.0 or patients with significant postprandial excursions independent of the A1C level.

Another interesting offshoot of the UKPDS trial was that 53% of patients using monotherapy with a sulfonylurea required insulin treatment within 6 years to achieve progressive glycemic control. The AACE recommends therapeutic assessments every 2–3 months until glycemic goals are obtained.

LIPID CONTROL

Several primary and secondary prevention trials are of importance.

Primary Prevention

1. The Air Force/Texas Coronary Atherosclerosis Prevention Study (AFCAPS/TexCAPS) – This study randomly assigned patients with average cholesterol levels (221 mg/dl), LDLs (150 mg/dl), and lower than normal HDLs (36 mg/dl for men and 40 mg/dl for women) to lovastatin, 20–40 mg daily, or placebo and followed then for an average of 5.2 years. Hundred and fifty-five of these patients were diabetic. In this study, lovastatin led to a relative risk reduction of 0.56% for any arteriosclerotic event (fatal or non-fatal myocardial infarction, unstable angina, or sudden death) and an absolute risk reduction of 0.04. Despite LDLs at closing of 115 mg/dl and HDLs of 39 mg/dl, the differences in the diabetics were not statistically significant [23].
2. The Antihypertensive and Lipid Lowering Treatment to Prevent Heart Attack Trial-Lipid Lowering Trial (ALLHAT-LLT) randomly assigned patients 55 years of age and older who had hypertension and at least one other risk factor to pravastatin 40 mg daily or placebo. There were 3,638 diabetics in the subgroup analysis. The relative risk reduction was 0.89 for coronary heart disease [24].
3. The Helsinki Heart Study (HHS) randomly assigned men aged 40–55 with elevated non-HDL cholesterol levels to gemfibrozil, 600 mg two times daily or placebo.

The mean total cholesterol was 290 mg/dl and the mean HDL was 47.6 mg/dl. There were 135 patients with diabetes in this study and the incidence of CHD was 3.45% in the gemfibrozil group and 10.5% in the placebo group at 5 years. The relative risk was 0.32 and the absolute risk was 0.07. Neither was statistically significant [25].

4. The landmark Heart Protection Study (HPS) included both primary and secondary prevention data in diabetic patients who were at risk for cardiovascular disease. The objective of this study was to study the effects of a fixed dose of simvastatin across a wide range of lipid abnormalities ranging from those below at and above goal. This study enrolled 3,982 diabetic patients and treatment with simvastatin, 40 mg, led to reduced risk for CHD events of statistical significance with relative risk reductions of 0.74 and absolute risk reductions of 0.05. This provided the first extensive clinical evidence supporting an LDL goal of <100 mg/dl in type-2 diabetics [20].

5. The Prospective Study of Pravastatin in the Elderly at Risk (PROSPER), randomly assigned men and women 70–82 years of age with a history of cerebral or peripheral vascular disease to pravastatin 40 mg daily or placebo. In the primary prevention group, 396 patients had diabetes. In this study, pravastatin led to a trend toward harm with interaction between the diabetes and the treatment group suggesting that patients with diabetes did substantially worse than those without diabetes [26].

6. The Anglo-Scandinavian Cardiac Outcome Trial-Lipid Lowering Arm (ASCOT-LLA) randomly assigned patients aged 40–79 years with CHD, but with hypertension to atorvastatin 10 mg daily. In the diabetes subgroup, 2,532 patients who had hypertension and at least two other risk factors had lower event rates of 3.6% in the control group and 3.0% in the intervention group. The absolute and relative risk reductions were not significant in the diabetes group [27].

The Collaborative Atorvastatin Diabetes Study (CARDS) evaluated 2,838 patients with type-2 diabetes, aged 40–75 years, without high LDL cholesterol, to determine the efficacy of 10 mg of atorvastatin to placebo in the primary prevention of major cardiovascular events [28]. The average duration of follow up was 3.9 years. The primary end point was time to first occurrence of acute coronary events, coronary revascularization, and stroke. Atorvastatin reduced acute coronary heart disease events by 36%, coronary revascularizations by 31%, and rate of stroke by 48%. Treatment with atorvastatin would be expected to prevent at least 37 major vascular events per 1,000 such people treated for 4 years. However, the Atorvastatin Study for Prevention of Coronary Heart Disease Endpoints in Non-Insulin Dependent Diabetes Mellitus (ASPEN) trial evaluated the benefits of ten of atorvastatin in a mixed primary and secondary cardiovascular disease cohort consisting of 2,410 type-2 diabetics in a 4-year double blinded, comparison with placebo. This trial did not find a statistically significant reduction in fatal and non-fatal myocardial infarction, non-fatal stroke, or composite cardiovascular death [29].

Secondary Prevention

1. The landmark Scandinavian Simvastatin Survival Study (4S) randomly assigned patients with coronary disease to simvastatin, 20 mg or placebo. Two hundred and two diabetics were included in a subgroup analysis. This study had the highest event rate of any of the control groups studied indicative of a very high risk population. Statistically significant absolute and relative risk reductions of 0.23 and 0.50, respectively, were seen. Of all the

data, the 4S trial was particularly impressive. The Simvastatin Survival Study represented the first randomized double blinded placebo control mortality study that was empowered to look at the effects of long-term simvastatin therapy, and total mortality and coronary events in patients with a previous MI and/or angina pectoris, and mild to moderate elevations in serum cholesterol [30].

Of all the lipid trials, these patients were at greatest risk of an event when we look at event rates in the placebo group. This involved 4,444 men and women age 35–70 years of age involving 94 clinical centers in five countries. These patients had established history of myocardial infarction and/or angina pectoris. Triglyceride levels were less than 221 mg/dl and total cholesterol ranged from 212 to 309 mg/dl. Treatment with simvastatin significantly improved survival over a median of 5.4 years. The risk of total mortality was reduced by 30%. The risk of coronary mortality was reduced by 42% by the end of the study. This 42% reduction accounted for improvement in overall survival. The risk of major coronary events was reduced by 34% at the end of the study. Major coronary events included coronary death and non-fatal death, myocardial infarction, or resuscitated cardiac arrest.

When we look at the post hoc subgroup analysis in the simvastatin trial, the results are even more remarkable. The post hoc subgroup analysis included 202 diabetic patients at baseline with a mean age of 60 years. Seventy-two percent of these patients were males. In this diabetic group, 12% were treated with insulin, 39% were on oral hyperglycemic drugs, and 50% were on diet therapy alone. Mean baseline glucose levels were 154.9 mg/dl in the placebo group and 154.2 mg/dl in the simvastatin group. Total cholesterol was 259.9 mg/dl in the placebo group, 259.5 mg/dl in the simvastatin group. LDL was 185.6 mg/dl in the placebo group and 186.0 mg/dl in the simvastatin, and triglycerides 157.7 mg/dl in the placebo group and 149.7 mg/dl in the simvastatin group.

Over the course of the trial, reductions in the simvastatin treated diabetic patients were 27% in total cholesterol, 36% in the LDL cholesterol, and improvement of 7% in the HDL, and a decrease of triglycerides of 11%. The major eye opener was the reduction in coronary events. The risk of major coronary heart disease events was significantly reduced by 54% in patients with diabetes with a P-value of 0.002!

There are equally significant reductions for the risk of any coronary heart disease events with a P-value of 0.015 and any atherosclerotic event with a P-value of 0.018. The 6-year probability of escaping a major coronary disease event was 50.7 in the placebo group and 75.1% in the simvastatin group representing a 55% risk reduction in the diabetic cohort.

This was even more impressive than the 32% risk reduction in the non-diabetic cohort. The risk of major coronary heart disease events was significantly reduced in diabetic patients and the risk of any coronary heart disease was also substantially reduced to a statistically significant degree.

The diabetic patients included in the 4S trial tended to have a longer duration of coronary heart disease and higher prevalence of chest pain on exertion than their non-diabetic cohorts.

From the basis of the data from the Simvastatin Survival Study, the potential benefit of simvastatin treatment for 6 years in 100 patients would prevent an expected major coronary heart disease event in 9 out of 29 non-diabetic patients compared to 24 out of 49 diabetic patients, showing a significant benefit in addition to the lipid lowering effects by using this particular agent in the diabetic patient population.

This post hoc subgroup analysis on diabetic patients provided the first trial based evidence that cholesterol lowering significantly and convincingly reduced the risk of major coronary heart disease events and other atherosclerotic events in diabetic patients [31].

The treatment effect did not appear to depend on baseline total cholesterol or LDL cholesterol levels. This data has suggested that the clinical benefit was greater in diabetic patients than non-diabetic patients because of their increased risk.

In addition to this study, an expanded 4S diabetes post hoc subgroup analysis trial was published by Haftner in the journal *Diabetes*, in 1998 [32]. In this study, subjects with known baseline fasting glucoses were evaluated using updated 1997 ADA diagnostic criteria. This added an additional 281 subjects to the diabetic sub-cohort. In addition to the 202 diabetes subjects previously identified, an additional 281 subjects met the ADA criteria having fasting glucoses greater than 126 mg/dl.

Of the remaining individuals, 678 made the criteria for impaired fasting glucose (fasting glucose between 110 and 125 mg/dl) and 3,237 patients still were within normal range. Interestingly, the event rate in the placebo groups was similar to the data obtained in previous cohorts showing that the patients with normal fasting glucoses had a 5-year event rate of approximately 26%. Those with impaired fasting glucose had an event rate of 30%. Those with diabetes with elevated fasting glucoses had an event rate of 32% and those patients who were known to be diabetic had a 5-year event rate of 45%.

Compared to the 335 placebo treated impaired fasting glucose subjects, the 343 simvastatin treated impaired fasting glucose subjects had significantly reduced coronary mortality with a relative risk reduction of 56% and a relative risk reduction of 46% in total mortality, a 40% risk reduction of major coronary events, and a 43% reduction in revascularizations, all of which were statistically significant. The study also demonstrated improved survival with reduced major coronary events and fewer revascularizations in the simvastatin treated 4S patients with impaired fasting glucose. The 251 simvastatin treated diabetic patients had significantly fewer major coronary events and revascularizations compared to placebo with a reduction of coronary events of 42% and revascularizations 47% in the diabetic cohort [33].

In fact, if we look at all the coronary heart disease prevention trials with statins in diabetic patients, including the HPS, data with simvastatin in the 4S trial in terms of coronary heart disease risk reduction demonstrates more robust and statistically significant reductions than seen with any other statin trial to date [34].

2. The Lescol Intervention Prevention Study (LIPS) was conducted in patients who had undergone percutaneous coronary intervention. Patients were randomly assigned to fluvastatin 80 mg daily or placebo. Two hundred and two patients were diabetic and demonstrated an absolute risk reduction of 0.16 with a relative risk reduction of 0.53 in preventing coronary heart disease events [35].

3. The Long Term Intervention with Pravastatin in Ischemic Disease (LIPID) trial randomly assigned patients with known heart disease to pravastatin 40 mg daily or placebo. Seven hundred and eighty-two patients in the subgroup were diabetic. There was a relative risk reduction of 0.84 and absolute risk reduction of 0.04 for cardiovascular events, but neither was significant [36].

4. The PROSPER trial randomly assigned elderly patients (>70 years of age) to pravastatin [37]. The secondary prevention arm involved 227 patients with diabetes. During a

follow-up period of 3 years, pravastatin reduced the composite risk of coronary events, coronary death, and fatal or nonfatal stroke compared to placebo [*38*].

5. The Post Coronary Artery Bypass Graft (Post-CABG) trial randomly assigned patients who had undergone coronary artery bypass grafting to aggressive LDL (60–85 mg/dl) or moderate (130–140 mg/dl) targets. Lovastatin was used and 116 patients had diabetes. Aggressive lowering led to non significant reductions in absolute and relative risks [*39*].

6. The Cholesterol and Recurrent Events (CARE) trial randomly assigned patient with previous myocardial infarction to pravastatin 40 mg daily or placebo. Here, 586 patients were diabetic with an absolute risk reduction of 0.08 and a relative risk reduction of 0.78 [*40*].

7. The HPS looked at the effects of simvastatin in 20,536 patients between the ages of 40 and 80 with coronary artery disease, myocardial infarction in the past, hypertension or diabetes. In this trial, over 8,000 patients were diabetic. No dose adjustments were given and the relative risk reduction was 0.89 for any cardiovascular event with the absolute risk reduction of 0.04, which were statistically significant. These individuals were all given simvastatin 40 mg with no titration. This study demonstrated that this dose safely reduced the risk of heart attack, stroke, and revascularization by approximately one-third, while the number needed to treat for major vascular events was seven in diabetic patients. Another important conclusion from the HPS trial was that reduction rates in major vascular events decreased even below the previously held threshold level of 100 mg/dl of LDL, demonstrating that lower is better for LDL reduction in both the diabetic and non-diabetic patient population [*41*].

8. The Veterans Administration High Density Lipoprotein Cholesterol Intervention Trial (VA-HIT) targeted male patients with the low HDL and low LDL syndrome.

   HDLs were less than 40 mg/dl and the LDLs were less than 140 mg/dl. This enrolled only those with documented coronary disease. In the diabetes subgroup, the relative risk for cardiovascular events was 0.76 and the absolute risk reduction was 0.08. Including patients with undiagnosed diabetes reduced risks further to relative risk of 0.68 and absolute risk reduction of 10% [*42*].

9. Treating to New Targets (TNT) consisted of 10,001 participants of whom 1,500 were diabetics with an LDL<130 mg/dl to evaluate whether intensive lipid lowering therapy would benefit patients with stable coronary artery disease. Patients were randomized to 10 or 80 mg of atorvastatin daily and followed for 4.9 years. For the diabetic participants, atorvastatin 80 mg reduced cardiovascular disease events by an additional 25% compared to ten of atorvastatin while lowering LDL levels 22% more than the 10 mg dose. This trial lent further support to achieving an LDL goal of <70 mg/dl in diabetic patients with known cardiovascular disease [*43*].

   (a) The Fenofibrate Intervention and Event Lowering in diabetes (FIELD) is the largest clinical endpoint trial of fibrate therapy in diabetic patients. This was a 5 year trial of 9,795 well controlled type-2 diabetics with a mean A1C of 6.9%, 78% of whom did not have prior known cardiovascular disease. This trial demonstrated that treatment with fenofibrate 200 mg daily did not significantly reduce the risk of nonfatal myocardial infarction and coronary death. There was a statistically significant reduction of 11% relative risk reduction in total cardiovascular events and slowed the progression of microalbuminuria [*44*]. A post hoc subgroup of those without prior or known cardiovascular disease showed that fenofibrate therapy resulted in statistically significant relative reductions in nonfatal myocardial infarction and coronary death in addition to a small, but statistically significant increase in the incidence of pulmonary embolism of 6 events/10,000 patient-years. This trial also demonstrated a significant 30% relative reduction in the need for first retinal laser therapy, reducing macula and pan-retinal laser treatment with a reduction in progression of diabetic retinopathy from baseline, but not primary prevention of retinopathy [45].

(b) The Diabetes Atherosclerosis Intervention Study (DAIS) enrolled 731 men and women with type-2 diabetes and demonstrated that fenofibrate treatment reduced the angiographic progression of coronary artery disease in type-2 diabetics over a 3-year period of time with pre and post treatment coronary angiograms, with a 6% reduction in LDL, 29% reduction in triglycerides, and 7% increase in HDL [46].

(c) The Coronary Drug Project (CDP) studied lipid lowering drugs in 8,341 men with a previous myocardial infarction from 1966 to 1974. Oral hypoglycemic agents were taken by 5.2% of the study population. Those treated with niacin had a statistically significant 29% reduction in myocardial infarction, a 17% reduction in combined coronary death and myocardial infarction, and a 24% decrease in stroke compared to placebo [47]. In a post hoc analysis, niacin reduced the incidence of 6-year myocardial infarction and 15-year total mortality in patients with and without metabolic syndrome. In 2002, additional analysis according to different levels of baseline and follow-up glucose revealed that niacin's beneficial effect was homogeneous for non-fatal myocardial infarction and all cause mortality across levels of fasting and 1-h glucose, with the most beneficial effect seen in patients who experienced the largest increase in glucose levels during the first year of the study.

(d) The Stop Atherosclerosis in Native Diabetes Study (SANDS) evaluated the effects of aggressive LDL lowering on CIMT in patients with type-2 diabetes. The cohort of 499 American Indian (Pima) men and women 40 years of age and older and were randomized to one of two groups: statins alone or statins plus ezetimibe. Two treatment groups also were present in this trial; the more aggressive treatment arm with an LDL of less than 100 mg/dl and the less aggressive (standard) group at an LDL of less than 130 mg/dl [48].

The non-HDL cholesterol levels were 30 mg/dl higher in each group. This study showed that comparable reductions in LDL and non-HDL cholesterol resulted in similar benefits on carotid intimal media thickness regardless of the therapy used, demonstrating that those patients who lowered non-HDL cholesterol below 70 mg/dl and LDL less than 100 mg/dl had a nearly identical regression in carotid intima media thickness. Also of note was the fact that CIMT increased in those patients who were titrated to a less aggressive goal of less than 100 mg/dl for LDL and less than 130 mg/dl for non-HDL cholesterol.

CIMT serves as an important surrogate marker for increased risk of cardiovascular events (myocardial infarction and stroke) and is frequently increased in prediabetic and diabetic individuals. A long-term follow-up evaluation of the Cholesterol Lowering Atherosclerosis Study (CLAS) showed that for every increase of CIMT by 0.03 mm/year, relative risk for any coronary event was 3.1 and for coronary death 2.2 [49].

CIMT is correlated with systolic blood pressure, LDL cholesterol, and postprandial glucose. Data from the Insulin Resistance Atherosclerosis Study (IRAS) showed that insulin resistance, associated with increased carotid artery intimal medial thickness is a reliable predictor of coronary heart disease [50].

Treatments with the alpha glucosidase inhibitors voglibose and acarbose have independently been shown to reduce CIMT by 0.006 and 0.008 mm/year respectively. Repaglinide treatment reduced CIMT by 0.029 mm/year compared to the sulfonylurea and glyburide, which reduced CIMT by 0.005 mm/year. In addition, repaglinide reduced the postprandial glucose peak compared to glyburide (148 ± 28 vs. 180 ± 32 mg/dl) [51].

The cardinal principal to be understood in reducing mortality in patients with diabetes is the reduction in ischemic and cardiovascular events. Arteriosclerotic complications from diabetes are responsible for 80% of diabetic mortality and 75% of this is due to cardiovascular disease.

Diabetes predisposes the individual to diffuse atherosclerotic cardiovascular disease, increases the severity of atherosclerotic deposition, and enhances the prevalence of multivessel cardiovascular disease making these vessels less amenable to PTCA (percutaneous transluminal coronary angioplasty).

The ongoing Framingham Heart Study shows that the data for diabetic women is even more alarming than men with the relative risk for heart failure, claudication, coronary heart disease, and total cardiovascular disease. Both diabetic men and women are more likely to have a first myocardial infarction and die within the first 5 years of a myocardial infarction than their non-diabetic cohorts [52].

The East/West Study published in the *New England Journal* in 1998 showed that the incidence of myocardial infarction in the diabetic was equal to that for a second MI in a non-diabetic patient [53]. While subsequent MI in the diabetic patient occurred in 45% of the 1,059 diabetic patients studied compared to 19% of the non diabetics over a 7-year period of time, the Minnesota Heart Survey indicated that the risk of death is 40% higher in diabetic individuals who had a myocardial infarction than non-diabetic individuals after 6 years of follow-up and diabetic individuals are more likely to have heart failure with acute myocardial infarction [31].

There are several potential mechanisms of atherogenesis in diabetes including abnormalities in apoprotein and lipoprotein particle distribution, procoagulant state, enhanced insulin resistance and hyperinsulinemia, glycosylation and advance glycation of proteins in the plasma arterial wall, hypertension, hormone growth factor and cytokine enhanced smooth muscle cell proliferation and foam cell formation, local tissue ischemia, and hypoperfusion with enhanced elaboration of angiotensin II and impaired nitric oxide release.

Proteins in the vessel wall like collagen, elastin, and fibrin may be come glycosylated and these glycosylated proteins acquire properties that are quite different from those of nonglycosylated proteins. Diabetes poses a constant oxidative stress at the tissue level with glycated low density lipoprotein more easily oxidized than non glycated low density lipoprotein.

As insulin resistance increases, so does the procoagulant state. Insulin resistance is associated with elevated circulated levels of free fatty acids These elevated free fatty acid levels have an effect on the liver, enhancing triglyceride content of VLDL particles, increasing the circulated levels of apolipoprotein B, and increasing overall VLDL levels.

Triglyceride rich VLDL particles exchange triglyceride for cholesterol with HDL, which leads to enhanced removal of apolipoprotein A-1 by the kidney, allowing the HDL particle to be more susceptible to metabolism and removal. The abnormal VLDL particles effect the composition of LDL because of the exchange of triglyceride for cholesterol.

The net result is the formation of small dense LDL particles and a suppression of the HDL, particularly the HDL-2 fraction. It is the HDL-2 that participates more in reverse cholesterol metabolism. Clearly, the over production of small dense LDL and reduction in HDL enhances arterosclerotic formation resulting in decreased infinity for the LDL receptor, increased vascular permeability, enhances susceptibility of oxidation and conformational changes in the apolipoprotein B, enhancing arteriosclerotic deposition. LDL lowering has been shown to have a beneficial effect on endothelial function in hypercholesterolemic patients with important implications for myocardial ischemia, stroke, and overall cardiovascular wellness [31].

Improvement in endothelial function is critical to managing arteriosclerotic vascular disease as increased degradation of nitric oxide is a key factor in promoting endothelial abnormalities.

Oxidative stress and local tissue injury enhance the production of angiotensin II, which promotes increased catabolism of nitric oxide and vasoconstriction. Angiotensin II mediated generation of free radicals enhances the upregulation of leukocyte adhesion molecules, and chemotaxis in cytokines making the endothelium more likely to be a collection locale for inflammatory cells and macrophages, which degenerate into foam cells with progressive accumulation of LDL.

In order to achieve the multiple lipid goals in the diabetic patient, combination therapy is required for many patients. However, more telling data from randomized clinical trials is needed to evaluate cardiovascular risk reduction. The ratio of triglycerides to high density lipoprotein has been proposed by some as a surrogate marker of not only insulin resistance in patients with metabolic syndrome, but cardiovascular risk. Triglyceride/HDL ratios greater than 2.75 in men and 1.65 in woman are associated with the metabolic syndrome with 80% sensitivity and 78% specificity. In addition, patients with the association of high triglycerides and low HDL are more likely to have an increased amount of apolipoprotein B particles with preponderance of small, dense atherogenic LDL. Clearly, the levels apolipoprotein B and HDL cholesterol are important markers of risk in the type-2 diabetic, while not to be overlooked is the role of non-HDL cholesterol with many authors believing that this parameter has a greater association with arteriosclerotic vascular risk than LDL.

Despite all the benefits of statin therapy, a large potential benefit remains for improved lipid control and reduction in outcomes in these patients with a large residual risk consisting in statin treated patients with diabetes compared to non-diabetics. In primary prevention trials, the cumulative event rate for 4.5 years for major coronary events is 8% in diabetic compared to 6% in non-diabetics. These statistics are even more striking in the secondary prevention trials with the cumulative coronary event rate 27% for diabetics and 17% for non-diabetics [37]. The lipid arm of the ACCORD trial showed that the combination of fenofibrate and simvastatin did not reduce the rate of nonfatal myocardial infarction, nonfatal stroke, or fatal cardiovascular events compared with simvastatin alone in this study of 5,518 patients with type-2 diabetes. Hence this data does not support the routine use of combination therapy with fenofibrate and a statin for the purpose of reducing cardiovascular risk in patients with type-2 diabetes [54].

Hypertension

Hypertension and diabetes mellitus frequently coexist with a prevalence of greater than 50% in those with type-2 diabetes, increasing with advancing age, while hypertension is found in approximately 25% of type-1 diabetics. In type-1 diabetes, hypertension is a complication of diabetic nephropathy while hypertension frequently exists at the time of diagnosis of type-2 diabetes and is associated with the metabolic syndrome. Clearly, however, uncontrolled diabetes enhances the risk of renal damage in either disease. In addition, the presence of renal disease is associated with a dramatic increase in risk of macrovascular disease.

Type-2 diabetes exerts it devastating effects at the cellular level with vascular dysfunction, exhibiting impaired endothelial independent and dependent vasodilatation.

Impaired endothelium dependent vasodilatation results from downstream signaling changes of cyclic guanosine monophosphate in the vascular smooth muscle cells and enhanced production of reactive oxygen species. Other factors involved include decreased production of prostacyclin, decreased bioavailability of nitric oxide, and increased production of thromboxane, endothelin-1, and cyclooxygenase dependent vasoconstrictors. All of these mechanisms are influenced or mediated by hyperinsulinemia, dyslipidemia, hyperglycemia, and the pro-thrombotic state. Increased insulin resistance, associated with endothelial dysfunction and hyperinsulinemia, activates the phosphatidyl inositol kinase pathway, the protein kinase pathway, and tyrosine kinases on the cell surface receptors, which ultimately activate the RAS. Insulin resistant individuals demonstrate sympathetic overactivity and impaired nitric oxide vasodilatation. The hypertension and vascular disease characteristics of type-2 diabetes may be enhanced or even initiated by increased endothelin-1 production mediated by hyperinsulinemia and various pro-inflammatory cytokines like interleukin-8 and interleukin-beta, which are prevalent in the metabolic syndrome.

Blockage of the angiotensin II type I receptor has been shown to improve endothelial function and diminish endothelial adhesiveness. Angiotensin II promotes sodium retention, vasoconstriction, slows progression of glomerular injury at the renal level, induces cardiac and vascular myocyte hypertrophy, fibromuscular proliferation, and endothelial cell apoptosis [55]. Hence, ACE inhibitors and angiotensin receptor blockers (ARBs) are the drugs of choice in hypertensive diabetics to prevent cardiovascular events.

With this in mind, the concept of therapy with ACE inhibitors and ARBs to lower blood pressure, reduce proteinuria, and reduce overall risk including congestive heart failure has received considerable attention, since these drugs target the angiotensin II mediated abnormalities associated with enhanced cardiovascular disease. Renin-angiotensin system (RAS) blockade promotes the recruitment and differentiation of pre-adipocytes and subsequent increased formation of insulin sensitive adipocytes that inhibit lipid deposition, while also having beneficial effects on endothelial function, inflammation, and oxidative stress, attenuating endothelial dysfunction induced by hyperglycemia.

Valsartan has been shown to improve flow mediated vasodilatation and inhibit the release of tumor necrosis alpha and interleukin-6 from leukocytes in a milieu of hyperglycemia, while cardiovascular oxidative stress in rodents with diabetes has been reduced by lisinopril. ACE inhibitor therapy has also been shown to reduce cardiomyocyte loss and hypertrophy and perivascular fibrosis often seen with diabetes. RAS blockade with losartan or perindopril prevented fatty acid induced endothelial dysfunction.

Based on their different mechanisms of action, ACEs and ARBs can have synergistic effects. ACE inhibitors block the conversion of angiotensin I to angiotensin II, but also inhibit the breakdown of vasodilatory bradykinin. This increase in bradykinin promotes the release of nitric oxide. The ARBs block the binding of angiotensin II to its receptor site [56].

Although not proven in clinical trials, prolonged treatment with ACE inhibitors can cause angiotensin II escape, enhancing angiotensin II production via the alternative pathways using enzymes such as tissue plasminogen activator, chymase, and cathepsin G. Blockage of the binding of angiotensin II to its receptor site by the ARBs prevents the detrimental actions of this substance, including accelerated atherogenesis, smooth muscle proliferation, myocardial hypertrophy, and vasoconstriction.

The therapeutic combination of an agent that decreases production of angiotensin II, inhibits breakdown of bradykinin, and prevents binding of angiotensin II to its receptor site can offer significant advantages. Combination of both types of agents has been investigated in a number of clinical trials in myocardial infarction, hypertension, heart failure, and renoprotection.

Two of the largest clinical trials in patients with hypertension involved adding losartan to enalapril and valsartan to benazepril. A pilot study by Azizi et al. of 177 hypertensive patients off medication for 7 days prior to therapy and studied for 6 weeks showed no significant effect on blood pressure compared to monotherapy. A 10-week trial by Stergiou evaluated 20 patients and showed reductions in both systolic and diastolic blood pressure in the combination group compared to monotherapy [57].

These trials involved a small number of patients, were of short duration, and had no other concomitant combination comparisons. Hence, the data need further evaluation before any conclusions can be derived with regard to hypertension.

The efficacy of ACE inhibitors and ARBs in reducing cardiovascular events and the development of type-2 diabetes has been evaluated in several clinical trials.

The Heart Outcomes Prevention Evaluation (HOPE) demonstrated that ten ramipril treatment for 4.5 years significantly reduced the risk stroke, myocardial infarction, and overall cardiovascular mortality and morbidity in individuals 55 years of age and older in high risk patients and those with diabetes [58]. A 2.6-year extension of the HOPE trial, HOPE-The Ongoing Outcomes (HOPE-TOO) showed that these cardiovascular benefits were maintained [59]. Overall, combining these two trials, patients were evaluated over a 7.2-year period of time and demonstrated that ramipril treated patients had an absolute risk reduction of 3.6% (24.2–20.6%) and a relative risk reduction of 14.9% in the combined occurrence of stroke, myocardial infarction, and cardiovascular death compared to placebo ($P=0.0002$). In addition, there was a statistically significant relative risk reduction of 31% in the development of new onset diabetes in patients taking ramipril compared to placebo ($P=0.0006$).

The Captopril Prevention Project (CAPPP) had a cohort of over 10,000 individuals to evaluate the effectiveness of this ACE inhibitor in reducing cardiovascular mortality and morbidity. In this study, there was a reduction of 50% in fatal cardiovascular events in those treated with captopril compared to conventional therapy (diuretics and beta blockers) [60]. A sub-analysis revealed that hypertensive diabetics in this study experienced a 66% lower rate of fatal and nonfatal myocardial infarction compared to conventional therapy.

A meta-analysis published in the *American Journal of Cardiology* by Andraws and Brown included 13 prospective randomized placebo or active controlled trials involving

93,451 patients taking ACE inhibitor or ARB therapy and reported a 26% risk reduction in new onset diabetes with a 27% reduction in developing diabetes with those individuals who were hypertensive [61]. Another pooled analysis by McCall, Craddock and Edwards covering over 23,000 patients with hypertension also demonstrated a decreased relative risk of new onset diabetes [45].

The Reduction of Endpoints in Noninsulin-dependent Diabetes Mellitus with the Angiotensin-II Antagonist Losartan (RENAAL) trial evaluated the benefits of losartan in 1,513 patients with diabetic nephropathy [62]. This trial demonstrated that losartan treatment resulted in a 16% reduction in the risk of end-stage renal disease, doubling of serum creatinine concentration or death independent of blood pressure control, while reducing the risk of proteinuria by 35% ($P<0.001$) and end-stage renal disease by 28%. Scheen reported a meta-analysis of ten randomized clinical trials revealing a 22% relative risk reduction of new onset diabetes with ARB or ACE therapy with a similar risk reduction in those with hypertension (22%).

The effect of dual therapy with an ACE and an ARB, although of questionable benefit for enhanced blood pressure lowering does produce benefits at the cellular level in reducing left ventricular mass, transforming growth factor beta, and improving diastolic dysfunction independent of blood pressure control.

Increased urinary albumin excretion is associated with an increased risk for cardiovascular events and nephropathy in both diabetic and non-diabetic patients. Rossing and others in the journal *Diabetes Care* evaluated the renoprotective effects of combining an ACE inhibitor (enalapril, captopril, or lisinopril) with an ARB (candesartan) in patients with diabetic nephropathy [63]. In this small analysis of 20 patients, dual RAS blockade resulted in a 28% reduction in albuminuria compared with ACE inhibitor monotherapy independent of blood pressure control.

The Candesartan and Lisinopril Microalbuminuria Study (CALM) evaluated 199 patients with type-2 diabetes. Mean reductions in urinary albumin and diastolic blood pressure was greater in the combination group than with either therapy alone after 24 weeks.

The Ongoing Telmisartan Alone and in Combination with Ramipril Global Endpoint Trial (ON-TARGET) analyzed the cardioprotective benefits of ramipril, telmisartan, or both in 25,600 ethnically diverse patients aged 55 years or older at high risk for cardiovascular disease [64]. At a median follow-up of 56 months, outcomes were essentially the same for ramipril and telmisartan. Thus, in a patient population similar to the HOPE trial, telmisartan demonstrated non inferiority. Another arm of this trial revealed that combination therapy was equivalent to monotherapy with ramipril for the primary outcomes of cardiovascular mortality, stroke, acute myocardial infarction, and hospitalization for heart failure, despite reduction in systolic blood pressure of 2–3 mmHg with the combination treatment. This trial was the first to establish that telmisartan was equally effective as the ACE inhibitor, ramipril for cardiovascular risk reduction in this high risk patient population.

Data from the Prevention of Events With Angiotensin Converting Enzyme Inhibition (PEACE) trial demonstrated that fewer patients in the trandalopril group developed diabetes compared to placebo, while the Losartan Intervention For Endpoint Reduction in Hypertension (LIFE) trial, showed that less patients with left ventricular hypertrophy developed diabetes if they received this ARB than those treated with atenolol.

The Australian National Blood Pressure (ANBP-2) trial showed a 33% reduction in the new onset of diabetes in the enalapril treated group compared to those with hydrochlorthiazide [65].

The North of Sweden Efficacy Evaluation (ALPINE) study demonstrated that antihypertensive therapy based on even a low dose of hydrochlorthiazide was associated with a worsening of glucose tolerance, while new onset of diabetes was reduced by 87% if candesartan combined with an angiotensin receptor blocker was compared with a group treated with atenolol and hydrochlorthiazide [66].

The Candesartan in Heart Failure Assessment of Reduction in Mortality and Morbidity (CHARM) study, few patients develop new onset diabetes compared to the placebo group, while a 40% reduction in the incidence of new diabetes when an ACE inhibitor was added to candesartan compared to placebo in the CHARM-ADDED trial [67].

The Valsartan Antihypertensive Long term Use Evaluation (VALUE) trial also demonstrated a 23% lower incidence of new onset diabetes in patients treated with valsartan compared to amlodipine [68].

The Nateglinide and Valsartan in Impaired Glucose Tolerance Outcomes Research (NAVIGATOR) study represents one of the largest trials to evaluate the effect of interventions to prevent cardiovascular disease and diabetes [69]. Nine thousand and ninety-two had undiagnosed type-2 diabetes, while 11,853 had unrecognized impaired glucose tolerance in over 43,000 cohorts. In this huge trial, valsartan reduced the progression to diabetes in individuals with impaired glucose tolerance and cardiovascular disease, but did not reduce cardiovascular events. Patients were followed for a mean of 5 years for the development of diabetes and 6.5 years for cardiovascular disease. The cumulative incidence of diabetes was 36.8% in the placebo group compared to 335 in the valsartan group. This trial provides compelling evidence of the effects of RAS system blockade and the subsequent development of type-2 diabetes. This trial also demonstrated that, among individuals with impaired glucose tolerance and cardiovascular risk factors or known cardiovascular disease, treatment with nateglinide did not reduce cardiovascular outcomes or the incidence of diabetes.

The Telmisartan Randomized Assessment Study in ACE Intolerant Subjects, (TRANSCEND) study, in which 35.7% of the 5,926 patients were diabetic, was designed to replicate the HOPE trial in high risk patients intolerant of ACE inhibitors [70]. TRANSCEND demonstrated a reduction of 13% compared to placebo for the risk of myocardial infarction, stroke, and overall cardiovascular mortality and morbidity, but no change in heart failure event rates or renal benefits.

The first cardiovascular outcome trial to prepare the use of two different fixed dose antihypertensive regimens, benazepril plus amlodipine vs. benazepril plus hydrochlorothiazide on cardiovascular endpoints in patients with high cardiovascular risk along with the presence of diabetes was the ACCOMPLISH (Avoiding Cardiovascular Events through Combination therapy in Patients Living with Systolic Hypertension) trial. About 11,506 patients, 60.4% of whom had diabetes, were randomized in a double blinded trial [71]. The benazepril–amlodipine combination was superior to the benazepril-hydrochlorthiazide combination in reducing cardiovascular events despite similar blood pressure reductions. Diabetic patients in this trial were more likely to have metabolic syndrome with higher levels of fasting glucose and lower levels of HDL compared to the non-diabetic cohorts. The incidence of previous myocardial infarctions and stroke was also higher in diabetic subset. In this trial, 42.8% of diabetic patients had blood pressure levels of <130/80 following 36 months of treatment and 75% of all patients attained blood pressures <140/90 mmHg. At the time of enrollment, 97.2% of patients were already being treated for hypertension with 74.7% taking two or more classes of anti-hypertensives, although only 37.5% had baseline blood pressures less than 140/90 mmHg with untreated hypertensives having systolic pressures equal to or >160/90 mmHg. In addition, the high rate of blood pressure control in both groups gives added credence to the Joint National Committee on Prevention, Detection, Evaluation and Treatment of High Blood Pressure (JNC7) recommendation of initiating combination therapy in patients with stage II hypertension with blood pressure levels equal to or greater than 20/10 mmHg above the desired goal.

Aliskiren (TEKTURNA) has been demonstrated to have renal protective effects in hypertensive type-2 diabetics with nephropathy concomitantly being treated with an angiotensive receptor blocker. In a study of 1,892 eligible patients, 805 were randomized into a 3-month open label trial [72]. Treatment was then initiated with losartan 100 mg daily along with other anti-hypertensive medications to achieve an optimal blood pressure of less than 130/80. Six hundred patients were then randomized, equally divided between losartan alone and losartan plus aliskiren 150 mg daily with the primary outcome being reduction in albumin to creatinine ratio.

By the end of the study period, the aliskiren group exhibited a 20% statistically significant reduction (P value less than 0.001) in their mean urinary albumin to creatinine ratio compared to placebo. In addition, a reduction in albuminuria of greater than 50% was seen in 24% of the aliskiren group compared to only 12.5% of the placebo group. The difference is systolic blood pressure was 2 mmHg and the diastolic was 1 mmHg in the aliskiren group. However, this difference was not statistically significant.

This data provides encouraging information to suggest that duel therapy to block the renin-angiotensin-aldosterone system with both a renin inhibitor and ARB may demonstrate additive or even synergistic effects.

Combination of an ACE inhibitor and an ARB in myocardial infarction was evaluated in the VALIANT trial [73]. Here, a valsartan and captopril combination was compared to either treatment alone in patients with myocardial infarction complicated by systolic dysfunction. Combination therapy did not improve survival compared to monotherapy.

The evidence in heart failure is more impressive. Three trials, the Valsartan Heart Failure Trial (Val-HeFT), CHARM, and the Randomized Evaluation of Strategies for Left Ventricular Dysfunction (RESOLVD) trial evaluated combination ACE/ARB combinations.

The Val-HeFT trial evaluated the addition of valsartan to Class II cardiac patients receiving beta blockers, ACE inhibitors, or diuretics [74]. Valsartan added to ACE inhibitor and beta blocker therapy seem to trend toward worsening outcomes with no benefits in blood pressure reduction. The combination of ACE and ARB, ACE and beta blocker, and ARB and beta blocker did show a benefit, however, with reduction in hospitalization for heart failure and reductions in all cause mortality and morbidity.

The CHARM added trial, similarly structured to the Val-HeFT trial evaluated patients in Class II–III. Here, the triple combination of ACE, ARB, and beta blocker did show a benefit in systolic dysfunction, but not diastolic dysfunction with reduced cardiovascular death and hospital admissions for worsening CHF [57].

The Randomized Evaluation of Strategies for Left Ventricular Dysfunction (RESOLVD) pilot study looked at enalapril and candesartan alone and in combination in Class II–III cardiac patients. Here, combination therapy resulted in a decrease in brain natriuretic peptide and blood pressure with no significant differences in hospitalizations for congestive heart failure, quality of life, or exercise tolerance. High doses of the ACE and ARB resulted in better outcomes [75].

Combination therapy and its renoprotective effects in diabetics have been evaluated in several studies. Rossing showed that adding an ACE to an ARB resulted in an average of 5–10 mmHg reduction, a 25% reduction in albuminuria, and a slight increase in glomerular filtration rate, although other studies have not demonstrated any beneficial effects in proteinuria reduction or reduction in blood pressure with combination therapy [76].

Although these clinical trials suggest that some short term advantages exist with combination therapy, (reduced proteinuria and blood pressure) the effects on long-term morbidity and mortality remain to be demonstrated. Certainly more complete inhibition of the RAS provides some theoretical benefits with demonstrated improvement in heart failure and the diabetic hypertensive patient.

The blood pressure arm of ACCORD evaluated the safety of lowering cardiovascular risk in diabetic patients since this risk is graded and continuous across the entire range of systolic blood pressure [77]. Although current JNC7 recommendations indicate a systolic blood pressure goal of 130 mmHg, minimal evidence from randomized controlled trials actually support these recommendations. In this trial, intensive therapy targeted a systolic blood pressure of less than 120 mmHg, while standard therapy targeted a systolic blood pressure of 140 mmHg. The researchers found that despite achieving systolic blood pressure of less than 119.3 mmHg in the intensive therapy group and 133.5 in the standard therapy group, there were no significant differences in primary endpoints of nonfatal myocardial infarction, nonfatal stroke, or death from cardiovascular causes.

The International Verapamil SR/Trandolapril (INVEST) study assigned 6,400 patients (27% of whom were diabetic) who had known coronary artery disease to blood pressure therapy based on either a calcium channel blocker or a beta-blocker plus an ACE inhibitor and/or thiazide diuretic [78]. Those with systolic blood pressure >140 mmHg were listed as "uncontrolled" while those lower than 130 mmHg were listed as "tight control." Those that were in between received a classification of "usual control." After a mean of 2.7 years, the uncontrolled group has a combined risk of myocardial infarction, death, and stroke 50% higher than the usual control group and the tight control group. All cause death, however, was increased in the tight control group. So that while tighter blood pressure control seems to benefit younger patients with diabetes and no known cardiovascular disease, it may not be as beneficial in high risk patients with moderate to advanced cardiovascular disease.

Clearly when and if combination therapy is used, careful monitoring of blood pressure, renal function, and serum potassium are critical.

THROMBOSIS PREVENTION

An important concept in enhanced diabetic risk is the production of advanced glycation end products. These are found in the vessel wall of diabetic patients, which have demonstrated a strong association with diabetic complications. When lipoproteins become glycosylated, the glycation matrix within the lining of the vessel wall changes the behavior of arterial smooth muscle cells, macrophages, and endothelial cells.

In a study in *Diabetes Care*, serum advanced glycation end product levels were significantly elevated by 76% in patients with Type-2 diabetes. Plaque rupture and clot formation over the plaque is the terminal event just prior to MI with 68% of myocardial infarctions occurring with less than 50% occlusion of the vessels [79].

With rupture of a plaque, clot forms and it is the clot that completely occludes the lumen which leads to myocardial infarctions. Diabetic patients are more likely to have vascular plaque because of the glycosylation of matrix proteins or because of abnormalities of matrix protein due to their exposure to these glycosylated proteins.

As the result of their procoagulant state, diabetic patients are more prone to forming adhesive clots. Vulnerable plaques have large lipid cores within fibrous caps and microphage enrichment especially at the periphery of the lesion. The macrophages secrete enzymes that degrade the fibrous cap allowing rupture. The cytokines and the activated smooth muscle cells that characterize vascular plaque tend to be increased in diabetic patients. This underscores the importance of aspirin therapy in the Type-2 diabetic [79].

Since diabetes is considered a coronary risk equivalent establishing the same risk of death as established coronary disease, diabetic patients should receive at least 81 mg of aspirin on a daily basis. Recent data has supported increasing this to 325 mg based on inherent aspirin resistance in some patients [80].

This therapy has been shown to be safe in diabetics, does not promote the progression of ophthalmic disease, and ophthalmologic studies have not demonstrated any association between aspirin use and worsening of retinopathy. In fact, some studies have shown a benefit of aspirin reducing the rate of microaneurysms in the early stages of diabetic retinopathy.

There also has not been demonstrated any increased risk of vitreous hemorrhage in proliferative diabetic retinopathy patients. In the Early Treatment of Diabetic Retinopathy Study (ETDRS) there was a 17% reduction in cardiovascular mortality and morbidity in diabetic patients taking aspirin, hence even though aspirin did not alter the course of diabetic retinopathy long-term, it did not have any detrimental effect on existing disease [1].

Aspirin rapidly and irreversibly inhibits synthesis of thromboxane, which is a potent vasoconstrictor and platelet aggregant. A 325 mg dose of aspirin every other day reduced the risk of myocardial infarction in diabetics in the U.S. Physician's Health Study.

In the Hypertension Optimal Treatment trial, 75 mg of aspirin daily reduced the risk of myocardial infarction by 36% and diminished overall cardiovascular risk by 15% in 4 years in older diabetic patients [81].

Meta-analyses have shown that aspirin reduces cardiovascular events by 25% in diabetic patients who have had a myocardial infarction or stroke [82]. Table 4 summarized the role of aspirin therapy in the type-2 diabetic.

Table 4
Aspirin therapy in diabetes

Indicated for primary prevention in type-2 diabetes

Indicated for secondary prevention in those with established macrovascular disease

Dose ranges 81–325 mg

Clopidogrel can be used for aspirin allergic patients

From U.S. Preventive Task Force [87]

Clopidogrel, 75 mg daily, was as effective as 325 mg of aspirin daily to reduce the risk of ischemic stroke, vascular death, or myocardial infarction in the CAPRIE trial (Clopidogrel vs. Aspirin in Patients at Risk of Ischemic Events). A sub-group analysis of the diabetics in this trial revealed an annual combined vascular event rate of 17.7% for aspirin and 15.6% for clopidogrel [83].

At the present time, prophylactic use of anticoagulants or fibrinolytics in type-2 diabetics is not supported in the literature with low dose warfarin failing to benefit diabetic patients in the Post Coronary Artery Bypass Graft Trial [84].

Aspirin is currently indicated for the reduction of the combined risk of death in non-fatal MIs in patients with a previous infarct, unstable angina, diabetes; reduction of the combined risk of sudden death and myocardial infarction in patients with chronic stable angina; and reduction of vascular death in patients with suspected acute myocardial infarction. It is also indicated for the reduction of death and stroke in patients who have had an ischemic stroke or transient ischemia of the brain due to fibrin platelet emboli.

There is an ongoing debate as to the appropriate dose of aspirin for prevention of cardiovascular events in the type-2 diabetic. Aspirin is indicated for diabetic individuals 40 years of age and older to attenuate vasoconstriction and inhibit platelet aggregation with current recommendation ranging from 81 to 325 mg. Ogawa and others reporting for the Japanese Primary Prevention of Atherosclerosis With Aspirin for Diabetes (JPAD) trial investigators in the *Journal of the American Medical Association* (*JAMA*) found that low dose aspirin (81–100 mg daily) did not reduce the risk of cardiovascular events [85]. Various meta-analyses have looked at this issue and found little benefit above 325 mg and an additional risk of gastrointestinal bleeding. Aspirin can inhibit cyclo-oxygenase in doses as low as 20 mg daily.

The inhibition of platelet aggregation by aspirin may be reduced with elevated A1C and low HDL levels as is seen in diabetics. A different dosage may be indicated due to increased platelet turnover, accelerated atherosclerosis, and higher fibrinogen levels The Antithrombotic Trialists Collaboration carried out a meta-analyses of 195 randomized trials (144,051 cohorts) involving anti-platelet agents, of which 65 involved only aspirin [86]. This study showed a tendency towards increased risk reduction for vascular events in the low dose range (75–150 mg) compared to the intermediate (160–325 mg) and high dose ranges (500–1,500 mg). In 2006, the American Heart Association and the ADA recommended 75–162 mg daily for primary prevention of heart disease for diabetic patients greater than 40 years of age or possessing additional risk factors for cardiovascular disease who have no contraindications for its use. The American Heart Association recommends using aspirin for cardiovascular protection in those individuals with a 10-year risk for cardiovascular events from 6 to 10%. As with any treatment modality, benefits must outweigh the risks of bleeding with aspirin. Based on these recommendations the U.S. Preventive Services Task Force (USPSTF) issued the following recommendations published in the March edition of the *Annals of Internal Medicine* [87]:

1. Men aged 45–79 years should use aspirin to reduce the risk of myocardial infarction provided that the risks of gastrointestinal bleeding are not prohibitive.
2. Women aged 55–79 years should use aspirin for ischemic stroke prevention if the benefits outweigh the risks of gastrointestinal hemorrhage.
3. Current level of evidence is not sufficient to recommend aspirin for cardiovascular prevention in individuals greater than 80 years of age.

The Task Force also did not recommend routine use of aspirin in non diabetic individuals under the age of 45 (men) and 55 (women).

The Clopidogrel for High Atherothrombotic risk and Ischemic Stabilization, Management and Avoidance (CHARISMA) trial sought to determine whether a clinical benefit could be determined for adding clopidogrel to patients already receiving low dose aspirin [88]. This study randomized 15,603 patients with an average age of 64 (30% female). Seventy-eight percent had documented cardiovascular disease and approximately 16% were either type-1 or type-2 diabetics who represented 80% of a "multiple risk factors only" arm. The overall data and even the subgroup analysis of those in the multiple risk factors revealed no benefit of adding clopidogrel, but a significant increase in gastrointestinal bleeding.

The Management of Atherothrombosis with Clopidogrel in High Risk Patients with Recent Transient Ischemic Attacks or Ischemic Stroke (MATCH) trial sought to determine the combined effects of aspirin and clopidogrel on reduction of second stroke in 7,599 individuals. Inclusion criteria were those with a transient ischemic episode or stroke within 3 months of randomization [89]. Seventy percent of the cohorts in this trial were diabetics. MATCH did not demonstrate any clinical benefit in adding clopidogrel to aspirin in a population with lacunar stroke or diabetic microangiopathy, but an increased risk of major bleeding. Although there has been some debate about the design of the trial with high risk patients, caution was advised against using this combination in diabetic patients.

The Prevention Regimen for Effectively Avoiding Second Strokes (PRoFESS) trial compared aspirin/dipyridamole ER (ERDP) with clopidogrel for secondary stroke prevention in those with noncardiometabolic ischemic stroke [90]. This study, involving 20,333 (28% diabetics) showed no difference in the two arms to prevent recurrent stroke, myocardial infarction, or death. Interestingly, in the diabetic subset on post hoc analysis, hazard ratios favored aspirin/ERDP over clopidogrel.

For diabetic patients with stenting for cardiovascular disease, a 2-year study by Lasala and others reviewed 7,492 patients receiving paclitaxel (TAXUS) Express stents (2,112 with medically treated diabetes). This report revealed that the paclitaxel eluting stents decreased the risk of restenosis in diabetic patients with a low risk of myocardial infarction compared to bare metal stents. Paclitaxel has been shown to inhibit smooth muscle cell proliferation and migration even in hyperglycemic and insulin resistant individuals [91].

MULTIPLE RISK FACTOR REDUCTION

Control of blood pressure plays a critical role in preventing the macro and microvascular complications of diabetes and a major contributor to excess mortality and morbidity due to end stage renal disease, stroke, and cardiovascular catastrophe.

The Hypertensive Optimal Treatment (HOT) trial evaluated the effect of calcium channel blockers in 18,790 hypertensive patients (8% of who were diabetic). Overall the results were that intensive blood pressure control randomized to the goal less than 80 mmHg did much better than those randomized to less than 90 mmHg. The study demonstrated significant improvements in major cardiovascular events for the diabetes subgroup with reduction of major cardiovascular events of 24.4% in the group with diastolic blood pressures less than 90 mmHg to 11.9 major cardiovascular events in the group with diastolic blood pressures equal to or less than 80 mmHg.

This represented the first significant trial that showed that lowering of diastolic blood pressure was statistically significant in a diabetic subcohort with prevention of 1.5 myocardial infarctions per 1,000 patients treated for 1 year and 2.5 myocardial infarctions per 1,000 patient years in diabetics when blood pressure were reduced to a mean of 82.6 mmHg.

The *New England Journal of Medicine* in 1998 published the results of the Appropriate Blood Pressure Control study (ABCD). This was designed to compare moderate blood pressure control with a target diastolic of 88–90 mmHg to more aggressive blood pressure control with a target diastolic blood pressure of 75 mmHg. The agents used in this study were dihydropyridine, nisoldipine, compared to the ACE inhibitor enalapril [92].

In this study, enalapril resulted in a statistically significant reduction of myocardial infarction and cardiovascular mortality compared to nisoldipine. The nisoldipine treated group experienced 25 myocardial infarctions compared to five in the enalapril group, where overall vascular mortality was 50% less in the ACE inhibitor group.

In a study of isolated systolic hypertension in Europe (SYST-EUR) investigators prospectively evaluated the effects of antihypertensive therapy in 492 patients with type 2-diabetes and isolated systolic hypertension. Risk reduction in the cardiovascular end points ranged from 55 to 76% in the diabetic cohort and no increased risk of major cardiovascular events was seen in the diabetic group compared with the non diabetics.

The UKPDS blood pressure subset showed that a difference of 10/5 mmHg (144/82 vs. 154/87 mmHg) was associated with statistically significant reductions in risk of 24% in combined microvascular and 32% in diabetes related deaths as well as 44% reduction in stroke. There was no difference according to the class of medication used [92].

A meta-analysis of four major clinical trials in patients with type-2 diabetes randomized to an ACE inhibitor or an alternative drug showed similar superior performances for the ACE inhibitor. The relative risk reduction in the ABCD trial was 0.43% of the ACE inhibitor compared to the dihydropyridine.

The Captopril Prevention Project trial (CAPPP), captopril vs. the combination of a diuretic beta-blocker resulted in a relative risk reduction of 0.59 for cardiovascular events for the ACE inhibitor captopril.

In the FACET trial (Fosinopril vs. Amlodipine Cardiovascular Events Trial), risk reduction was 0.49% for the ACE group. In the UKPDS comparing captopril vs. the beta-blocker atenolol, the risk reduction was more robust at 1.29%. Meta-analysis of the ABCD, CAPPP, and FACET trials showed reduction of 0.49% in cardiovascular events for the ACE inhibitor compared to all other agents used. This further broke down into 63% reduction in myocardial infarction with a *P*-value of less than 0.001, a 51% reduction in cardiovascular events with a *P*-value less than 0.001, and a 62% reduction in all cause mortality with a *P*-value of 0.01 [93].

The HOPE trial, which was a non-hypertensive trial, showed the superiority of the ACE inhibitor ramipril at 10 mg, with statistically significant reductions in myocardial infarctions, stroke, and overall cardiovascular mortality and morbidity independent of blood pressure effect and medications that were concomitantly used including aspirin, statins, and other anti-hypertensive drugs. This data was especially impressive in the diabetic subgroup with 22% reductions in combined cardiovascular events that were statistically significant. In addition, the HOPE trial demonstrated a 24% reduction in total mortality, a 24% reduction in overt nephropathy, and a 17% reduction in revascularization all of which were statistically significant. Curiously, these benefits were not seen when a smaller trial looked at the 5 mg dose of ramipril for risk reduction in a similar patient population.

The benefit of beta-blockers in diabetic patients post myocardial infarction was evaluated in the *European Heart Journal* in 1990, which included a large multi-centered cohort of 2,024 patients including 340 diabetics. In this study, beta-blocker use was an independent predictor of 1-year cardiac survival following hospital discharge for all diabetics. In this study, the 1-year survival was decreased with no beta-blockers compared to the diabetics who had taken beta-blockers [65].

According to JNC-7, beta-1 selective agents are beneficial as part of multi-drug therapy in diabetics being especially helpful in hypertensive diabetics with ischemic heart disease, with recurrent myocardial infarction being significantly reduced in the beta-blocker treated population. In the Metoprolol CR/XL Randomized Intervention Trial in congestive Heart Failure (MERIT-HF) diabetic sub-population, death plus hospitalization due to heart failure was reduced by 29% in the first year with less hypoglycemia than the non selective beta blockers.

Exciting recent developments have highlighted the importance of the peroxisomal proliferators activated receptors (PPARs), especially the TZDs, in risk reduction. Fibrates are ligands for PPAR-alpha, while the TZDs are ligands for PPAR-gamma. A critical aspect of the atherosclerotic process is the central role of inflammation.

Adhesion molecules like the vascular cell adhesion molecule-1 (VCAM-1), which contributes to the entry of inflammatory cells into the arterial wall, while the ATP-binding cassette A-1 (ABCA-1) helps the efflux of cholesterol out of the endothelium and limits cholesterol accumulation.

Cytokines, like tumor necrosis alpha and interferon gamma, are released by inflammatory cells in atherosclerotic plaque, while matrix degrading enzymes and metalloproteinases can weaken the fibrous cap precipitating plaque rupture.

Animal models of atherosclerosis have demonstrated that the TZDs can inhibit macrophage accumulation reducing atherosclerosis, while improving lipid profiles and reducing the levels of various inflammatory markers.

Activation of the PPAR system is associated with various pleiotropic benefits especially in those individuals with diabetes and metabolic syndrome. TZD activation of PPAR-gamma reduces high sensitivity C-reactive protein (hs-CRP), decreases inflammation, and increases adiponectin levels, inhibiting atherosclerosis, and preventing restenosis.

The positive influence of this class on lipid subfractions and reduction in hyperplasia in the vascular intima supports their potential for cardiovascular benefit. Once a patient has been deemed a candidate for TZD therapy, pioglitazone is the drug of choice based on the current data and the less favorable lipid and cardiovascular profile of rosiglitazone.

According to new practice guidelines released by the American College of Physicians, lipid lowering therapy should be used for prevention of cardiovascular mortality and morbidity in all patients with type-2 diabetes and known coronary disease and to prevent macrovascular disease and its complications for primary prevention in diabetic men and women, regardless of their cholesterol level [94].

The HPS involved almost 6,000 patients with diabetes, while almost 2,000 of these diabetic patients also had known coronary disease. Significant benefit was derived by simvastatin therapy at any level of LDL. The diabetics without known coronary disease, had a lower amount of risk reduction, but still received significant benefit.

Physicians should not delay in starting treatment with statins in the diabetic patient and can consider use of fibrate therapy for patients with low LDL cholesterols and low HDL levels without being on statins. Meta-analyses have shown that statin use reduces major cardiovascular events by 22–24% in diabetics with similar relative risk reductions in primary and secondary prevention, but doubles the absolute risk reduction for those with known coronary heart disease.

For the primary prevention trials reviewed, the number needed to treat to prevent one cardiovascular event over an average of 4.3 years was 34.5, and 13.8 for 4.9 years in a secondary prevention situation.

In the UKPDS trial, the stratification priorities for coronary heart disease risk reduction were:

1. LDL
2. HDL
3. Hemoglobin A1C
4. Systolic blood pressure
5. Smoking

Patients with diabetes are at increased risk for all forms of ischemic stroke, but interestingly no high quality evidence supports stroke risk reduction with improved glycemic control. Major randomized clinical trials have demonstrated no significant reduction in the risk of ischemic stroke or any macrovascular outcome when glucose control alone was evaluated. Multifactorial risk reduction strategies are important for stroke reduction for all patients, especially the diabetic subset [1].

This involves:

1. Therapuetic lifestyle changes – especially smoking cessation, avoidance of excessive alcohol, and regular exercise
2. Hypertensive control – effective control of systolic and diastolic blood pressure will reduce stroke risk
3. Lipid lowering therapy – treatment with statins has been shown to reduce the risk of stroke in diabetics
4. Anti-platelet medication – the FDA recommends aspirin doses of 50–325 mg daily for primary stroke prevention, with aspirin combined with extended release dipyridamole or clopidogrel for secondary prevention
5. Tight glycemic control – reducing fasting glucose below 100 mg/dl, 2-h postprandial glucose below 140 mg/dl, and A1C less than 6.5%. Table 5 summarizes the benefits to better glycemic control in landmark studies of type-1 and type -2 diabetics

Table 5
A1C lowering reduces complications of type-1 and type-2 diabetes

	DCCT (%)	KUMAMOTO (%)	UKPDS (%)
A1C	9.1–7.3	9.4–7.1	7.9–7.0
Retinopathy	−63	−69	−(17–21)
Nephropathy	−54	−70	−(24–33)
Neuropathy	−60	–	–
Macrovascular disease	−41[a]	–	–

From UKPDS Group [21], DCCT Research Group [100], and Ohkubo [101]
[a]Not statistically significant

The Steno-2 study enrolled 160 patients with type-2 diabetes and microalbuminuria from the Steno Diabetes Center in Denmark [95]. The patients, with an average age of 55 years, were placed in two management groups – conventional and intensive therapy. The intensive group all received ACE inhibitors (ARBs if ACE intolerant), aspirin, dietary intervention, more than 30 min of exercise weekly, smoking cessation, tight control of glucose (<6.5%), blood pressure (<130/80 mmHg), and lipids (total cholesterol <175 mg/dl and triglycerides <150 mg/dl). Most outcomes in the intensive strategy group were consistently better than the conventionally managed patients. The primary outcomes of composite cardiovascular death, nonfatal myocardial infarction, coronary revascularization, nonfatal stroke, amputation, or peripheral surgery was reduced by 53% in the intensive therapy group, whereas nephropathy was reduced by 61%, retinopathy by 58%, and autonomic neuropathy by 3% after a follow up of 7.8 years. This study demonstrated the value of intensive, target driven therapy that addresses multiple risk factors. It is this type of aggressive lipid, blood pressure, and glycemic control that is associated with more benefit and risk reduction than traditional, less intensive approaches.

Proper care of the lower extremities is critical in caring for the diabetic. Multiple causation factors including peripheral neuropathy which impairs sensation, leukocyte mobility and healing, arteriosclerotic disease of both large and small vessels, the effects of hyperglycemia on healing and leukocyte migration at the cellular level and atherogenic and thrombotic microemboli all contribute to increased risk for the diabetic extremity.

In addition, bone structure abnormalities that impair foot and ankle biomechanics are also risk factors for the development of severe ulcers of the feet. Chemical and structural abnormalities enhance the risk for ulcerations and tend to increase with age.

Diabetics, 1.8 million, will develop a serious foot ulcer sometime during their life time which equates to over 15% of the estimated diabetics in this country. Many of these ulcerations lead to loss of tissue and amputation. In this country alone, 45% of all non-traumatic amputations are the result of diabetes. One-third of all diabetic ulcers occur beneath the big toe due to repetitive stress, local tissue ischemia, and loss of nerve sensation.

An interesting review by Rith-Najarian and Reiber, blames two structural abnormalities playing a critical role in predisposition to foot ulcers, which include limited joint motion in the first toe and tightened Achilles tendon [96].

Nonetheless in addition to these issues, the physician must not underestimate the importance of glycemic control, peripheral neuropathy, and thrombotic and atherogenic arteriosclerotic vascular disease in the etiology of progression of ulcerations in the lower extremities.

Type-2 diabetes represents a monumental challenge for the primary care physician. The diabetic is at significant risk for arteriosclerotic vascular disease and all of its complications as well as the microvascular disasters associated with the continued and progressive hyperglycemic state.

Diabetics are less likely to survive their first myocardial infarction and aggressive primary care prevention is essential and includes dietary management, exercise, smoking cessation with specific pharmacologic measures treating lipids to goal, including LDL cholesterol, HDL cholesterol and triglycerides, strict blood pressure control with blood pressure lowering to 125/75 mmHg with any evidence of end-organ disease and 130/85 mmHg otherwise, tight glycemic control achieving hemoglobin A1C less than 6.5%, postprandial sugars less than 140 mg/dl, and minimizing postprandial excursions to less than 40 mg/dl along with the judicious use of aspirin to inhibit platelet aggregation, reducing the risk of stroke, myocardial infarction, and other arterial thrombotic disasters.

The use of ACE inhibitors – particularly ramipril – in the diabetic patient, has been well established and should be considered for all these patients not only as a treatment for hypertension, but for overall risk reduction [97]. The ARB, telmisartan, has now been shown to have similar data for risk reduction and should be used in those patients who cannot tolerate an ACE inhibitor.

It is only with this multifaceted approach and targeting all risk factors aggressively that the physician and patient can bond together to reduce risk in this devastating disease.

The key to managing cardiovascular risk in diabetic patients is to treat and address all risk factors simultaneously. This includes proper glycemic control, blood pressure control, lipid control, and the use of aspirin in all individuals greater than 40 years of age unless aspirin is contraindicated.

Prevention of diabetic retinopathy includes, annual dilated retain examination, maintenance of blood pressure less than 130/80 mmHg, tight glycemic and lipid control. Neuropathy management involves tight glycemic and hypertension control with judicious use of analgesics, antidepressants, and or anticonvulsants.

For diabetic nephropathy, aggressive glycemic and blood pressure control are critical along with ACE inhibitor and/or ARB therapy and lipid control. For the diabetic foot, regular self and professional examinations, wound debridement and protection with topical recombinant human platelet derived growth factor when indicated.

SUMMARY

Overall risk reduction in the diabetic patient involves an aggressive, multifactorial approach to inhibit macro and microvascular disease. This involves early treatment with statins and ACE inhibitors (particularly ramipril with normal left ventricular function) or ARBs for macro and microvascular disease prevention.

REFERENCES

1. Spanheimer RG. Reducing cardiovascular risk in diabetes. Which factors to modify first? Postgrad Med 2001;109:26–36.
2. Duckworth WC, McCarren M, Abraira C. Glucose control and cardiovascular complications: the VA diabetes trial. Diabetes Care 2001;24:942–945.
3. Holman RR, Paul SK, Bethel MA, Matthews DR, Neal HA. Ten year follow up of intensive glucose control in type-2 diabetes. N Engl J Med 2008;359(15):1577–1589.
4. Patel A, MacMahon S, Chalmers J. Intensive blood glucose control and vascular outcomes in patients with type-2 diabetes. The ADVANCE Trial. N Engl J Med 2008;358:2560–2572.
5. Gerstein HC, Riddle MC, Kendall DM. Glycemia treatment strategies in the Action to Control Cardiovascular Risk in Diabetes (ACCORD) trial. Am J Cardiol 2007;99:34i–43i.
6. Magee MF, Isley WL. Rationale, design, and methods for glycemic control in the Bypass Angioplasty Revascularization Investigation 2 Diabetes (BARI 2) trial. AM J Cardiol 2006;97:20G–30G.
7. Weintraub W, Spertus J, Kolm P, Maron D, Zhang Z. Effect of PCI on quality of life in patients with stable coronary artery disease. N Engl J Med 2008;359:677–687.
8. Greenfield S, Billimek J, Pelligrini F, Franciosi M. Comorbidity affects the relationship between glycemic control and cardiovascular outcomes in diabetes. Ann Intern Med 2009;151(12):854–860.

9. Evans JMM, Ogston SA, Emslie-Smith A, Morris AD. Risk of mortality and adverse cardiovascular outcomes in patients treated with metformin and sulfonylureas. Diabetologia 2006;49:930–936.

10. Johnson J, Majumda S, Simpson S, Toth E. Decreased mortality with metformin compared to sulfonylurea monotherapy in type-2 diabetes. Diabetes Care 2002;25(12):2244–2248.

11. Shaya FT, Lu Z, Sohn K, Weir MR. Thiazolidinediones and cardiovascular events in high risk patients with type-2 diabetes mellitus. P T 2009;34(9):490–501.

12. Winkelmayer W, Setoguchi S, Levin R, Solomon D. Comparison of cardiovascular outcomes in elderly patients who initiated rosiglitazone vs pioglitazone therapy. Arch Intern Med 2008;168(21):238–275.

13. Dormandy JA, Charbonnel B, Eckland DJ. The PROACTIVE Study; pioglitazone in secondary prevention of macrovascular events in patients with type-2 diabetes. Curr Diab Rep 2006;6(1):45–46.

14. Nissen S, Wolsky K. The effect of rosiglitazone on the risk of myocardial infarction and death from cardiovascular causes. N Engl J Med 2007;356:2457–2471.

15. Singh S, Loke Y, Furberg C. Long term risk of cardiovascular events with rosiglitazone. JAMA 2007;298(10):1189–1195.

16. Psaty BM, Furberg K. Rosiglitazone and the risk of myocardial infarction (The RECORD trial). N Engl J Med 2007;357:67–69.

17. Lincoff A, Wolsky K, Nichols S. Pioglitazone and the risk of cardiovascular events in patients with type-2 diabetes. JAMA 2007;298:1180–1188.

18. Nissen S, Wolsky S, Nichols K, Nesto R. Comparison of pioglitazone and glimepirideon progression of coronary atherosclerosis in patients with type-2 diabetes. The PERISCOPE Trial. JAMA 2008;299(13): 1561–1573.

19. Giugliano D, Esposito K. Pioglitazone vs. glimpeiride and carotid intima media thickness. JAMA 2007;297(12):1315–1316.

20. Collins R, Armitage J, Parish S, Sleigh P, Peto R, Heart Protection Study Collaborative Group. MRC/BHF Heart Protection Study of cholesterol lowering with simvastatin in 5963 people with diabetes. Lancet 2003;361:2005–2016.

21. United Kingdom Prospective Diabetes Study (UKPDS) Group. Intensive blood glucose control with sulfonylureas or insulin compared with conventional treatment and risk of complication in patients with type-2 diabetes. Lancet 1998;352:837–853.

22. Malmberg K. The DIGAMI trial. Study of intensive insulin treatment on long term survival after acute myocardial infarction. BMJ 1997;314:1512–1515.

23. Downs JR, Clearfield M, Weis S. Primary prevention of acute coronary events with lovastatin in men and women with average cholesterol levels results of the AFCAPS/TexCAPS. JAMA 1998;279:1615–1622.

24. ALLHAT Officers and Coordinators for the ALLHAT Collaborative Research Group. The ALLHAT Trial. Major outcomes in moderately hypercholesterolemic, hypertensive patients randomized to pravastatin vs. usual care. JAMA 2002;288:2998–3007.

25. Koskinen P, Manttari M, Manninen V. Coronary heart disease incidence in NIDDM patients in Helsinki Heart Study. Diabetes Care 1992;15:820–825.

26. Shepherd J, Baluw GJ, Murphy MB. Prospective Study of Pravastatin in the Elderly at Risk. Pravastatin in elderly individuals at risk of vascular disease (PROSPER). Lancet 2002;360:1620–1630.

27. Sever PS, Dahlof B, Poulter NR. Prevention of coronary and stroke events with atorvastatin in hypertensive patients who have average or lower than average cholesterol concentrations, in the ASCOT-LLA trial. Lancet 2003;361:1149–1158.

28. Colhoun HM, Betteridge DJ, Durrington PN. Primary prevention of cardiovascular disease with atorvastatin in type-2 diabetes in the Collaborative Atorvastatin Diabetes Study (CARDS). Lancet 2004;364: 641–642.

29. Knopp RH, D'Emden M, Smilde JG, Pocock SJ. Efficacy and safety of atorvastatin in the prevention of cardiovascular end points in subjects with type-2 diabetes. The ASPEN Trial. Diabetes Care 2006;29:1478–1485.

30. Scandinavian Simvastatin Survival Study Group. Randomised trial of cholesterol lowering in 4444 patients with coronary heart disease: the Scandinavian Simvastatin Survival Study (4S). Lancet 1994;344:1383–1389.

31. Garber AJ. Attenuating cardiovascular risk factors in patients with type 2 diabetes mellitus. Am Fam Physician 2000;62:2633–2642.

32. Haffner SM. Management of dyslipidemia in adults with diabetes. Diabetes Care 1998;21:160–178.
33. Ginsburg HN, Plutzky J, SobelBE. A review of metabolic and cardiovascular effects of oral antidiabetic agents: beyond glucose lowering. J Cardiovasc Risk 1999;6:337–347.
34. Tikkanen MJ, Laakso M, et al. Treatment of hypercholesterolemia and combined hyperlipidemia with simvastatin and gemfibrozil in patients with NIDDM. Diabetes Care 1998;21:477–481.
35. Serruys PW, deFeyterp P, Macaya C (2002) Fluvastatin for prevention of cardiac events following successful first percutaneous coronary intervention. The LIPS trial. JAMA 287:3215–3222.
36. The Long Term Intervention with Pravastatin in Ischemic Disease (LIPID) Study Group. Prevention of cardiovascular events and death with pravastatin in patients with coronary heart disease and a broad range of initial cholesterol levels. N Engl J Med 1998;339:1349–1357.
37. McKenney J. Pharmacologic options for aggressive low density lipoprotein cholesterol lowering: benefits versus risks. Am J Cardiol 2005;96 (suppl):60E–66E.
38. Shepherd J, Blauw GJ, Murphy MB. PROSPER Study Group. Prospective Study of Pravastatin in the Elderly at Risk. Lancet 2002;360:1623–1630.
39. Knatterud GL, Rosenberg Y, Campeau L. Long term effects on clinical outcome of aggressive lowering of low density lipoprotein cholesterol levels and low dose anticoagulation in the post coronary bypass graft trial. Circulation 2000;102:157–165.
40. Sacks FM, Pfeffer MA, Moye LA. The effect of pravastatin on coronary events after myocardial infarction in patients with average cholesterol levels. Cholesterol and Recurrent Events trial Investigators. N Engl J Med 1996;335:1001–1009.
41. Dunn FL. Hyperlipidemia in diabetes mellitus. Diabetes Metab Rev 1990;6:47.
42. Robins SJ, Rubins HB, Faas FH. Veterans Affairs HDL intervention Trial. Insulin resistance and cardiovascular events with low HDL cholesterol. The VA-HIT. N Engl J Med 1999;341:410–418.
43. La Rosa JC, Grundy SM, Waters DD. Treating to new targets investigators. Intensive lipid lowering with atorvastatin in patients with stable coronary disease. N Engl J Med 2005;352:1425–1435.
44. Keech A, Simes RJ, Barter P, FIELD Study Investigators. Effects of long term fenofibrate therapy on cardiovascular events in 9795 people with type-2 diabetes mellitus (the FIELD study). Lancet 2005;366:1849–1861.
45. McCall KL, Craddock D, Edwards K. Effect of angiotensin-converting enzyme inhibitors and angiotensin II type-1 receptors blockers on the rate of new onset diabetes mellitus: a review and pooled analysis. Pharmacotherapy 2006;26(9):1297–1306.
46. Gladstone PSJ, McLaughlin PR, Syvanne M, Steiner G. DAIS Investigators. Micronized fenofibrate decrease progression of coronary heart disease in type-2 diabetes. The DAIS Trial. Circulation 2000;102 (suppl II):II-409.
47. Canner PL, Berge KG, Wenger NK. Fifteen year mortality in Coronary Drug Project patients: long term benefit with niacin. J Am Coll Cardiol 1986;8:1245–1255.
48. Howard B, Roman M, Devereaux R, Fleg J, Galloway J, Henderson J, Howard WJ. Effects of lower targets for blood pressure and LDL cholesterol on atherosclerosis in diabetes; the SANDS Trial. JAMA 2008, 299(14):1678–1689.
49. Blankenhorn DH, Nessin SA, Johnson RL, Sanmarco ME, Azen SP, Cashin-Hemphill L. Beneficial effects of combined colestipol-niacin therapy on coronary atherosclerosis and coronary venous bypass grafts. JAMA 1987;257:3233–3240.
50. Rao AK, et al. Platelet coagulation activity in diabetes mellitus. Evidence for relationship between platelet coagulant hyperactivity and platelet volume. J Lab Clin Med 1984;103:82–92.
51. Esposito K, Giugliano D, Nappo F, Marfella R. Regression of carotid atherosclerosis by control of postprandial hyperglycemia in type-2 diabetes mellitus. Circulation 2004;110:214–219.
52. Betteridge DJ. Diabetes, lipoprotein metabolism and atherosclerosis. Br Med Bull 1989;45:285–311.
53. Imanishi M, Yoshioka K, et al. Glomerular hypertension as one cause of albuminuria caused by angiotensin converting enzyme inhibitor in early diabetic nephropathy. Kidney Int Suppl 1997;63:S198–S200.
54. The Accord Study Group. Effects of combination lipid therapy in type-2 diabetes mellitus. N Engl J Med 2010;362(17):1563–1574.
55. Dandona P, Aljada A. A rational approach to pathogenesis and treatment of type 2 diabetes mellitus, insulin resistance, inflammation and atherosclerosis. Am J Cardiol 2002;90 (suppl)27G–33G.
56. Stergiou GS, Skeva II, et al. Additive hypotensive effect of angiotensin converting enzyme inhibition and angiotensin receptor antagonism in essential hypertension. J Cardiovasc Pharmacol 2000;35:937–941.

57. McMurray JJ, Ostergren J, et al. Effects of candesartan in patients with chronic heart failure and reduced left ventricular systolic function taking angiotensin converting enzymes inhibitors: the CHARM added trial. Lancet 2003;362:767–771.

58. Arnold JM, Yusuf S, Young J. Prevention of heart failure in patients in the Heart Outcomes Prevention Evaluation (HOPE) Study. Circulation 2003;107(9):1284–1290.

59. Bosch J, Lonn E, Pogue J, Arnold JM, Dagenais GR, Yusuf S, HOPE-TOO Study Investigators. Long term effects of ramipril on cardiovascular events and on diabetes; results of the Hope study extension. Circulation 2005;112(9):1339–1346.

60. Niskanen L, Hedner T, Hansson L, Lanke J, Nikalson A, CAPPP Study Group. Reduced cardiovascular morbidity and mortality in hypertensive diabetic patients on first line therapy with an ACE inhibitor compared with a diuretic/beta blocker based treatment regimen: a subanalysis of the Captopril Prevention Project. Diabetes Care 2001;24(12)2091–2096.

61. Andraws R, Brown DL. Effect of inhibition of the renin-angiotensin system on development of type-2 diabetes mellitus (meta-analysis of randomized trials). Am J Cardiol 2007;99(7):1006–1012.

62. Brenner BM, Cooper ME, de Zeeuw D, RENAAL Study Investigators. Effects of losartan on renal and cardiovascular outcomes in patients with type-2 diabetes and nephropathy. N Engl J Med 2001;345(12): 861–869.

63. Rossing K, Jacobsen P, Pietraszek L, Parving HH. Renoprotective effects of adding angiotensin II receptor blocker to maximal recommended doses of ACE inhibitor in diabetic nephropathy; a randomized double blind crossover trial. Diabetes Care 2003;26(8):2268–2274.

64. Yusef S, Teo KK, Pogue J, ON TARGET Investigators. Telmisartan, ramipril, or both in patients at high risk for vascular events. N Engl J Med 2008;358(15):1547–1559.

65. Mehler PS, Jeffers BW, et al. Associations of hypertension and complications in non-insulin dependent diabetes. Am J Hypertens 1997;10:152–161.

66. Lindholm LH, Kartman B, Carlberg B, Persson M. Cost implications of development of diabetes in the ALPINE study. J Hypertens Suppl 2006;24(1):S65–S72.

67. McMurray JJ, Ostergren J, Swedberg K. Effects of candesartan in patients with chronic heart failure and reduced left ventricular systolic function taking angiotensin converting enzyme inhibitors; The CHARM Added trial. Lancet 2003;362:767–771.

68. Julius S, Kjeldsen SE, Weber M, VALUE Trial Group. Outcomes in hypertensive patients at high cardiovascular risk treated with regimens based on valsartan or amlodipine. The VALUE randomized trial. Lancet 2004;363(4926):2022–2031.

69. The NAVIGATOR Study Group. Effect of valsartan on the incidence of diabetes and cardiovascular events. N Engl J Med 2010;362:1477–1490.

70. Yusuf S. Effects of angiotensin receptor blocker telmisartan on cardiovascular events in high risk patients intolerant to angiotensin converting enzyme inhibitors: a randomized controlled trial. Lancet 2008. DOI: 10.1016/S0140-6736(08)61242-8.

71. Kjeldsen SE, Jamerson KA, Bakris GL. For Avoiding Cardiovascular Events Through Combination Therapy in Patients Living with Systolic Hypertension investigators. Predictors of blood pressure response to intensified and fixed combination treatment of hypertension: the ACCOMPLISH study. Blood Press 2008;17(1):7–17.

72. Parving HH, Persson F, Lewis JB, Lewis EJ, Hollenberg NK. Aliskiren combined with losartan in type-2 diabetes with nephropathy. N Engl J Med 2008;35823:2433–2446.

73. Pfeffer MA, et al. Valsartan, captopril or both in myocardial infarction complicated by heart failure, left ventricular dysfunction or both. N Engl J Med 2003;349:1893–1906.

74. Cohn JN, Tognoni G. A randomized trial of the angiotensin-receptor blocker valsartan in chronic heart failure. N Engl J Med 2001;345:1667–1675.

75. McKelvie RS, Yusuf S, et al. Comparison of candesartan, enalapril and their combination in congestive heart failure. Randomized Evaluation of Strategies for Left Ventricular Dysfunction. (RESOLVD) pilot study. Circulation 1999;100:1056–1064.

76. Rossing P, Parving H, de Zeeuw D. Renoprotection by blocking the RAAS in diabetic nephropathy – fact or fiction? Nephrol Dial Transplant 2006;21(9):2354–2357.

77. The ACCORD Study Group. Effects of Intensive blood pressure control in type-2 diabetes mellitus. N Engl J Med 2010;362(17):1575–1586.

78. Pepine C, Handberg E, Cooper-DeHoff R, Marks R. A calcium antagonist versus a non calcium antagonist hypertension treatment strategy for patients with coronary artery disease. The INVEST Trial. JAMA 2003;290(21):2805–2816.

79. Schneider DJ, Sobel BE. Diabetes and Thrombosis. Contemporary Cardiology: Diabetes and Cardiovascular Diseases. Totowa: Humana Press; 2001:149–167.

80. Aronow H, Califf R, Harrington R, Vallee M, Graffagnino C, Shuaib A. Relation between aspirin dose, all cause mortality, and bleeding in patients with recent cerebrovascular or coronary ischemic events (from the BRAVO Trial). Am J Cardiol 2008;102:1285–1290.

81. Hansson L, Zanchetti A, Carruthers SG. Effects of intensive blood pressure lowering and low dose aspirin in patients with hypertension. The HOT trial. Lancet 1998;351:1755–1762.

82. Bhatt DL, Marso SP, Hirsch AT, Ringleb PA, Hcke W, Topol EJ. Amplified benefit of clopidogrel versus aspirin in patients with diabetes mellitus. Am J Cardiol 2002;90:625–628.

83. Colwell JA. Position statement: aspirin therapy in diabetes. Diabetes Care 2003;26 (suppl 1):S87–S88.

84. The Post Coronary Artery Bypass Graft Investigators. The effect of aggressive lowering of low density lipoprotein cholesterol levels and low dose anticoagulation on obstructive changes in saphenous vein coronary artery bypass grafts. N Engl J Med 1997;336(3):153–163.

85. Ogawa H, Nakayama M, Morimoto T, Uemora S, Kanauchi M. Low dose aspirin for prevention of primary events in patients with type-2 diabetes: The JPAD trial. JAMA 2008;300(18):2134–2141.

86. Antithrombotic Trialists' Collaboration. Collaborative meta-analysis of randomized trials of antiplatelet therapy for prevention of death, myocardial infarction, and stroke in high risk patients. BMJ 2002;324:71–86.

87. U.S. Preventive Services Task Force. Aspirin for the prevention of cardiovascular disease: recommendation statement. Ann Intern Med 2009;150(6):396–404.

88. Bhatt DL, Fox KA, Hacke W, Berger PB, Black HR, Boden WE, Cacoub P, Cohen EA. Clopidogrel and aspirin versus aspirin alone for the prevention of atherothrombotic events. The CHARISMA trial. N Engl J Med 2006;354:1706–1717.

89. Amarenco P, Donnan G. Should the MATCH results be extrapolated to all stroke patients and affect ongoing trials evaluating clopidogrel plus aspirin? Stroke 2004;35:2606–2608.

90. Sacco RL, Diener HC, Yusuf S. Aspirin and extended release dipyridamole versus clopidogrel for recurrent stroke. N Engl J Med 2008;359(12):1238–1251.

91. Kirtane AJ, Dawkins SG, Colombo A, Grube E, Popna JJ. Paclitaxel eluting coronary stents in patients with diabetes mellitus: pooled analysis from 5 randomized trials. J Am Coll Cardiol 2008;51(7):708–715.

92. Gress TW, Nieto FJ, et al. Hypertension and antihypertensive therapy as risk factors for type 2 diabetes mellitus. Atherosclerosis risk in communities study. N Engl J Med 2000;342;905–912.

93. Fogari R, Zoppi A, et al. Comparative effects of lisinopril and losartan on insulin sensitivity in the treatments of non diabetic hypertensive patients. Br J Clin Pharmacol 1998;46;467–471.

94. Ridker PM, et al. C-reactive protein, the metabolic syndrome, and risk of cardiovascular events: a 8 year follow up of 14,719 initially health American women. Circulation 2003;107:391–397.

95. Vaag AA. Glycemic control and prevention of microvascular and macrovascular events in the Steno 2 study. Endocr Pract 2006;12 (suppl 1):89–92.

96. Rith-Najarian SJ, Reiber GE. Prevention of foot problems in persons with diabetes. J Fam Pract 2000;49:S30–S39.

97. HOPE Study Investigators. Effects of ramipril in cardiovascular and microvascular outcomes in people with diabetes mellitus: results of the Hope and Micro-Hope Trials. Lancet 2000;355:253–259.

98. Krentz AJ, Bailey CJ. Oral anti-diabetic agents. Drugs 2005;65(3):385–411.

99. Nathan DM, Buse MB, Davidson JB. Medical management of hyperglycaemia in type-2 diabetes; a consensus algorithm. Diabetologia 2009;52(1):17–30.

100. DCCT Research Group. The DCCT trial. N Engl J Med 1993;329:977–986.

101. Ohkubo Y. The Kumamoto trial. Diabetes Res Clin Pract 1995;28:103.

SUPPLEMENTARY READINGS

Agarwal R. Add on angiotensin receptor blockade with maximized ACE inhibition. Kidney Int 2001; 59:2282–2289.

Ardaillou R. Angiotensin II receptors. J Am Soc Nephrol 1999;10 (suppl):S30–S39.

Azizi M, Linhart A, et al. Pilot study of controlled blockade of the renin-angiotensin system in essential hypertensive patients. J Hypertens 2000;18:1839–1147.

Chaturvedi N, Sjolle AK, Stephenson JM, et al. Effect of lisinopril on progression of retinopathy in normotensive people with type 1 diabetes. Lancet 1998;351:28–31.

Carvalho CR, et al. Effect of captopril, losartan and bradykinin on early steps of insulin action. Diabetes 1997;46:1950–1957.

Colwell JA. Treatment for the procoagulant state in type 2 diabetes. Endocrinol Metab Clin North Am 2001;30:1011–1030.

Dzau VJ. Mechanism of protective effects of ACE inhibition on coronary artery disease. Eur Heart J 1998;19 (suppl):12–16.

Estacio RO, Schrier RW. Antihypertensive therapy in type 2 diabetics: implications of the appropriated blood pressure control in diabetics (ABCD) trial. Am J Cardiol 1998;82:9R–14R.

Frick MH, Elo H. Primary prevention trial with gemfiborzil I middle aged men with dyslipidemia. N Engl J Med 1987;317:1237–1245.

Ginsberg HN. Effects of statins on triglyceride metabolism. Am J Cardiol 1998;81:32B–35B.

Haffner SM, Lehto S, Ronnemaa T, Pyorala K, Laakso M. Mortality from coronary heart disease with type-2 diabetes and nondiabetic subjects with and without previous myocardial infarction: implications for treatment of hyperlipidemia in diabetic subjects without prior myocardial infarction. N Engl J Med 1998;339:229–234.

Hiatt WR. New treatment options in intermittent claudication. Int J Clin Pract Suppl 2001;119:20–27.

Jain A, Varma A, Mole R. Digital amputations in the diabetic foot. J Diabetic Foot Complications 2010;2(1)3.

Knobl P, Schernthaner G, et al. Hemostatic abnormalities persist despite glycemic improvement by insulin therapy in type 2 diabetics. Thromb Haemost 1994;71:692–697.

Kodama M, et al. Antiplatelet drugs attenuate progression of carotid intima thickness in subjects with type 2 diabetes. Thromb Res 2000;97:239–245.

McGill JB, et al. Factors responsible for impaired fibrinolysis in obese and diabetic patients. Diabetes 1994;43:104–109.

Menys VS, Bhatnagar D, et al. Spontaneous platelet aggregation in whole blood is increased in insulin dependent diabetics. Atherosclerosis 1995;112:115–122.

Mogensen CE, et al. Randomized controlled trial of dual blockade of renin-angiotensin system in patients with hypertension, microalbuminuria, and non-insulin dependent diabetes: the candesartan and lisinopril microalbuminuria (CALM) study. BMJ 2000;321:1440–1444.

New JP, Bilous RW. Insulin sensitivity in hypertensive type 2 diabetic patients after 1 and 19 days with trandolapril. Diabetes Med 2000;17:134–141.

Reid CM, Ryan P, Nelson M. General practitioner participation in the second Australian National Blood Pressure Study (ANBP2). Clin Exp Pharmacol Physiol 2001;28:663–667.

Rossing K, Christensen PK, et al. Dual blockade of the rennin-angiotensin system in diabetic retinopathy. Diabetes Care 2002;25:95–100.

Torlone E, Britta M, Rambotti AM, et al. Improved insulin action and glycemic control after long term angiotensin-converting enzyme induction in subjects with arterial hypertension and type 2 diabetes. Diabetes Care 1993:16:1347–1355.

Unger T. Neurohormonal modulation in cardiovascular disease. Am Heart J 2000;139:S2–S8.

Unger T. The Ongoing Telmisartan Alone and in Combination with Ramipril Global Endpoint Trial program. Am J Cardiol 2003;91;28G–34G.

15 Diabetes in Special Populations

Key Words: Mental health, Type-2 diabetes in children, Diabetes in women, Acquired immune deficiency syndrome (AIDS), Hemodialysis, Foot problems, Perioperative and post-operative glycemic control, Skin disease in type-2 diabetic patients

MENTAL HEALTH AND TYPE-2 DIABETES

Major depressive disorders and depressive symptoms not only occur frequently with diabetes, but in many patients, mental health symptoms and even depression go unrecognized or incorrectly diagnosed [1]. Even among those that undergo successful treatment, close to 80% will experience relapsing symptoms within 5 years. Diabetic patients at higher risk for depression include those of female gender, poor social support system, lower education, low socioeconomic status, and unmarried status. Clinical research has revealed that having type-2 diabetes increases the risk of depression and depression is an independent risk and predictive factor for the quantity and severity of type-2 diabetes complications. Depression early in life also increases the risk for unhealthy lifestyle, obesity, sedentary existence, and addictive habits – especially smoking. In addition, patients with

From: *Current Clinical Practice: Type 2 Diabetes, Pre-Diabetes, and the Metabolic Syndrome*
Edited by: R.A. Codario, DOI 10.1007/978-1-60327-441-8_15
© Springer Science+Business Media, LLC 2011

depression and type-2 diabetes are far more likely to be non-compliant with medications, glucose self monitoring, and therapeutic life style changes [1].

Both psychotherapeutic and pharmacologic interventions are effective, with anti-depressants being the first line of therapy with selective serotonin reuptake inhibitors, serotonin norepinephrine reuptake inhibitors, and bupropion. Therapeutic interventions have shown promising results in improving diabetes control and adherence to therapeutic life style changes.

Physicians should be aware of some important side effects on lipids and glycemic control inherent in some psychotropic medications like risperidone (Risperdal), clozapine (Clozaril), olanzapine (Zyprexa), aripiprazole (Abilify), ziprasidone (Geodon), and quetiapine (Seroquel) and individualize treatment to maximize benefits and reduce unwanted metabolic side effects.

Routine screening for depression is recommended by the American Diabetes Association (ADA) especially for non-compliant individuals. Patients who present with depression should be monitored on a regular basis for the development of diabetes, pre-diabetes, and the metabolic syndrome.

Drugs that possess anti-cholinergic properties may have a direct effect on pancreatic islet cells, impacting insulin secretion via the muscarinic M3 receptors which innervate the beta cells. These effects can have an impact in those patients with mental disorders and who are overweight, dyslipidemic, diabetic, or pre-diabetic. Many of the atypical antipsychotic medications function as M3 receptor antagonists, inhibiting insulin secretion by the beta cells by binding to the M3 receptors in the pancreas [2].

In order to maintain euglycemia, a balance must exist between the effects of hyperglycemic hormones, like growth hormone corticosteroids, epinephrine, and glucogon, and the hypoglycemic hormones like insulin. Insulin secretion is increased by parasympathetic stimulation, with vagus nerve fibers exerting control over the endocrine and exocrine function of the pancreas by connecting with the intra-pancreatic ganglia.

During feeding, intra-pancreatic nerve terminals release acetylcholine, the principal parasympathetic neurotransmitter, which subsequently binds to the M3 receptors in the beta cells resulting in an increase in nutrient-induced insulin secretion. Insulin cells have been found to contain high concentrations of enzymes involved in the degradation of acetycholine (acetycholinesterase) and its synthesis (choline transferase). Reports of severe hyperglycemia with ketoacidosis following treatment with atypical antipsychotics have fostered further research into the effects of these agents on insulin secretion [3].

Transgenic rodents with either an overexpression of the pancreatic M3 receptors or an absence of those receptors have been observed to produce opposite effects on insulin secretion. Marked decreases in insulin secretion and subsequent glucose intolerance occur in the absence of beta cell M3 receptors, while lower glucose levels and overproduction of insulin are demonstrated with over expression of these receptors. Both olanzapine and clozapine have been demonstrated to block muscarinic receptor activation of insulin secretion, with even low concentrations of 10–100 nmol/L significantly impairing cholinergic mediated insulin secretion [4].

These potent muscarinic antagonist effects were not seen with risperidone, haloperidol, or ziprazodone. Hence, the choice of an antipsychotic medication can have significant effects on glucose metabolism. The hyperglycemic effects of clozapine and olanzapine have even been demonstrated in the absence of weight gain. Other antipsychotics exhibiting high M3 receptor binding affinity with the subsequent increased capacity for inducing glucose intolerance are the first generation antipsychotics, chlorpromazine and thioridazine. Other medications with high affinity include antidepressants paroxetine, imipramine, doxepin, and amitriptyline. Those with intermediate affinity include first generations antipsychotic agents perphenazine, fluphenazine, trifluoperazine, and pimozide and second generation agents aripiprazole and quetiapine. First generation agents thiothixene and haloperidol and second generation agents risperidone and ziprasidone have low affinity [5].

A 2004 consensus development conference made recommendations concerning therapeutic use of first generation and second generation antipsychotics, highlighting increased risk of developing diabetes in patients treated with olanzapine and clozapine, and recommending taking a family history for the presence of diabetes, dyslipidemia, hypertension, obesity, and cardiovascular disease at baseline followed by regular monthly measurements of waist circumference, weight, and blood pressure in addition to baseline and quarterly measurements of fasting plasma glucose and lipid profiles [6].

In addition, the effect of weight gain caused by anti-depressives is a well recognized troublesome side effect. High binding affinities for the M3 receptors have also included anti-depressants like amitriptyline, doxepin, eliperdine, and paroxetine demonstrating increased propensity for weight gain, whereas fluoxetine, sertraline, venlafaxine, and bupropion have demonstrated lower binding affinities for the M3 receptors and have decreased propensity for causing obesity during long term use.

Weight gain induced by psychotropic agents should be considered as an imposition because of the increased risk of metabolic syndrome, diabetes, hypertension, and their subsequent complications. Within the anti-depressant class, desipramine, nortriptyline, paroxetine, and protriptyline have the capacity for inducing mild weight gain with the potential change of 1–5 pounds/year. In the antipsychotic class, not only fluphenazine, haloperidol, paliperidone, and perphenazine but also the anti-seizure mood stabilizer, carbamazepine, may induce mild weight gain [7].

Moderate weight gain of 6–10 pounds/year may be seen with the antidepressants amitriptyline, doxepin,imipramine, mirtazapine, phenelzine, and tranylcypromine as well as the antipsychotic drugs risperdone, thioridazine, and quetiapine and the mood stabilizer, anti-seizure medication gabapentin. Moderate to severe weight gain of 11–15 pounds has been seen with the mood stabilizer lithium and valproate, with severe weight gain of greater than 15 pounds/year seen with clozapine and olanzapine. The antidepressants bupropion and fluoxetine along with the anti-seizure medicine topiramate have been associated with weight loss up to 5 pounds/year, with some patients responding with even greater weight reductions [8].

Weight gain in early stages of treatment with psychotrophic drugs may be a harbinger of future weight gain and can be a problem in those patients who are overweight prior to treatment. Depression, of course, is a known risk factor for obesity, diabetes, and metabolic syndrome, with their joint occurrence being even more common than the predicted prevalence rate for the various individual syndromes.

The weight gain induced by many of these agents is usually the result of appetite stimulation and clinicians should be aware of the risks vs. benefits when selecting psychotrophic agents, avoiding those drugs that may induce weight gain in patients with metabolic syndrome, glucose intolerance, or obesity unless clinical circumstances dictate otherwise.

TYPE II DIABETES IN CHILDREN

Alarmingly, the incidence of metabolic syndrome, obesity, and type-2 diabetes is increasing rapidly in children and adolescents. Early diagnosis, encouragement of therapeutic lifestyle changes, and pharmacotherapy when appropriate are the cornerstones of managing this increasing problem. Sixteen percent of new cases of diabetes in children were diagnosed in 1994 compared to 45 percent of the total cases of diabetes diagnosed in 1999, with Native American, Hispanic, and African American children being at higher risk for the development of type-2 diabetes [9]. Insulin resistance characteristic of the type-2 diabetic paradigm is common in patients with polycystic ovaries, positive family history, sedentary lifestyle, obesity, and predisposing ethnic background, with girls being 1.7 times more likely to develop type-2 diabetes than boys.

According to data from the Third National Health and Nutrition Examination survey from 1988 to 1994, 4.2% of adolescents were known to have metabolic syndrome, while 25% of obese children between the ages of 4 and 10 and 21% of obese adolescents between the ages of 11 and 18 years were found to have impaired glucose tolerance [10]. By 1999, the percentage of new case of type-2 diabetes was up to 45% in some areas of the United States and by the year 2000, 16% of youth were characterized as being overweight with a body mass index (BMI) greater than the 95th percentile for gender and age. Obesity, hypertension, and glucose intolerance in childhood are strongly associated with increased rates of premature death. Children who are overweight and have a pre-disposing ethnic group (American Indian, African American, Hispanic, Asian American, or Pacific Islander) along with a family history of type-2 diabetes should be screened at the onset of puberty and every 2 years thereafter, with a fasting blood sugar and a 2 h glucose tolerance test for those individuals with fasting sugars between 100 and 124 mg/dl and A1C greater than 5.9.

Various factors have contributed to the development of type-2 diabetes, for example, insulin resistance, obesity, and metabolic syndrome in children, sedentary lifestyle, unhealthy high fat and carbohydrate laden foods, and high fructose corn syrup soft drinks, as well as intrauterine factors with a higher incidence of type-2 diabetes in the offspring of mothers with gestational diabetes, of low birth weights, and of small head circumference. Not to be overlooked as well are inherited factors including race, ethnicity, and family history as 85% of children diagnosed with diabetes have family members with the disease [11]. Puberty is associated with various physiologic alterations and developmental changes including enhanced growth hormone secretion and sex hormone elaboration which increase insulin resistance. In addition, 15% of teenage girls with polycystic ovarian syndrome have diabetes, with one-third having impaired glucose tolerance, and with diabetes more common in young females than males with a female/male ratio of 1.7/1.0 [12].

Hypertension is a significant co-morbidity with type-2 diabetes in children and adolescents, representing a major risk factor for arteriosclerotic vascular disease and subsequent nephropathy. Hence, blood pressure, lipid, and vascular abnormalities should be screened for and treated aggressively in the pediatric population. Insulin and metformin are approved for diabetes treatment in children, insulin being especially appropriate for diagnostic uncertainties between type 1 and type 2 diabetes in this age group. It should be appreciated that the presence of diabetic ketoacidosis or ketosis alone does not necessarily rule out type 2 diabetes. C-peptide levels and islet cell and anti-insulin antibodies along with glutamic acid decarboxylase antibodies help to differentiate type-1 from type- 2 diabetes.

The ADA screening guidelines for type 2-diabetes require that (1) the person has a BMI greater than the 85th percentile for age and sex, (2) weight greater than 120% of ideal for height, and (3) weight greater than the 85th percentile for height plus any two of the following risk factors: (a) ethnicity of Pacific Islander, Hispanic, Latino, Asian American, Black, or American Indian, (b) family history of type-2 diabetes in a first or second degree relative, (c) mother with a history of gestational diabetes, and (d) signs of insulin resistance or other conditions that are usually associated with insulin resistance including dyslipidemia (hypertriglyceridemia with decreased HDL, polycystic ovary syndrome, hypertension, and acanthosis nigricans) [*13*].

The ADA also recommends regular screening every 2 years beginning at the age of 10 or at the onset of puberty with fasting plasma glucose as the preferred test. A1C levels of >6.5% are now accepted as being diagnostic for diabetes. Pre-diabetes is defined as a fasting blood glucose level of 100–125 mg/dl, with diabetes diagnosed with a fasting plasma glucose level of 126 mg/dl repeated on a subsequent day. It is to be appreciated that insulin and C-peptide levels can be low at the time of diagnosis in children with either type-1 or type-2 diabetes and some patients can actually have elements of both types [*14*].

Children with type-2 diabetes who are overweight and are insulin resistant may on occasion have pancreatic islet cell antibodies typically associated with type-1 diabetes. This has been termed double, mixed, or hybrid diabetes. In these situations, measurements of C-peptide levels or islet cell antibodies in addition to insulin and glutamic acid decarboxylase antibodies for 1 year or more after the diagnosis can prove helpful. Many type-2 children and adolescents will seek medical attention because of a variety of complaints, including sleep apnea, dyslipidemia, obesity, hypertension, amenorrhea, sluggishness, headaches, or physical abnormalities like acanthosis nigricans and polycystic ovarian syndrome.

Treatment of children and adolescents with type 2 diabetes focuses on decreasing insulin resistance in the face of advancing physical growth and sexual maturity. This is best achieved with a team concept involving not only the patient but also the family and diabetes educators to counsel both the patient and the family about daily physical activity and healthy eating habits as well as self monitoring of blood glucose levels. Unfortunately, diet and exercise alone are effective in less than 10% of patients with type-2 diabetes and oral medication is usually required. Insulin is used more often in children than in adults with type-2 diabetes as significant insulin deficiency usually exists in adolescents who are symptomatic at presentation. The DPP-IV inhibitors and the GLP-1 agonists (incretin mimetics) have not been approved for use in children or adolescents.

However, other oral agents including sulfonylureas, meglitinides (glinides), biguanides (with metformin the drug of choice for polycystic ovarian syndrome and diabetes), alpha-glucosidase inhibitors, and thiazolidinediones (TZDs) are all being used with variable success in monotherapy or in combinations.

DIABETES IN WOMEN

Background

The current epidemic of obesity and the increase in type-2 diabetes have had a profound effect on health care in women in the United States. Alarmingly, there has been a 70% increase in type-2 diabetes among women between the ages of 30–39 from 1990 to 1998, especially in the Hispanic Mexican American and African American population. It is estimated that nearly 2 million reproductive age women in the United States have type-2 diabetes, with about 30% of these cases as yet undiagnosed [15].

The common risk factors for the development of type-2 diabetes include sedentary life style, diets rich in saturated fat, trans fat, and excessive calories, inherited factors, and obesity (BMI>25 kg/m^2) [16]. In the United States alone, over 50% of women 20 years or more of age are overweight. Close to 60% of these engage in little or no physical activity. This excess body weight contributes significantly to insulin resistance, subsequent impaired glucose tolerance, and ultimately increased risk for developing diabetes and other health problems.

Type-2 diabetes is primarily a vasculopathic disease that begins decades before its clinical diagnosis, with the macrovascular complications beginning in the pre-diabetic stage characterized by the group of risk factors termed the metabolic syndrome. It is important for primary care physicians to understand, recognize, and treat this condition to prevent the development of type-2 diabetes.

The National Cholesterol Education Program (NCEP) ATP-3 guidelines [17] list three or more of the following as diagnostic of metabolic syndrome: waist circumference equal to or greater than 40 in. in men, equal to or greater than 36 in. in women, triglycerides equal to or greater than 150 mg/dl, HDL cholesterol less than 40 mg/dl in men or less than 50 mg/dl in women, systolic blood pressure equal to or greater than 130 mmHg or diastolic blood pressure equal to or greater than 85 mmHg, and a fasting blood sugar equal to or greater than 100 mg/dl.

The Diabetes Prevention Project (DPP) [18] randomized 3,234 non-diabetic individuals, 25 years of age or older, with impaired glucose tolerance and fasting glucose between 95 and 125 mg/dl to a placebo, a life style modification program, a goal of 7% weight loss, and 150 min of physical activity weekly or metformin 850 mg twice daily. In this study, 68% of the participants were women, with 45% being members of minority groups. Life style intervention reduced the incidence of type-2 diabetes by 58% compared to placebo, while the metformin intervention resulted in a 31% reduction in development of type-2 diabetes.

Clearly therapeutic life style changes can have a major impact not only in treating this condition, but also preventing progression to type-2 diabetes. The NCEP ATP-3 criteria may not be consistently predictive in all ethnic and gender groups with differences existing among Whites, African Americans, and Hispanic Americans. The prevalence of the metabolic syndrome is significantly higher in Mexican American women at 27% while in African American and White women the incidence is approximately the same 20–23% [19].

Among men of age 45–65, the incidence is 8.3/100 persons in Whites, 14.1 for African Americans, and 13.7 for Hispanics. However, in women of age 45–65, the rate is 6.7 for Whites, 16.6 for African Americans, and 13.2 for Hispanics. With aging, however, come more significant disparities [20].

The incidence of diabetes between the ages of 65 and 74 in men is 16.4/100 persons for Whites, 23.0 for African Americans, and 23.5 for Hispanics while the rates in women are 12.8 for Whites, 25.4 for African Americans, and 23.8 for Hispanics. Alarmingly, there has been a 33% increase in the overall prevalence of diabetes in the past 30 years, while the rate has tripled in African Americans [21]. In 1999, the diabetes age adjusted death rate per 100,000 was 18.4 among Asian Americans, 22.8 among White Americans, 33.6 among Hispanic Americans, 50.1 among African Americans, and 50.3 among Native Americans [22].

This disparity is even more striking in cardiovascular disease where African Americans are dying at the rate of 336.5/100,000 vs. Whites at approximately 263/100,000.

Data from the Third National Health and Nutrition Examination Survey indicated that the prevalence of type-2 diabetes is higher among non-Hispanic black women and Mexican American women than in non-Hispanic White women, with 4–6% of United States women older than 50 having undiagnosed diabetes [23]. This disease attacks nearly 10% of women older than 65 and 20% older than 80.

Early diagnosis is critical to prevent and delay the macro and microvascular complications of this disease. Macrovascular disease begins with impaired glucose tolerance, while microvascular disease begins with the onset of type-2 diabetes. The ADA recommends screening for women with one or more of the following risk factors: (1) obesity (BMI > 25 kg/m²), (2) minority-ethnicity (Hispanic American, Asian American, Pacific Islander, Native American, and African American), (3) family history of diabetes, (4) sedentary life style, (5) preeclampsia, (6) gestational diabetes mellitus (7) large for gestational age at birth, delivering a child equal to or greater than 9 pounds, (8) cigarette smoking, (9) high saturated fat diet, (10) polycystic ovary syndrome, and (11) dysmetabolic syndrome, also known as syndrome X or metabolic syndrome [24].

Prevention of Type-2 Diabetes

Several large scale clinical trials have been performed to evaluate the prevention of type-2 diabetes in women at high risk. In addition to the previously cited Diabetes Prevention Program Study, a Finnish trial randomized 522 obese women and men with BMIs exceeding 31 kg/m² to either intense training and dietary restriction or a less intense training program [25]. The mean rate reduction was 7% in the intensive group compared to 1% in the non-intensive group after 3.5 years, with a 58% reduction in the relative risk of type-2 diabetes in the weight loss group.

The Diabetes Prevention Program showed that therapeutic life style changes resulted in 58% risk reduction compared to 31% risk reduction with metformin [26]. The Troglitazone in the Prevention of Diabetes (TRIPOD) Study looked at obese women with a history of gestational diabetes mellitus treated with short term troglitazone after delivery and then followed for 2 years [27]. This trial was subsequently discontinued when troglitazone was removed from the market but resumed with pioglitazone as the Pioglitazone in Prevention of Diabetes (PIPOD) trial. The data here were impressive, indicating significant reduction in the risk of developing diabetes when these patients were placed on a thiazolidinedione. Hence, diet and exercise can play a critical role in the prevention of type-2 diabetes in women at risk for developing the disease.

Gestational Diabetes

Glucose intolerance, with the onset or first recognition during pregnancy, is referred to as gestational diabetes. Approximately 200,000 cases each year or 7% of all pregnancies are complicated by this condition [28]. It is customary to perform risk assessment testing during the first prenatal visit. Patients with family history of diabetes, marked obesity, previous history of gestational diabetes, and glucosuria are considered high risk and should receive glucose testing as soon as possible and retested if necessary at the 24 to the 28th week of pregnancy.

Patients considered at low risk who do not require glucose testing are younger than 25 years of age, normal weight before pregnancy, and with no known diabetes in first degree relatives, no history of abnormal glucose tolerance test or poor obstetric outcomes, or no ethnic predisposition [29].

Initial screening for this condition consists of plasma glucose measurement 1 h after the administration of a 50 g oral glucose load. If the 1-h glucose is equal to or greater than 140 mg/dl, then an oral glucose tolerance test should be performed using 75 g of glucose. Under these circumstances (75 g glucose load) a 1-h glucose equal to or greater than 180 mg/dl or a 2-h glucose equal to or greater than 155 mg/dl establishes a diagnosis of gestational diabetes [30].

It is important to diagnose gestational diabetes in women as there is an increased risk of fetal macrosomia, neonatal hypoglycemia, polycythemia, hypocalcemia, jaundice, and intrauterine fetal death along with maternal hypertension and increased need for cesarean deliveries with this condition and with women who are diabetic before becoming pregnant [31]. In addition, women who manifest gestational diabetes are at increased risk for development of type-2 diabetes after pregnancy, with a 50% incidence 10 years after delivery. These women should all undergo oral glucose tolerance test 6 weeks after delivery [32]. Thiazolidinedione therapy, weight loss, dietary changes, and exercise are all important to decrease the risk of developing type-2 diabetes.

Gestational diabetic patients have a 50% lifetime risk for developing type-2 diabetes, with the risk being increased with the degree of abnormality of postpartum glucose tolerance test, obesity, and gestational age at the time of diagnosis. Weight reduction, exercise, and diet are important aspects of therapy to correct lifestyle changes and prevent the onset of type-2 diabetes. Data from the TRIPOD and the subsequent PIPOD studies have suggested an encouraging role for pioglitazone in the prevention of diabetes in this patient population. However, this drug is currently not approved for this particular use.

At the 6 week post partum visit, patients who had gestational diabetes should be reevaluated with a 75-g, 2-h glucose tolerance test, although some centers are simply using a fasting glucose test.

MACROVASCULAR DISEASE

In the United States, more than 9 million women have diabetes with 10% in the type-1 category [33]. The association of diabetes with risk in women is so significant that this disease erases any protective female advantage for coronary heart disease. Initial reports in the Framingham study in 1979 demonstrated that men and women had a similar risk for coronary heart disease [34]. It is significant to note, however, that the risk for coronary heart disease in women with diabetes is five times the risk in women without diabetes. Regrettably, the prevalence of coronary heart disease mortality in women is also increasing. A review in the *Journal of the American Medical Association* in 1998 reported a 36% decline in coronary heart disease mortality in non-diabetic men compared to a 27% decline in women [35]. However, in diabetic women, there was an increase in coronary heart disease of 23%.

Not only are women with diabetes at a greater risk for coronary heart disease but they also experience more adverse outcomes after experiencing an acute cardiovascular event. Both early (28 days) and late (2 years) mortality are greater in women than in men with diabetes [36].

Various interrelated factors contribute to the acceleration of coronary heart disease risk in diabetic women. These include low social and economic status, higher rates of depression, central obesity, and more severe elevations in circulating lipids and blood pressure along with a greater tendency for poor glycemic control [37]. Wide fluctuations in range of glucose are a significant contributing factor for macro and microvascular disease complications in women with diabetes. Various factors can influence glycemic control in women including menstrual irregularity, insulin sensitivity, pregnancy, variability in glucose control throughout the perimenopausal period, a higher frequency of eating disorders, and use of hormonal contraception.

Low HDL cholesterol and high triglycerides clearly have a greater adverse impact on risk for vascular disease in women compared to men [38]. In addition, elevations in both systolic and diastolic blood pressure occur more frequently in diabetic women than in men, independent of body fat distribution, fasting insulin, age, or body weight.

The presence of hypertension increasingly aggravates the risk for vascular complications in diabetes [39]. In the United States, the majority of women with type-2 diabetes are overweight, and weight gain increases the risk for type-2 diabetes and coronary heart disease in women. Greater adverse metabolic risk profiles are associated with a waist to hip ratio greater than 0.76. This correlates even greater than the presence of gynecoid or peripheral obesity [40]. In addition, women with diabetes have a higher prevalence of depression and are more likely to be of a lower social economic status than individuals without diabetes.

The ADA currently recommends that all women greater than 45 years of age be screened with a fasting glucose test on a regular basis preferably yearly [41]. Individuals at high risk, who should be screened more frequently and at an earlier age, include those with a history of gestational diabetes or positive family history, or are members of racial or ethnic groups with high prevalence rates or obesity.

Those individuals with signs and symptoms consistent with the existence of polycystic ovary syndrome (acne, hirsutism, infertility, and irregular menses) are also at greater risk. This syndrome affects 5% of pre-menopausal women, 20% of whom have either overtly abnormal glucose tolerance or impaired glucose tolerance. Over 40% of these women are obese when presenting to their physicians [42].

The Diabetes Prevention Program stressed the importance of weight reduction and exercise to reduce the likelihood of developing diabetes and to improve overall glucose tolerance [43]. The use of metformin was effective to a lesser degree in women with a BMI greater than 35 kg/m^2.

Hence, all primary care providers should encourage their female patients to avoid sedentary behavior, and restrict fat intake and obesity. Institution of a regular exercise program consisting of 35 min of physical activity 3–4 times weekly has been associated with improved glucose tolerance and weight reduction in conjunction with a prudent dietary program.

Clinical trials have clearly demonstrated that it is not the intensity but the duration of exercise that is important [44]. In addition, multiple short periods of exercise in the form of brisk walking also produce beneficial cardiorespiratory fitness and weight loss. As diabetes is a coronary artery disease risk equivalent, medical management must stress reduction of all risk factors by including glycemic, lipid, and hypertension control, along with inhibition of platelet aggregation.

Randomized controlled clinical trials have shown that hormone replacement therapy carries no benefit either in primary or secondary prevention of cardiovascular disease.

An increase in overall cardiovascular disease events and combined endpoints in the Women's Health Initiative study [45] prompted early discontinuation, while a greater frequency of recurrent cardiovascular disease events in the Heart and Estrogen/Progestin Replacement Study (HERS) trial [46] in patients who were randomized to hormone replacement therapy compared to placebo during the first year highlighted the risks of hormone replacement therapy. In addition, in the Women's Angiographic Vitamin and Estrogen or WAVE trial [47], cardiovascular benefits were not demonstrated with hormone replacement therapy in postmenopausal women with established coronary disease but rather an increase in cardiovascular events was seen.

In the HERS trial, hormone replacement therapy did reduce the incidence of diabetes by 35%. However, despite this observation, hormone replacement therapy is not recommended for any woman with or without diabetes as part of a therapeutic strategy for the primary or secondary prevention of coronary heart disease [48].

It should also be noted that diabetic patients who have had a myocardial infarction increase their risk of a second infarction by 45%. Data from Molberg, published in Circulation in 1999 from the Diabetes Mellitus, Insulin-Glucose Infusion in Acute Myocardial Infarction (DIGAMI) trial revealed that 232 women admitted to the hospital with acute myocardial infarction improved survival up to 3.4 years after discharge with the early institution of intensive insulin therapy [49]. In this study, admission blood glucose levels were the strongest predictor of a fatal outcome. It has also been established that beta-blockers improve long term survival and decrease the risk of recurrent myocardial infarction both in diabetic and in non-diabetic individuals [50].

In 1999, Chen reported statistically significant differences in 1 year mortality for insulin and non-insulin dependent diabetic patients given beta-blockers compared to those not given beta-blockers after sustaining a myocardial infarction [51]. In the Glycemic Effects in Diabetes Mellitus (GEMINI) trial, the alpha/beta-blocker carvedilol was shown to be superior to metoprolol in terms of its lipid and microalbuminuric lowering effects in diabetic patients [52].

Screening for Coronary Heart Disease

According to the ADA Consensus Development Conference, stress testing should be performed in any individuals with diabetes who meet one of the following criteria [53]: (1) resting electrocardiogram suggestive of ischemia or infarction, (2) peripheral or carotid occlusive disease, (3) typical or atypical cardiac symptoms, (4) age equal to or greater than 35 years, planning a vigorous exercise program, and (5) two or more risk factors in addition to diabetes including total cholesterol greater than 240 mg/dl, HDL cholesterol less than 35 mg/dl, LDL cholesterol greater than 160 mg/dl, blood pressure greater than 140/90 mmHg, smoking, positive test for micro or macroalbuminuria, and family history of premature coronary disease. It is important to note that women have a higher rate of false/positive exercise stress tests than men, and a negative exercise stress test also has a lower negative predictive value. Hence, perfusion imaging, in combination with exercise testing, improves the accuracy in women. Symptoms of coronary artery disease in women tend to be different than in men, with shortness of breath and fatigue being more prevalent than chest discomfort [54]. The clinician should have a high index of suspicion in the diabetic female patient to enhance discovery of underlying ischemic heart disease.

Other Complications of Diabetes in Women

The genitourinary tract is significantly affected by diabetes in women [55]. Acute urinary tract infections have a positive correlation with increased glucose levels. The female diabetic patient is more prone to lower urinary tract infections as a result of recurrent vaginitis, diabetic microangiopathy, renal vascular disease, impaired leukocyte function, and diabetic neuropathy associated with neurogenic bladder or urinary retention [56].

Asymptomatic bacteriuria and structural abnormalities of the urinary tract are more common in women with diabetes and are more likely to be associated with significant upper urinary tract disease. Because of the risk of ascending infection, non-pregnant women with diabetes, as well as pregnant patients, should be treated for asymptomatic bacteriuria. Symptomatic pyelonephritis is 4–5 times more common in diabetic women vs. their non-diabetic counterparts. In addition, cystourethroceles and rectoceles are more common in women with diabetes as a result of vascular compromise and/or recurrent vaginitis [57]. Female patients should be educated about the importance of frequent voiding and complete emptying of the bladder with appropriate attention to even minor symptoms of a urological disorder.

Infections

The most common infections in female patients with diabetes are of urinary tract, respiratory tract, and skin [58]. Colonization and overgrowth of organisms can present a significant problem in the female patient, with group D streptococcal infections being more common in diabetic women. Anaerobic infections are much more likely, predisposing the patient to abscess formation, emphesematous complications, and necrotizing soft tissue infections because of defects in polymorphonuclear leukocytes and vascular compromise [59]. Localized soft tissue infections in the form of furuncles, impetigo, carbuncles, and cellulitis due to staph and beta-hemolytic strep are also commonly found in diabetic women. Vulvar abscesses in diabetics must be considered necrotizing fasciitis until proven otherwise. Any vulvar abscesses, cellulitis, or postoperative wound infections need to be aggressively evaluated and treated [60].

Gynecological Abnormalities

Recently, there has been a trend toward a higher incidence of condylomata acuminata in patients with diabetes but few definitive perspective data exist as of this time [61]. In addition, it is believed that human papilloma virus (HPV) may also be more prevalent in women with diabetes [62]. Vulvovaginal candidiasis is also increased in the diabetic women. Hyperglycemia increases the risk of candidiasis, in addition to high estrogen states, and use of antibiotics and systemic glucocorticoids. Hence, proper patient education about the appropriate undergarments and avoidance of tight clothes, such as pantyhose, should be considered.

In a study of women with diabetes with and without symptoms of vulvovaginal candidiasis, *Candida glabrata* was isolated most frequently (50% of cases) followed by *Candida albicans* (35%) [63]. The best in-office test for diagnosing vulvovaginal candidiasis is microscopy, but this can lack accuracy, missing up to 50% of cases, especially with *Candida glabrata*, which tends to lack hyphae formation.

Hence, the obtaining of proper cultures, in investigating not only recurrent infections, but also treatment failures, is important in managing this condition. Fortunately, topical imidazoles and triazoles are associated with cure rates of about 85–90%, although *Candida glabrata* and *Candida tropicalis* are less sensitive to standard imidazol antifungals [*64*]. Oral anti-mycotic agents can also be used for these infections. In type I diabetics, menarche age is increased by approximately 1 year, with irregular menses common especially in the face of uncontrolled diabetes. The prevalence of menstrual irregularities in the diabetic population can be twice that of controlled subjects. Cyclical changes occur in insulin and glucose requirements during the menstrual cycle, with variations of insulin dosages to achieve glycemic control occasionally demonstrating inconsistent results.

Risk Reduction in the Female Diabetic Patient

Only a comprehensive program of overall risk reduction can achieve optimal results in diabetic women. This includes careful attention to hypertension, dyslipidemia, hyperglycemia, and platelet aggregation. Antihypertensive therapy with an ACE inhibitor or angiotensin receptor blocker is indicated for patients with diabetes and blood pressures greater than 130/80 mmHg or microalbuminuria [*65*]. The Heart Outcomes Prevention Evaluation Study (HOPE) trial demonstrated the efficacy of ramipril in reducing the risk for myocardial infarction, stroke, and overall cardiovascular mortality and morbidity, and revascularization in individuals with diabetes greater than 55 years of age [*66*]. Women of child bearing age, who are not using contraception, should be warned about the harmful effects to developing fetuses of ACE inhibitor or angiotensin receptor blocker use and should discontinue these agents immediately on becoming pregnant. For lipid control, a target LDL cholesterol should be less than 100 mg/dl, with HDLs greater than 55 mg/dl in diabetic women.

Data from several large lipid lowering trials indicate the benefits of statin therapy in diabetic women with coronary disease [*67*]. There are relative risk reductions from 24 to 34% in non-diabetic women and 19–42% in the presence of diabetes. Hemoglobin A1C should be less than 6.5%, with postprandial sugars less than 140 mg/dl and fasting sugars less than 100 mg/dl. It is to be understood that the pursuit of the optimal A1C represents a continuum goal below 6.5% – not a threshold at this value.

The UKPDS demonstrated a 14% reduction in the risk for coronary heart disease for each 1% reduction in A1C, even below 6.5% [*68*]. In addition, an independent association in women has been described between A1C and the prevalence of coronary heart disease.

Aspirin therapy is indicated for diabetic individuals greater than 21 years of age to attenuate vasoconstriction and inhibit platelet aggregation [*69*]. The current recommendation is 160–325 mg of aspirin daily for type 2 diabetic patients, unless contraindicated by recent gastrointestinal bleeding, bleeding tendencies, or allergies. In the Hypertension Optimal Treatment (HOT) trial, 75 mg of aspirin daily reduced pooled cardiovascular risk by 15% and myocardial infarction by 36% [*70*]. In diabetic patients who have had a myocardial infarction or stroke, low doses can be as effective as high doses and can reduce cardiovascular events by as much as 25%.

In those patients who are allergic to aspirin, clopidogrel (Plavix) may be substituted. The Clopidogrel vs. Aspirin in Patients at Risk for Ischemic Events (CAPRIE) trial, showed clopidogrel to be equally effective as 325 mg of aspirin in reducing the risk of vascular death, ischemic stroke, or myocardial infarction [71]. Sub-analysis of the diabetic cohort in this trial showed clopidogrel to be particularly effective in patients with peripheral vascular disease.

The importance of addressing all four risk factors in the diabetic population was shown in the Steno-II trial which enrolled 160 patients with type-2 diabetes and microalbuminuria [72]. Patients with an average age of 55 years were placed in an intensive therapy group and a conventional therapy group. In the intensive group, all had ACE inhibitors, dietary intervention, aspirin, more than 30 min of exercise weekly, tight glucose control with A1C's less than 6.5, blood pressures less than 130/80 mmHg, total cholesterol less than 175 mg/dl, and triglycerides less than 150 mg/dl in addition to smoking-cessation.

Outcomes in the intensive strategy group were consistently better than that from the conventionally managed group, with primary outcomes of composite cardiovascular death, nonfatal myocardial infarction, coronary revascularization, nonfatal stroke, amputation, or peripheral vascular surgery reduced by 53% in the intensive strategy group, with neuropathy being reduced by 61%, retinopathy by 58%, and autonomic neuropathy by 3%.

PREGNANCY AND DIABETES

Because of the continuing increase in type-2 diabetes in adolescents and young adults, physicians should be aware that diabetes can present in three ways in the pregnant woman: (1) gestational diabetes in a woman who has never had diabetes before but develops hyperglycemia during pregnancy, (2) the known type-2 diabetic patient on oral agents and/or insulin who becomes pregnant, and (3) the type 1 diabetic patient.

The presence of diabetes enhances pregnancy risks, with increased risk of delivering a stillborn infant, caesarian delivery, complicated vaginal delivery (forceps or vacuum extraction), congenital malformations, neonatal hypoglycemia, fetal macrosomia with birth weights greater than 9 pounds, and shoulder dystocia as a result of entrapment of the fetal shoulder under the mother's pelvic bone. For those women who are diabetic before they become pregnant, prenatal care begins with glycemic control which reduces risk to the mother and the fetus.

With the management of other concomitant conditions, if present, like peripheral vascular disease, hypertension, and heart disease, it is also important to reduce pregnancy related complications. These may include the following:

1. Diabetic neuropathy – Treatment, here, may be largely ineffective and limited because of neonatal and fetal risks. The course of the ailment may be uncertain, with aggravation of carpal tunnel syndrome and lower extremity neuropathies being the most prevalent and tending to improve after delivery.
2. Diabetic nephropathy – The severity of hypertension and baseline renal function play an important role in the risk of worsening diseases. Microalbuminuria may worsen during pregnancy and improve postpartum with up to 45% developing preeclampsia. Doubling of the total urinary protein in a 24 h collection may occur. When proteinuria >300 mg/24 h is present at the inception of pregnancy with normal glomerular filtration rates (GFRs) and creatinine clearance >80 ml/min, 6% of women will develop renal failure several years after delivery, with 25–20% showing renal function decline during pregnancy. This pattern may not be drastically different from the non-pregnant diabetic patients with similar data. However, if renal function is abnormal at the beginning of pregnancy with creatinine clearances <80 ml/min, then up to 40% will show further decline during pregnancy while 50% will develop renal failure over the next several years.

3. Diabetic retinopathy – Background retinopathy may develop or worsen during pregnancy and usually improves or regresses postpartum. Risk factors for progression to neovascularization and proliferative retinopathy include hypertension, poor glycemic control during pregnancy, and the combined effects of growth factors secreted during pregnancy. When background retinopathy is present at the outset of pregnancy, the rate of progression to proliferative retinopathy depends on the severity of the retinopathy at baseline. The more severe the retinopathy, the higher the risk of progression is – with rates of progression varying from 6% with mild baseline background retinopathy to 38% with severe baseline retinopathy. Regular ophthalmologic examinations are critical during the course of the pregnancy, with some patients requiring laser photocoagulation.

As pregnancy enhances insulin resistance, women with type 2 diabetes may require insulin during this time even if they did not take insulin prior to pregnancy, while those already taking insulin require adjustment of their insulin doses. Even some women who have gestational diabetes may require insulin during their pregnancy.

In the United States, diabetes is found in 4% of all pregnant women, with 88% of these having gestational diabetes and the remaining 12% being either type 1 or type 2 [73]. Before 1940, diabetic women who became pregnant were faced with a substantial risk of congenital anomalies, perinatal mortality, and miscarriage as well as diabetic ketoacidosis and preeclampsia. With the development of insulin and the evolution of its use, creation and development of blood glucose monitors, and an enhanced knowledge of diabetes management in women during pregnancy, these risks have been decreased so that most women who are or become diabetic, can experience successful pregnancy, gestational development, and delivery. Nonetheless, fetal growth and development abnormalities do occur. As listed in Table 1, these include the following:

1. Fetal macrosomia – Even in controlled diabetic mothers, many newborns and fetuses are too large for their birth dates, with increased thorax or abdomen-to-head ratios and increased length due to increased fat stores. This process is set in motion with maternal hyperglycemia which causes fetal hyperglycemia resulting in fetal hyperinsulinemia which stimulates enhanced weight and size, with high fetal C-peptide levels in the amniotic fluid or cord sera. In addition other transplacental substrates may contribute to macrosomia such as the insulinogenic branched chain amino acids and lipids. Women with mean postprandial glucose levels in excess of 130 mg/dl show increase in the risk of macrosomia and birth trauma, while average postprandial glucose levels <110 mg/dl may result in small-for-date infants and impaired fetal growth.
2. Polyhydramnos – Excess volume of amniotic fluid >1,000 cc may cause significant discomfort or premature delivery and is often associated with fetal macrosomia. Several factors may be

Table 1
Fetal growth and developmental abnormalities in the gravid diabetic patient [98]

Fetal macrosomia

Polyhydramnos

Neural tube defects

Impaired growth

Intrauterine death

Birth defects

involved including amniotic fluid prolactin, glucose concentration in the amniotic fluid, excess fetal urine output, decreased fetal swallowing, and other unknown factors controlling intrauterine water transfer. This problem can be significantly abrogated with well controlled diabetes.

3. Neural tube defects – Infants of poorly controlled diabetic mothers have a higher incidence of neural tube defects (meningomyelocele, spina bifida, or anencephaly) which can usually be detected by ultrasound within the first 20 weeks of gestation. Elevated alpha-fetoprotein levels can be usually found at 14–16 weeks with this anomaly. Ultrasound examinations at 18–22 weeks are needed to detect congential heart deformities, with fetal growth and development being assessed by ultrasound at 26 and 36 week periods.

4. Impaired growth – Women with long standing diabetes and vascular disorders may harbor a fetus with significant growth restriction due to insufficient placental perfusion. Oligohydramnos and poor Doppler flow measurements are usually seen. Tight blood pressure and glycemic controls are imperative along with close fetal surveillance.

5. Intrauterine death – The incidence of fetal death is greater than 50% with maternal ketoacidosis and is also increased with preeclampsia, eclampsia, and pyelonephritis. Fetal hypoxia and hyperglycemia promote acidosis and a dysfunctional myocardium. Once again, glycemic control plays an important role in reducing risk.

6. Birth defects – Although perinatal deaths due to respiratory distress syndrome and still births have declined since 1970 when the rate was 5%, the incidence of fetal anomalies, including those incompatible with life, has risen to 50%.

The commonest congenital malformations seen in infants of diabetic mothers include caudal regression, situs inversus, renal anomalies (duplicated ureter, agenesis, cystic kidney), cardiac anomalies (ventricular septal defect, atrial septal defect, and transposition of great vessels), anencephaly, and spina bifida. These are all correlated with elevated A1C levels early in pregnancy [74].

Because of the continuing obstacles faced by the gravid patient with diabetes, effective management of hyperglycemia and appropriate counseling with the challenges of pregnancy are essential. It should be appreciated that the pregnant state and its production of human placental lactogen and human chorionic gonadotropin impair the sensitivity to insulin action resulting in enhanced insulin resistance. This can result in the development of type 2 diabetes in a woman who already has impaired insulin resistance and marginal insulin reserve.

Gestational diabetes usually does not develop until the second or third trimester of pregnancy as placental hormones increase with placental size. Women who have had diabetes before becoming pregnant with enhanced resistance will have increased insulin requirements during pregnancy and may even require insulin while their disease was managed either with diet or oral agents prior to pregnancy. Type-1 patients will also experience an enhanced need for insulin because of the glycemic effect of the placental hormones.

The subsequent gradual increase in placental function and size occurring in the second and third trimester may require weekly adjustments in insulin regimens since glucose is readily diffusable across the placenta; fetal hyperglycemia can result in complications both in utero and neonatally with compensatory fetal hyperinsulinemia, enhanced fat distribution in the fetal trunk, and subsequent larger size, decreasing the likelihood of vaginal birth. The fetus is also at risk for developing hypoglycemia because of enhanced insulin levels at birth [75].

It is important to appreciate that glycemic control during pregnancy will substantially reduce fetal neonatal risk, while 4 mg of folic acid is recommended not only throughout the first trimester but also prior to gestation for the diabetic mother to reduce the risk of neural tube defects and fetal abnormalities.

The initial step in normalizing glycemic control begins prior to conception for any diabetic woman as the risk for congenital anomalies and spontaneous abortion is increased during the first trimester of pregnancy for a woman with an elevated A1C, with the risk being 3–6 times greater in a woman whose A1C values are greater than 8.0% compared to a woman with lower values.

Poor glycemic control is likely to result in fetal macrosomia with birth weights more than 4 kg (10 pounds), in addition to enhanced risk for intrauterine fetal death which is increased in all patients with pre-gestational diabetes and enhanced in a milieu of poor glycemic control during the gestational period increasing the risks of preeclampsia, neonatal jaundice, and respiratory distress syndrome. Should the patient also develop nephropathy or hypertension in addition to poor glycemic control, low birth weight may result. In addition, the children of a diabetic woman experience an enhanced risk of insulin resistance, carbohydrate intolerance, and obesity – especially those with low birth weight and small size at birth [76].

It is important that a multi disciplinary approach be used in managing these patients, involving a certified diabetes educator, obstetrician, dietician, ophthalmologist, and primary care provider or endocrinologist.

Women who are diabetic (either type 1 or type 2) before becoming pregnant, have an increased risk of delivering children with skeletal abnormalities, renal disturbances (renal dysplasia and renal malformation), neural tube defects (anencephaly and spinal bifida), gastrointestinal abnormalities (abdominal wall defects and intestinal atresia), and cardiovascular disturbances (tricuspid atresia, trunk arteriosus, and transposition of the great vessels).

The United States Preventative Services Task Force supports universal screening in all pregnant patients, with approximately 94% of providers in the United States providing diabetic screening to their pregnant patients [77]. Some controversy still exists as to whether a 50-g glucose loading test or 100-g, 3-h glucose tolerance test should be used and what the cut off values should be.

The American College of Obstetricians and Gynecologists recommends a 50-g, 1-h glucose loading test for its practicality [32]. Using a threshold abnormality of 140 mg/dl with this 50-g glucose loading test, a 13% screening positivity will be achieved and 80% of gestational diabetics would be diagnosed. On lowering the threshold to 135 mg/dl, 98% of gestational diabetes can be diagnosed, with approximately 20% of patients screening positive. One hundred percent can be achieved using a screening value of 130 mg/dl, with 22% of individuals screening positive.

In addition, it should be noted that the testing and results may differ among certain ethnic groups, with 135 mg/dl having 95% sensitivity among African American women and with a somewhat lower value of 130–133 mg/dl for women of other ethnicities. By setting a goal at 140 mg/dl, the false positive rate can be reduced to less than 10% for White women while a goal of 135 mg/dl is set for African American women [78].

In general, the higher the cutoff rate is set, the greater the specificity is and the lower the sensitivity becomes. In women who have already been gestationally diabetic and are now presenting with prenatal care with another pregnancy, the 3-h oral glucose tolerance test using 100 g of anhydrous glucose should be used. This test should be performed after an overnight fast of 8–14 h with a 3 day unrestricted diet of greater than 150 g of carbohydrates per day.

The following are the normal thresholds: fasting glucose <95 mg/dl; 1 h <180 mg/dl; 2 h <155 mg/dl; and 3 h <140 mg/dl. A positive diagnosis of diabetes is made when two or more of these values are equal or exceeded. Risk factors for gestational diabetes include a prior macrosomic fetus, non-White ethnicity, obesity with a BMI greater than 25 kg/m^2, increased maternal age greater than 25 years, a prior history of gestational diabetes, a history of abnormal glucose tolerance, and a family history of type 2 diabetes in a first degree relative. Given the variability of the glucose loading test, most clinicians will use a threshold of 135 mg/dl providing 98% sensitivity.

The management of the pregnant woman involves self monitoring of blood glucose, diet, exercise, and education. Ideally, glucose levels should be measured in the fasting state and following each meal, with glycemic levels of less than 95 mg/dl in the fasting state and less than 140 mg/dl 1 h postprandially and 120 mg/dl 2 h postprandially. Ideally, carbohydrate counting can be an important point of management, with carbohydrate intake ranging from 30 45 g at breakfast to 45–60 g at lunch and dinner, with a 15–30 g evening snack. A simple 15 min walk after each meal will enhance postprandial glycemic control.

Exercise certainly is good therapy for expectant mothers – especially diabetic mothers. Current recommendations by the 2008 Physical Activity guidelines for Americans include the following: (1) at least 2 h and 30 min of moderate intensity aerobic activity per week for those women who are not regularly exercising, and (2) women already engaging themselves in regular vigorous physical or aerobic activity should exercise as long as their physical condition remains unchanged, but only with ongoing guidance from their health care professional [74].

A fetal ultrasound is often performed at 36 weeks of gestation to determine the presence of macrosomia, offering the patient an option for labor induction. However, it should be appreciated that induction can be associated with lower birth rates and has not been shown to reduce the risk of caesarian delivery. To achieve the desired glycemic controls, subcutaneous insulin is the standard of care. Although insulin overdose may lead to hypoglycemia in the pregnant woman, insulin itself does not cross the placental barrier. The metabolic problems and the increased fetal weight are due largely to complications of hyperglycemia, as glucose will traverse the placenta, stimulating insulin release within the fetus. Unless maternal or fetal complications arise in the interim, the delivery date goal should be 38–41 weeks to reduce neonatal morbidity. During labor, glucose values should be checked every 2 h with insulin administered preferably in a drip for values greater than 120 mg/dl.

Multiple acceptable insulin regimens exist and it is the judgment of the clinician and the efficacy of that regimen that determine which approach will be used. Some physicians utilize longer acting insulins like neutral protemine hagadorn (NPH) at bedtime supplemented by analog insulins to control post prandial hyperglycemia. Even regular insulin with its 30 min onset and 2 h peak can be more challenging to use than the analog insulin lispro. Although glargine and detimir insulin with their continuous long acting duration may be somewhat appealing to these patients, the lack of safety data for approval for use in the gestational diabetic patient reduces their role, if any, at this time.

Of the oral agents available, the alpha-glucosidase agents (acarbos and miglitol), glyburide, and DPP-IV inhibitors, saxagliptin and sitagliptin, as well as metformin extended release are all listed as category B. When glyburide was compared with conventional insulin therapy in 404 patients with gestational diabetes, there was no difference in neonatal outcomes [75]. Although there appeared to be a trend toward an increase in neonatal complications in the glyburide treated group, the study, however, was underpowered to actually demonstrate a difference between the two groups.

Jacobson reported one study of 584 women initially managed with insulin vs. glyburide [76]. In this study, there were higher rates of phototherapy use and preeclampsia in the neonates with no difference in birth weight. Mothers treated with glyburide have also demonstrated an increased risk of neonatal hyperglycemia and macrosomia, with approximately 20% of women treated with glyburide achieving satisfactory glycemic control.

Metformin will cross the placenta and should be avoided during pregnancy despite the fact that metformin extended release carries a Category B designation. A recent review in the *New England Journal of Medicine* compared metformin and insulin for the treatment of gestational diabetes [79]. This study randomized 751 women at 20–33 weeks of gestation to open treatment with either insulin or metformin, which could be supplemented with insulin if required. The primary outcome was a composite of birth trauma, need for further therapy, 5 min Apgar score less than 7, prematurity, neonatal hypoglycemia, or respiratory distress. Secondary outcomes included postpartum glucose tolerance, maternal glycemic control, maternal hypertensive complications, neonatal anthropometric measurements, and acceptability of treatment. The trial was designed to rule out a 33% increase in composite outcomes in women treated with metformin compared with those treated with insulin.

In this study, 363 women were assigned metformin with 46.3% receiving supplemental insulin and 92.6% continuing to receive metformin until delivery. The rate of primary composite outcome was 32.0% in the metformin group and 32.2% in the insulin group with a 95% confidence interval. Secondary outcomes did not differ significantly between the groups and no serious adverse events were associated with the metformin group. In addition, more women preferred metformin to the insulin treatment alone.

This study demonstrated that there was no increase in perinatal complications with metformin use compared to insulin in women with gestational diabetes. In addition, cord serum in the metformin group did not demonstrate a reduction in insulin concentration; however, these data were only available for half of the participants. Although the frequency of preterm birth was somewhat higher in the metformin group than in the insulin group, this was felt to be due to the rate of frequency of spontaneous rather than iatrogenic circumstances. Although the unrecognized effect of metformin on the labor process cannot be completely ruled out, this preterm birth rate increase was not associated with a higher rate of other complications.

In addition, in this particular study, there was no significant difference between those who required supplemental insulin and those who received metformin alone. However, those women who received combined treatment with insulin and metformin gained less weight and required less insulin than those taking insulin alone. It should be noted, however, that this trial was not blinded and was open labeled. Nonetheless, a 95% confidence interval suggests an increase in risk of less than 10% with metformin therapy and a post partum analysis supported the conclusion that metformin was inferior to insulin. Although these data are encouraging, further follow-up data are necessary with repeated trials, and analysis of the offspring. Long term safety data with metformin in this patient population are needed.

A review by Langer and others viewed 404 women with gestational diabetes demonstrating similar glycemic control of pregnancy outcomes in glyburide and insulin treated groups [*80*]. This trial, however, was not empowered to address neonatal complications. .

Another controversy centers on the elective Caesarian delivery in women with pregestational or gestational diabetes to prevent brachial plexus and shoulder injuries caused by vaginal delivery. The American College of Obstetrics and Gynecology suggests that an elective Caesarian is reasonable with fetal weights at 5.0 kg or greater [*81*]. A patient with diabetes has the same risk of delivering a child with shoulder dystocia as a non-diabetic patient with a fetus whose birth weight is 250 g higher. Hence, there are some who advocate a threshold of 4.2 kg to reduce the risk of brachial plexus injury. Maternal glucose levels greater than 150 mg/dl can be associated with intrapartum fetal hypoxia.

With the collaborative effort of the patient, physician, and physician extenders, diabetes during pregnancy have complications less than in the distant past. Although patient management is still clinically challenging, the desired goal of a healthy pregnancy and subsequent delivery is currently more achievable.

Summary

Early detection of diabetes in women is essential to prevent serious complications, with improved mortality and morbidity accomplished by aggressively controlling the multiple risk factors underlying the disease. It is only with this aggressive multifaceted approach that better survival and improved life quality can be achieved.

THE GERIATRIC PATIENT

In the 1999 and 2000 National Health and Nutritional Examination survey, 809 American adults greater than 65 years of age demonstrated a prevalence of undiagnosed diabetes in 6.9% and a prevalence of diagnosed diabetes of 15.3%. In the United States, over 50% of diabetics are greater than 60 years of age while 39.4% of type-2 diabetics are diagnosed at age 65 or older [*82*]. Prevalence of type-2 diabetes peaks between 65 and 74 years of age, while those individuals who had their diabetes diagnosed between the ages of 40 and 64 have a similar incidence of macrovascular disease but a greater incidence of microvascular disease and higher A1Cs than individuals who had their onset of diabetes at greater than age 65. In addition, those individuals with onset of diabetes after 65 years of age are less likely to receive oral medications, insulin, or both compared to those individuals who were diagnosed between the ages of 40 and 64. The prevalence of type-2 diabetes and metabolic syndrome increases with advancing age with the peak incidence of metabolic syndrome between 60 and 69 years of age, because of several factors including age related alterations in carbohydrate metabolism, decreased responsiveness of the beta cells to incretin hormones, impaired insulin response to glucose, and deficiencies in glucose disposal [*83*]. Coexisting illnesses, inflammatory conditions, medications, and age related obesity may also contribute to glucose intolerance. The lean, elderly diabetic patient exhibits impairments in glucose mediated insulin release, while the elderly, obese patient demonstrates insulin resistance. On rare occasions, islet cell antibodies may even be seen in lean individuals who develop latent autoimmune diabetes (LADA).

In addition, the glucagon response to hypoglycemia may be impaired in elderly individuals making them more prone to severe and even fatal reactions because of impairments in awareness of autonomic warning symptoms.

Previously, there were no clear cut screening recommendations for diabetes in individuals greater than 65 years of age who did not demonstrate classic symptoms of the disease. As diabetes has a serious impact on the quality of life in individuals in this age group, it is vital that primary care physicians screen aggressively for the onset of this disease, encourage therapeutic lifestyle changes, and prescribe medications that can delay or prevent the development of diabetes. Glycemic control is only one of many considerations in managing the care for those individuals over 60 years of age with type-2 diabetes. Compared to those who do not have diabetes, physiologic changes and the aging process may occur at a faster rate, enhancing the potential for earlier decline in functional and cognitive capacity and an increased risk of cataracts, hip fractures, infections, accelerated arteriosclerotic vascular disease, myocardial infarction, and stroke.

Hyperglycemia accelerates aging by generating the production of advanced glycation end products, oxidative stress, and vascular inflammation, while the physiologic age of a person with diabetes is 10 years more than the chronological age. Risk reduction principles include glycemic, lipid, and hypertension control, and minimizing prothrombotic and inflammatory factors.

Although individuals with a family history of diabetes are more likely to develop the illness as they grow older, the development of type 2 diabetes in the elderly patient is clearly a combination of psychologic, environmental, and genetic factors. Individuals who are inactive or obese and consume diets high in fat and low in complex carbohydrates have increased risk.

It is also important to appreciate that many patients may be given medications to treat hypertension or other disease states that may aggravate glycemic control promoting insulin resistance. Hence, proper monitoring of *all* medications (prescribed and not prescribed) including supplements and over the counter items is vital. Curiously, the older type-2 diabetic patients are less likely to have an increase in hepatic glucose output and are more prone to have impaired and dysregulated glucose metabolism with decreased insulin production and secretion compared to their middle aged counterparts. Older, leaner individuals demonstrate essentially normal insulin activity with significant impairment in glucose induced insulin secretion.

Because of these differences in the diabetic paradigm according to the age of onset of the disease, therapeutic approaches may be somewhat different. Patients diagnosed in middle age should be getting therapy that enhances insulin sensitivity along with medications that stimulate insulin secretion. The older, lean type-2 diabetic patients benefit from exogenous insulin or drugs that stimulate insulin secretion. Quite often, in patients greater than 65 years of age, the classic symptoms of hyperglycemia are not present and the condition is often diagnosed with a random blood test or the patient experiences a macrovascular complication. In addition, older patients with diabetes are more prone to manifesting urinary tract infections that can lead to acute papillary necrosis, necrotizing papillitis, hyperthermia, malignant otis externa, diabetic peripheral neuropathy, depression, and painful asymmetric weakness of the pelvic girdle muscles (diabetic amyotrophy). Because of the enhanced risk of hypoglycemia in the elderly patient population, short acting secretagogues like nateglinide, alpha-glucosidase inhibitors, and even reduced doses of DPP-4 inhibitors should be tried initially to minimize the risk of hypoglycemia. Metformin, alone or in combination with a secretagogue, can also be effective, provided that renal function is normal and the patient does not have a history of any disease process that generates acidosis (i.e., congestive heart failure, cor pulmonale, or liver disease).

Not to be underemphasized is the importance of therapeutic lifestyle changes as early as possible, as 25% of older individuals will demonstrate impaired glucose tolerance, with the risk of vascular complications increasing according to the duration of illness and the age of the patient. Glucose monitoring is a valuable tool to enhance glycemic control and is of particular value in the postprandial period, giving patients some insight as to the effect of their food intake on blood glucose.

Patients in this age group often have other particular challenges that include visual impairment, complex and worsening social situations, co-morbid medical conditions, and multiple medications. The benefit of tight glycemic control (A1C less than 7.0%) is extremely controversial in this patient population and may increase the risk of macrovascular complications of the disease, especially in individuals with multiple co-morbidities.

It is also important to understand that compared with community dwelling patients, the elderly nursing home diabetic patient may have a higher risk of renal disease, skin infections, nosocomial pneumonia, and macrovascular complications. These patients are more likely to develop urinary and soft tissue infections compared with their non-diabetic nursing home residents. Patients greater than 65 years of age with diabetes usually die of macrovascular disease complications at twice the rate of age matched controls who are non-diabetic [84].

With the presence of diabetes being one of the strongest predictors of functional decline, a poorer life quality is usually in the offing. The risk of micro and macrovascular complications increases with the age of the patient compared to non-diabetic controls. These risks are enhanced by the presence of co-morbid conditions like hypertension and dyslipidemia and enhanced by unhealthy lifestyles like cigarette smoking.

Advancing age also enhances the risk of severe or even fatal hypoglycemia as a result of the impaired secretion of counterregulatory hormones like glucagon. Impairments in psychomotor performance during a hypoglycemic attack reduce awareness of hypoglycemic symptoms and impair the patient's ability to rectify the low blood glucose. In addition, reduced cognitive performance and higher incidence of depression have been demonstrated in this patient population greater than 65 years of age.

Improvements in cognitive function have been reported with better glycemic control in this age population. However, further studies are needed to address the question on how to improve glycemic control and reduce risk for dementia in this age group. The Study to Prevent Non-Insulin Dependent Diabetes Mellitus (STOP – NIDDM) demonstrated that macrovascular events, as well as the incidence of diabetes, were reduced with the alpha-glucosidase inhibitor, acarbose.

Although agents like the TZDs and metformin have been effective in other studies in reducing the development of diabetes, their efficacy for this purpose in this age group has not been clearly demonstrated. They should only be used with caution because of an increased risk of congestive heart failure with TZD use and decreased renal function with the use of metformin.

The American Diabetes Association's diagnostic criteria for diabetes are not adjusted for age. Patients considered at risk or with suspicious elevations in random blood glucose should be given an oral glucose tolerance test. Although it is generally believed that blood glucose should be reduced in the elderly patient population, there is no data from randomized control trials, similar to the DCCT or UKPDS trials, indicating a reduction in long term complications with improved glycemic control. However, prospective studies have suggested improvement in neuropsychological function and a reduced risk in vascular complications. Studies like ACCORD and ADVANCE seem to indicate that cautious prudence should be exercised in lowering blood glucose particularly in those individuals at very high risk.

In general, the best predictor of outcomes in the older patient is the postprandial glucose test, but further studies would be needed to determine whether the focus should be on pre- or post-prandial blood glucose in this patient population. Risk factor modification is an essential part of management of the elderly diabetic patients, with angiotensin receptor blockers, angiotensin converting enzyme inhibitors, calcium channel blockers, and judicious use of low dose thiazide diuretics reducing the risk for major cardiovascular events.

Use of renin inhibitor agents like aliskiren in this patient population remains to be determined although encouraging results have been seen, particularly when this agent is used in combination with an ACE inhibitor or an angiotensin receptor blocker in both hypertension control and reduction of proteinuria. However, careful monitoring of renal function and ser potassium is necessary.

A recent review comparing miglitol with glyburide in this patient population demonstrated lower A1Cs with glyburide but a higher incidence of cardiovascular events, greater weight gain, and hypoglycemia [85]. Acarbose has also been shown to effectively reduce postprandial glucose in the elderly patient. Major side effects of these alpha-glucosidase inhibitors (miglitol and acarbose) are gastrointestinal and further studies are indicated to determine efficacy in the elderly patient.

Thiazolinediones should not be used in patients who have Class 3 or 4 heart failure, particularly in the elderly patient with significant valvular disease or diastolic dysfunction. When used judiciously, these agents can be effective in improving glycemic control in the elderly patient population. This patient group particularly should be observed closely for the presence of fluid retention. Because of the enhanced cardiovascular risks associated with rosiglitazone, pioglitazone is the thiazolidinedione of choice.

Both glipizide and glimepiride may be safer than glyburide in the elderly patient when a sulfonylurea is indicated as the use of glyburide can be associated with an increased risk of severe or fatal hypoglycemia because of its longer duration of action and active hepatic metabolites that are excreted renally. Glipizide, in particular, can be effective in those patients who have decreased renal function.

In general, the glinides (nateglinide and repaglinide) have a lower frequency of hypoglycemia in the aging population than glyburide, with nateglinide being the least likely to cause hypoglycemia. Further studies in this patient population are needed to confirm the therapeutic relevance of these agents, but they do remain attractive because of their rapid onset and relatively short duration of action, particularly in the case of nateglinide.

It should be appreciated that repaglinide, with its longer duration of action than that of nateglinide, is also metabolized via the cytochrome P450-3A4 system, raising the potential for drug interactions with other agents that are so metabolized.

Hyperglycemia is more frequently seen in elderly patients and is treated with once daily injections of NPH rather than with the use of insulin glargine or detimir, because of their slow and continuous sustained release.

Type 2 diabetes in this patient population represents unique challenges. Risk stratification, early diagnosis, and prevention are vital in reducing cardiovascular and microvascular complications.

TYPE-2 DIABETES AND ACQUIRED IMMUNE DEFICIENCY SYNDROME (AIDS)

Increased survival rates from infection with the human immunodeficiency virus-1 (HIV-1) have also resulted in an increased incidence of type-2 diabetes in this population. The increasing proportion of people infected with the AIDS virus and developing type-2 diabetes results from a complex interaction of multiple factors including body composition, family history, disease progression by HIV therapy, and treatment strategies, as well as concomitant hepatitis C infection (HCV). Estimates of HCV in patients with HIV-1 are close to 30%, with these individuals being at even greater risk for the lipodystrophy and insulin resistance associated with these coinfections than individuals who do not have HCV [86]. Coinfection with HIV-1 and HCV may have additive or even synergistic effects on hepatic lipid and glucose metabolism.

The metabolic disturbances and altered glucose homeostasis have become more prevalent with the use of potent highly active antiretroviral therapy (HAART), including that with nonnucleoside reverse transcriptase inhibitors (NNRTIs), protease inhibitors (PIs), ritonoavir boosted protease inhibitors, and nucleoside reverse transcriptase inhibitors (NRTIs). The Multicenter AIDS Cohort Study (MACS) demonstrated that 14% of HIV infected male patients using HAART had type-2 diabetes compared with 5% of HIV seronegative men while the rate of incidence of type-2 diabetes was 4.7 cases/100 person-years among HIV infected men using HAART compared with 1.4 cases/100 person-years among HIV seronegative men [87]. This suggested that the incidence of type-2 diabetes in men using HAART was greater than four times that in HIV seronegative men.

The stage of progression of HIV-1 infection and the viral replication rate directly affect glucose regulation and lipogenesis in the absence of antiretroviral therapy, while the PIs and the NNRTIs adversely affect insulin resistance. Advanced disease is accompanied by lower HDL and LDL levels and higher triglyceride and VLDL levels. Prior to the introduction of the highly active antiretroviral therapeutic agents, approximately 2% of HIV-1 treated patients were insulin resistant compared to 80% with the protease inhibitors [88].

Patients with HIV-1 infection may develop a variety of metabolic and glucoregulatory abnormalities including hypertriglyceridemia, hypercholesterolemia, lipodystrophy with abnormal fat distribution, reduced bone mineral density, and altered carbohydrate metabolism. Although the introduction of HAART therapy has resulted in significant reductions in mortality and morbidity with this disorder, this treatment may also increase cardiovascular and type-2 diabetes risk.

General rules for glycemic therapy in HIV-1 infected individuals involve initiation of treatment at the lowest possible dose and titration upward. Pentamidine treatment for opportunistic Pneumocystis pneumonia may be associated with hypoglycemia; hence, caution should be exercised when considering sulfonylureas. The American Diabetes Association recommends the use of an insulin sensitizing agent like metformin for patients at very high risk for developing type-2 diabetes – particularly the obese individuals. HIV-1 infected individuals treated with metformin had significant reductions in weight, fasting glucose, and visceral adipose tissue compared to placebo [89]. Rosiglitazone has been associated with beneficial effects on lipoatrophy, adiponectin levels, and insulin sensitivity compared to placebo, while pioglitazone has been associated with modest, beneficial improvements in thigh fat distribution in addition to lowering triglycerides.

Despite the positive effect of simvastain and atorvastatin in lowering both LDL cholesterol and triglycerides, bioavailability may increase by 267 and 343% respectively when used with PIs ritonavir and saquinavir by competing with the same enzyme system within the liver (P450-3A4), which can also occur with lovastatin. The bioavailability of pravastatin was reduced by 50% with these same two drugs. Fluvastatin has the lowest interaction potential within the statin class. Fibric acid derivatives and omega-3 acid ethyl esters work well for treating hypertriglyceridemia and low HDL levels with a low risk for drug interactions.

Therapeutic management of patients with HIV-1 infection and type-2 diabetes presents the clinician with unique challenges because of the pharmacologic drug interactions, while combining antiretroviral therapy with diabetes and dyslipidemia management, taking into consideration disease stages and the individual patient's demographic characteristics.

TYPE-2 DIABETES AND HEMODIALYSIS

Diabetes is the most common cause of renal failure worldwide, representing 44% of end stage renal disease (ESRD) in the United States Renal Data System in 2005 [90]. Uremia and dialysis can complicate glycemic control affecting clearance, secretion, and sensitivity of peripheral tissues to insulin. Various and opposing effects of ESRD can cause blood glucose levels to widely fluctuate, while most anti-diabetic drugs are excreted renally increasing the risk for hypoglycemia, so insulin constitutes the cornerstone of therapy in these patients.

Compensatory increase in insulin secretion due to insulin resistance is lacking in patients with ESRD because of secondary hyperparathyroidism, concomitant metabolic acidosis, and 1,25 dihydroxy-vitamin D deficiency. Improvement in acidosis, uremia, and phosphate handling that occurs with hemodialysis further impairs insulin secretion and alters its clearance. Dialysates with higher dextrose concentrations are usually reserved for peritoneal dialysis, with lower concentration used in hemodialysis. Hence, hyperglycemia is more common with peritoneal dialysis and hypoglycemia more common in hemodialysis. Reduction in renal gluconeogenesis and insulin clearance in ESRD patients may exert varying effects on the type-2 diabetic patients with significant insulin resistance and minimal beta cell function while hemodialysis alters the pharmacokinetics of anti-diabetic medications.

It is important to appreciate that A1C measurements may be falsely elevated in patients with ESRD, as elevated urea nitrogen enhances the formation of carbamylated hemoglobin, which is indistinguishable from glycosylated hemoglobin in an electrical charge based assay, while iron deficiency in recent blood transfusions, shortened life span of red blood cells, and treatment with erythropoietin stimulating agents may cause underestimation of the A1C. Other parameters like the serum fructosamine, which measures the average glucose over a 2 week period of time, may be more useful under these circumstances, although even this can be affected by altered protein metabolism.

Although the National Kidney Foundation Kidney Disease Outcomes Quality Initiative did not clearly establish a target A1C level for patients with diabetes and ESRD, levels of 6–7% are reasonable. Fasting glucose levels should be targeted at less than 100 mg/dl and postprandial glucose levels at less than 140 mg/dl unless persistent hypoglycemia occurs.

Several oral anti-hyperglycemic agents should not be used in patients with ESRD. Sulfonylurea medications are highly protein bound, but it is the unbound drug that exerts a clinical effect. Because of the high protein binding, dialysis will not effectively clear elevated levels of sulfonylurea drugs. Other drugs like beta-blockers, fibric acid derivatives, salicylates, and sulfonamides may displace sulfonylureas from albumin, increasing the risk of severe hypoglycemia. First generation sulfonylureas (chlorpropamide, acetohexamide, tolbutamide, and tolazamide) are excreted renally and are contraindicated in ESRD. Second generation agents glimepiride, glyburide, and glyclazide are metabolized hepatically with active metabolites excreted renally and should be avoided in ESRD. Glipizide is also metabolized hepatically, but its metabolites are inactive, so it can be used with caution at low doses (2.5–10 mg/day) in patients with ESRD. Sustained release preparations, however, should be avoided. Metformin is contraindicated in ESRD.

The meglitinides, repaglinide and nateglinide, are not recommended for patients on hemodialysis. Nateglinide is metabolized hepatically and excreted renally with active metabolites and a short duration of action, while repaglinide is longer acting and almost completely converted to inactive metabolites in the liver with less than 10% excreted by the kidneys.

TZDs do not accumulate in ESRD and require no dose adjustments. These agents, although not affected by ESRD and dialysis, should be used with caution in this patient population because of the potential for fluid retention and precipitation of heart failure.

The alpha-glucosidase inhibitors, acarbose and miglitol and their metabolites, attain high levels in renal failure and are not recommended to be used in ESRD.

GLP-1 agonists, exenatide and liraglutide, are excreted renally and should not be used in patients with a GFR less than 30 ml/min, with no dosage adjustment if the GFR is greater than 30 ml/min.

DPP-IV agents, saxagliptin and sitagliptin, can be used in patients with ESRD with dose reductions; Saxagliptin 2.5 mg can be used daily after dialysis, while sitagliptin 50 mg should be used in patients with a GFR of 30–50 ml/min and 25 mg for patients with a GFR less than 30 ml/min independent of dialysis timing.

Half of the daily insulin requirement is normally secreted at a steady basal rate of 0.5 units/kg/day, while the other half is secreted in a bolus fashion in response to feeding.

After being secreted into the portal system, insulin circulates through the liver where approximately 75% is metabolized and the remainder is renally excreted. Of the 25% that is excreted renally, 40% is actively secreted and metabolized into amino acids in the nephric tubules and 60% is filtered through the glomerulus, with less than 1% secreted as intact insulin [91]. Renal metabolism plays a major role for exogenous insulin metabolism in dialysis patients as first pass metabolism is bypassed hepatically. Once the GFR drops below 20 ml/min, less insulin is cleared renally and with the onset of uremia there is an additional attenuation of hepatic insulin metabolism. Hence, exogenous insulin requirements usually decrease in ESRD despite the enhanced insulin resistance due to renal failure. When the GFR is <50 ml/min, insulin dose should be reduced by 25% and by 50% if the GFR is <10 ml/min. The short (lispro, aspart, and glulisine) and long acting (levimir and glargine) analog insulins are preferred in ESRD with less risk of hypoglycemia.

FOOT PROBLEMS IN THE DIABETIC PATIENT

Meticulous care of the feet in the diabetic patient plays a critical role in avoiding amputations and other dreaded complications from this disease. Diabetic foot wounds represent the leading cause of lower extremity amputations in the United States [92]. Foot disorders in the type-2 diabetic patient can be caused by vascular ischemic, neuropathic, and developmental disorders from direct and indirect injury. Diabetic patients are at increased risk for amputation as shown by the multiple risk factors for this calamity listed in Table 2.

Cigarette smoking and diabetes represent two extremely strong risk factors for peripheral arterial disease (PAD). PAD is twice more common in diabetic patients than in non-diabetic individuals and four times more common in smokers than in non-smokers.

Vascular disorders can run the gamut from capillary basement membrane thickening due to microangiopathy to large vessel arteriosclerotic stenoses and occlusions. The net result is local tissue hypoxia worsened by the glycosylation and osmotic effects of hyperglycemia, resulting in insufficient perfusion to meet the metabolic requirements for wound prevention and healing which can be twenty times greater than requirements for maintenance of a steady state. Doppler studies measuring ankle-brachial index, pressure–volume recordings, and Doppler wave form analysis provide valuable information about the condition of the blood vessels. Ankle-Brachial Index (ABI) pressures less than 0.9 are consistent with ischemia, with ABIs less than 0.6 consistent with severe ischemia. Clinical features of the ischemic foot include diminished sensation with a pulseless, cool, or even cold extremity, and ulcerations on the margins of the heels and tips of toes with loss of subcutaneous fat on the plantar surface of the toes with pitting.

Neuropathic changes may result in muscle weakness causing gait deformities and loss of sensation, impairing wound recognition. This loss of painful sensation and the

Table 2
Foot related risk conditions with an increased risk for amputation

Bone deformities

Peripheral neuropathy

Altered biomechanics

Peripheral vascular disease

Previous history of amputation or ulcerations

Severe nail pathology

Increased persistent pressure conditions with erythema and hemorrhagic callus formation weakening of the bone structure of the foot (Charcot's joint) can lead to severe consequences when mechanical stress that normally causes pain results in tissue injury.

Boney abnormalities usually are found at the tarsal-metatarsal region, but can also involve the ankle and metatarso-phalangeal areas. Special shoes and fitted insoles can help accommodate the deformities and prevent ulceration. Vasomotor changes and arteriovenous shunting can cause neuropathic edema that can be seen with severe peripheral neuropathy.

Bunions, spurs, clawed toes, and bosses result from the bone's response to repetitive stresses, hereditary factors, and muscle abnormalities, resulting in and contributing to ulcerations and infections. These deformities are responsible for most diabetic foot wounds and found in many patients with this disease. Repetitive use stress and heel pressure sores can be particularly troublesome. When the heel of the foot rests against a firm surface for a prolonged period of time, perfusion can be compromised and bisters can result. If this occurs in a particularly under perfused tissue, apoptosis results, inducing ulcerations, cellulitis, and osteomyelitis.

Danger signs requiring urgent evaluation and treatment are the following:

1. Cellulitis, discoloration, and crepitus due to soft tissue gas formation
2. Pink, painful, and pulseless foot without gangrene
3. Redness, swelling, and pain in an otherwise painless foot may be a sign of a developing abscess
4. Cold, painful, immobile, pulseless extremity with lack of sensation indicates an arterial occlusion

Skin and nail care, appropriate footwear, and patient education and diligent surveillance are the cornerstones of prevention. Encourage patients to remove their shoes when presenting for an examination so that feet can be properly checked. Regular podiatric care and examination is crucial as proactive surgical procedures can correct deformities when they develop, before resulting in more deleterious consequences.

PERIOPERATIVE AND POSTOPERATIVE GLUCOSE CONTROL

Hyperglycemia during the perioperative and postoperative periods may inhibit vasodilatation, enhance thrombosis, and exacerbate infectious and vascular complications while impairing leukocyte phagocytosis, chemotaxis, and adherence. Attempts to control glucose during these periods have centered on subcutaneous sliding scale regimens or intravenous protocols. Sliding scale regimens are not recommended as the most effective way to control perioperative glucose that causes glycemic fluctuations and high rates of hyper and hypoglycemia compared to continuous intravenous infusion protocols. Another approach that has been tried has been glucose/insulin infusions with and without potassium as studied in the Diabetes and Insulin-Glucose Infusion in Acute Myocardial Infarction (DIGAMI) protocol where investigators made use of glucose/insulin infusions to lower glucose from 277 to 183 mg/dl in a patient with an acute myocardial infarction [49].

Insulin infusion protocols vary from institution to institution but clearly need to be started early, prior to unacceptably elevated glucose levels. Glucose levels should be checked hourly to ensure stability with insulin doses titrated to maintain control. Intensive glucose control in the postoperative period can increase the risk for hypoglycemia because of too much insulin and sudden changes in insulin sensitivity (infection resolution, pain control, intravascular fluid expansion, counterregulatory hormone responses, as well as quantity, type, route, and alterations in caloric intake).

Insulin therapy represents the best method for achieving glycemic control in the postoperative period because of its rapid effects, flexible dosing, and safety with hepatic, renal, and cardiorespiratory comorbidities. When well administered and closely checked, glucose control is usually achievable and risk of hypoglycemia is minimized. The most rapid and flexible way to manage hyperglycemia is through an insulin drip, which alleviates any variability in subcutaneously administered insulin.

Significant improvements in postoperative mortality and morbidity as well as decreased risk for wound infections can be achieved when glucose control is ensured with intravenous glucose protocols, improving myocardial function, and attenuating postoperative complications.

SKIN DISORDERS IN TYPE-2 DIABETES

As a consequence of the effects of diabetes on skin collagen and the microcirculation, cutaneous lesions can commonly occur in type-2 diabetes, while autoimmune lesions predominate in type-1 diabetes [93]. Not only can these lesions be annoying and unsightly, but they may also serve as a nidus for secondary infection while drugs used to treat diabetes – insulin and oral agents — may cause unwanted dermatologic side effects.

Dermatologic problems that can be seen in type-2 diabetes and summarized in Table 3 include the following:

1. Necrobiosis lipoidica diabeticorum – These are nonscaling plaques with an atrophic, yellow center, with erythematous raised borders, and with telangiectasias on the surface. These usually occur at a later age than in the type-1 diabetic, and may respond to tight glycemic control. They may also respond to topical and intralesional injections of steroids.

Table 3
Dermatological abnormalities seen in diabetic patients [95, 99]

Necrobiosis lipoidica diabeticorum
Achrochordons
Calciphylaxis
Diabetic dermopathy
Acquired perforating dermatosis
Onychomycosis
Thickened skin
Granuloma annulare
Eruptive xanthomata
Fungal infections
Bacterial infections
Reactions to oral agents, insulin

2. Acanthosis nigricans – These hyperpigmented velvet appearing lesions are usually related to high circulating insulin levels in insulin resistant states or formed as a complication of niacin or steroid therapy and endocrinopathies (Cushing syndrome, acromegaly), and in paraneoplastic states. The keratin laden superficial dermal epithelium creates the darkened color as a result of insulin like growth factor stimulation of dermal fibroblasts and kerationocytes. Exercise and weight reduction can result in improvement of these lesions which can be malodorous, macerated, or painful, but usually are asymptomatic.

3. Acrochordons (skin tags) – Pedunculated and small, these soft lesions can occur on the neck, axillae, and eyelids and can be easily removed with electrodessication, cryotherapy, or excision.

4. Calciphylaxis – This usually occurs in patients with kidney failure in areas that have thicker adipose tissue first with localized erythema and tenderness, subcutaneous nodules, or necrotizing painful skin lesions. This small vessel vasculopathy occurs in 1–4% of patients on dialysis and pathologically is characterized by intimal fibrosis, thrombosis, and proliferation with mural calcification. Fibrous proliferation is found in the capillaries, venules, and arterioles with medial wall calcification. Prognosis is poor and requires analgesic therapy. Glycemic control may lessen the likelihood of secondary infection.

5. Diabetic dermopathy – This is usually associated with pretibial papules and pretibial scarring, atrophy, and hyperpigmented macules. Although not pathognomonic for diabetes, these lesions can be seen in up to 70% of diabetic patients as well as 20% of nondiabetics. These lesions, often harbingers of abnormal glucose tolerance and microvascular complications, can also be found on the lateral malleoli, thighs, and forearms. Some lesions respond spontaneously with no known effective treatment.

6. Acquired perforating dermatosis (APD) – This is characterized by dome shaped nodules and papules (2.0–10 mm) with hyperkeratotic plugs involving the dorsal surface of the hands, trunk, and extremities. These can be seen in up to 10% type-2 diabetic patients on dialysis. Intralesion or topical steroids may provide some relief.

7. Yellow nails – This is usually seen in elderly type-2 diabetic patients or in patients with onychomycosis. This discoloration, resulting from glycosylation end products, is usually found in the distal end of the hallux toenail.

8. Thickened skin – This can manifest itself as (1) thickening of the epidermis and dermis measurable by ultrasound, increasing with age and also involving the fingers and hands, (2) diabetic scleroderma involving a peau d'orange thickening in the dermis of the neck and upper back, found in 2.5–14% of type-2 diabetic patients, more commonly in women than in men, (3) Huntley papules or pebbled knuckles characterized by multiple, grouped lesions on the periungual surface, knuckles, and the extensor surface of the fingers found in 20–30% of all diabetic patients, and (4) diabetic hand syndrome which can occur in 8–50% of type-2 diabetic patients, characterized by Dupuytren contractures and palmar fascial thickening with stiffness of the proximal interphalangeal and metacarpophalangeal joints [94]. No known treatment exists for thickened skin.

9. Granuloma annulare – Although this has often been linked to a harbinger of type-2 diabetes, no known association has been clearly established for this idiopathic disorder. This is characterized by oval or ring shaped lesions with a slightly raised erythematous border. Histologically, the dermis demonstrates focal collagen degeneration, abundant mucin, and collagenous bundles surrounded by histiocytes. No known treatment exists with the lesions resolving spontaneously.

10. Eruptive xanthomata – These yellow papules which can itch and cause discomfort, usually occur on the buttocks and the extensor surfaces of the extremities. These are found in patients with hypertriglyceridemia, tend to resolve with treatment, and result from impaired clearance of chylomicrons and VLDL because of impaired lipoprotein lipase activity [95].

11. Fungal infections – These include the following: (1) Mucormycosis – an anaerobic cellulitis caused by Phycomycetes, usually found in the sinuses but can also involve the brain and lungs in type-2 diabetic patients with prolonged hyperglycemia, often accompanied by *Clostridium* superinfection. This is diagnosed by biopsy and treated with surgical debridement combined with intravenous antifungal and antibiotic therapy. (2) Candida – this can be a sign of undiagnosed diabetes particularly when presenting with perleche in children and intercrural, intertrigonous, or vaginal monilia infections. Candidal balanitis can be seen in uncircumsized male patients. Treatment resolves with topical or oral antifungal treatment, but can reoccur if underlying diabetes remains undiagnosed. (3) Trichophyton – this can present as no inflamed White, powdery scaling over the palms and soles of the palms and soles of the feet (*T. rubrum*) or as superficial, scaling, macerated lesions with red borders between the digits of the hands or feet ("Athlete's feet"). This *T. mentagrophytes* infection usually responds to topical or even oral antifungal medications.

12. Bacterial infections like impetigo, ecthyma, erysipelas, folliculitis, and carbuncles can be more severe and reoccurring in diabetic patients and respond to improved glycemic control and topical or oral antibiotics. Erythrasma, which can often be confused with acanthosis nigricans or intertrigonous monilia, is caused by *Corynebacterium minutissimum* and shows a characteristic coral fluorescence with Wood's light. This usually results from sweating and friction, and is treated successfully with topical and oral antibiotics.

13. Lesions due to oral hypoglycemic agents – (a) Sulfonylureas (SFUs) – this can be present with a wide variety of lesions including maculopapular eruptions, urticaria, exfoliative dermatitis, erythema nodosum, photosensitivity, and generalized erythema and photosensitivity. These occur more commonly with the first generation SFUs and respond to withdrawl of the offending medication.(b) Metformin – reactions include leukocytoclastic vasculitis, psoriasiform drug eruptions, urticaria, and pruritus. (c) Acarbose – isolated cases of eythema multiforme and acute, generalized exanthematous pustulosis have been documented [96].

14. Lesions due to insulin – (a) Analogs – Iisolated case reports of vitiligo and IgE mediated anaphylaxis have been seen with lispro, and local injection site irritation with detimir and glargine can occur [97]. (b) Allergic reactions can occur in less than 1% of patients, taking the form of delayed hypersensitivity reactions and immediate local or generalized eruptions. Arthus immune complex reactions resulting in serum sickness have been rarely reported with biphasic insulin preparations.

Appropriate recognition is vital to render appropriate treatment along with dermatologic consultation.

RESOURCES

American Association of Diabetes Educators
444 North Michigan Avenue,
Suite 1240,
Chicago, IL 60611, USA;
www.diabetesnet.com/aade.html

American college of Sports Medicine
P.O. Box 1440,
Indianapolis, IN 46206-1440, USA;
http://www.acsm.org

American Diabetes Association (ADA)
ADA National Service Center,
1600 Duke Street,
Alexandria, VA 22314, USA;
www.diabetes.org

American Dietetic Association
216 West Jackson Boulevard,
Chicago, IL 60606-6995, USA

American Heart Association
7320 Greenville Avenue,
Dallas, TX 75231, USA

Council for the Advancement of Diabetes
Research and Education
www.cadre-diabetes.org

Diabetes Action Research and Education Foundation
426 C Street, NE,
Washington, DC 20002, USA;
daref@diabetesaction.org, diabetesaction.org

Division of Diabetes Translation
National Center for Chronic Disease Prevention and Health Promotion
Centers for Disease Control and Prevention
Mail Stop K-10,
4770 Buford Highway NE,
Atlanta, GA 30341-3717, USA;
www.cdc.gov/diabetes

Indian Health Service IHS Headquarters West
Central Diabetes Program
5300 Homestead Road NE;
Albuquerque, NM 87110, USA;
www.ihs.gov

International Association for Medical Assistance to Travelers
417 Center Street,
Lewiston, NY 14092, USA

International Diabetes Center
3800 Park Nicollet Boulevard,
Minneapolis, MN 55416, USA;
www.idcdiabetes.org

International Diabetes Federation
1 Rue DeFacqz,
1000 Brussels, Belgium;
www.idf.org

International Diabetic Athletes Association
1647 West Bethany Home Road #B,
Phoenix, AZ 85015, USA

Joslin Diabetes Center
One Joslin Place,
Boston, MA 02215, USA;
www.joslin.org

Juvenile Diabetes Foundation International
120 Wall Street,
19th Floor, New York, NY 10005-40001, USA;
www.jdfcure.org

Mayo Clinic Health Oasis
Mayo Foundation for Medical education and Research
200 First Street NW,
Rochester, MN 55905, USA;
www.mayohealth.org

National Diabetes Education Initiative
A division of Physicians World Communications Group
400 Plaza Drive,
Secaucus, NJ 07094, USA;
www.ndei.org

National Diabetes Education Program
c/o National Diabetes Information Clearinghouse,
I Information Way,
Bethesda, MD 20892-3560, USA;
ndic@aerie.com, http://niddk.nih.gov/health/diabetes/diabetes.htm

National Eye Institute
National Eye Health Education Program
2020 Vision Place,
Bethesda, MD 20892-3655, USA;
www.nei.nih.gov

National Health Council
Suite 500,
1730 M Street NW,
Washington, DC 20036, USA;
www.nhcouncil.org

National Institute of Diabetes and Digestive and Kidney Diseases
National Institute of Health
31 Center Drive, MSC 2560,
Bethesda, MD 20892-2560, USA;
www.niddk.nih.gov

National Kidney Foundation
Suite 1100,
30 East 33rd Street,
New York, NY 10016, USA;
www.kidney.org

National Kidney and Urologic Diseases Information Clearinghouse
3 Information Way,
Bethesda, MD 20892-3580, USA;
nkudic@aerie.com, http://www.niddk.nih.gov

National Stroke Association
9707 East Easter Lane,
Englewood, CO 80112, USA;
www.stroke.org

Office of Minority Health Resource Center
P.O. Box 37337,
Washington, DC 20013-7337, USA

Pennsylvania Diabetes Academy
777 East Park Drive,
P.O. Box 8820,
Harrisburg, PA 17105-8820, USA

Taking Control of Your Diabetes
1100 Camino Del Mar,
Suite B,
Del Mar, CA 92014, USA;
www.tcoyd.org

The Diabetic Traveler
P.O. Box 8223 RW,
Stamford, CT 06905, USA

Weight Control Information Network
1 Win Way,
Bethesda, MD 20892-3665, USA;
WINNIDDK@aol.com, http://www.niddk.nih.gov

REFERENCES

1. Knol MJ, Twisk JW, Beekman AT, Heine RJ, Snoek FJ, Pouwer F. Depression as a risk factor for type-2 diabetes mellitis. Diabetologia. 2006;49:837–845.
2. Jindal RD, Keshavan MS. Critical role of M3 muscarinic receptor in insulin secretion. J Clin Psychopharmacol. 2006;26(5):449–450.
3. Gilon P, Henquin JC. Mechanisms and physiological significance of the cholinergic control to pancreatic beta cell function. Endocr Rev. 2001;22(5):565–604.
4. Gautam D, Han SJ, Hamdan FF. A critical role for beta cell M3 muscarinic acetylcholine receptors in regulating insulin release and blood glucose homeostasis in vivo. Cell Metab. 2006;3(6):449–461.

5. Renuka TR, Robinson R, Paulose GS. Increased insulin secretion by muscarinic M1 and M3 receptor function from rat pancreatic islets in vivo. Neurochem Res. 2006;31(3):313–320.

6. American Diabetes Association; American Psychiatric Association; American Association of Clinical Endocrinologists; North American Association for the Study of Obesity. Consensus development conference on antipsychotic drugs, obesity and diabetes. Diabetes Care. 2004;27(2):595–601.

7. Fava M. Weight gain and antidepressants. J Clin Psychiatry. 2000;61(suppl 11):37–41.

8. Ackerman S, Nolan LJ. Bodyweight gain induced by psychotropic drugs. Incidence, mechanisms, and management. CNS Drugs. 1998;9:135–151.

9. Fagot-Campagna A, Pettitt DJ, Englegau MM, Burrows NR, Geiss LS, Valdez R. Type-2 diabetes among North American children and adolescents. J Pediatr. 2000;136:664–672.

10. Ogden CL, Carroll MD, Curtin LR, McDowell MA, Tabak CJ, Flegal KM. Prevalence of overweight and obesity in the United States 1999-2004. JAMA. 2006;295(13):1549–1555.

11. Molnar D. The prevalence of the metabolic syndrome and type-2 diabetes mellitus in children and adolescents. Int J Obes Relat Metab Disord. 2004;28(suppl 3):570–574.

12. Legro RE, Kunselman AR, Dodson WC. Prevalence and predictors of risk for type-2 diabetes mellitus and impaired glucose tolerance in polycystic ovary syndrome. J Clin Endocrinol Metab. 1999;84:165–169.

13. Weiss R, Dziura J, Burgert TS. Obesity and the metabolic syndrome in children and adolescents. N Engl J Med. 2004;350:2362–2374.

14. American Diabetes Association. Type-2 diabetes in children and adolescents: consensus statement. Diabetes Care. 2000;23:381–389.

15. Vinicor F. Diabetes and Women's Health Across the Life Stages: A Public Health Perspective. Atlanta: Centers for Disease Control, US Department of Health and Human Services; 2002.

16. Narayan KM, Boyle JP, Thompson TJ, Sorenson SW, Williamson DF. Lifetime risk for diabetes mellitus in the United States. JAMA. 2003;290(14):1884–1890.

17. Expert Panel on Detection, Evaluation, and Treatment of High Blood Cholesterol in Adults. Executive Summary of the Third Report of The National Cholesterol Education Program (NCEP) Expert Panel on Detection, Evaluation, and Treatment of High Blood Cholesterol in Adults (Adult Treatment Panel III). JAMA. 2001;285(19):2486-2497.

18. Knowler WC, Barrett-Connor E, Fowler SE. Reduction in the incidence of type 2 diabetes with lifestyle intervention or metformin. N Engl J Med. 2002;346(6):393-403.

19. Ford ES, Giles WH, Dietz WH. Prevalence of the metabolic syndrome among US adults: findings from the third National Health and Nutrition Examination Survey. JAMA. 2002;287:356–359.

20. Isomaa B, Almgren P, Tuomi T. Cardiovascular morbidity and mortality associated with the metabolic syndrome. Diabetes Care. 2001;24:2486–2497.

21. Jack L, Boseman L, Vinicor F. Aging Americans and diabetes. A public health and clinical response. Geriatrics. 2004;59:14–17.

22. Smedley BD, Stith AY, Nelson AR. Unequal Treatment: Confronting Racial and Ethnic Disparities in Health Care. Washington, DC: National Academic Press; 2003.

23. Harris MI, Flegal KM, Cowie CC. Prevalence of diabetes, impaired fasting glucose, and impaired glucose tolerance in US adults. The Third National Health and Nutrition Examination Survey. Diabetes Care. 1998;21:136–144.

24. American Diabetes Association. Standards of medical care in diabetes. Diabetes Care. 2004;27(suppl 1):S15–S35.

25. Tuomilehto J, Lindstrom J,Eriksson JG. Prevention of type 2 diabetes mellitus by changes in lifestyle among subjects with impaired glucose tolerance. N Engl J Med. 2001;344:1343–1350.

26. Kanaya AM, Narayan KM. Prevention of type 2 diabetes: data from recent trials. Prim Care. 2003;30:511–526.

27. Buchanan TA, Xiang AH, Peters RK. Prevention of type 2 diabetes by treatment of insulin resistance: comparison of early vs. late intervention in the TRIPOD study. Diabetes. 2002;51(suppl 2):A35.

28. Moses RG. The recurrence rate of gestational diabetes in subsequent pregnancies. Diabetes Care. 1996;19(12):1348–1350.

29. Dornhorst A, Rossi M. Risk and prevention of type 2 diabetes in women with gestational diabetes. Diabetes Care. 1998;21(suppl 2):B43–B49.

30. Expert Committee on the Diagnosis and Classification of Diabetes Mellitus. Report of the Expert Committee on the Diagnosis and Classification of Diabetes Mellitus. Diabetes Care. 2000;23(suppl 1):S4–S19.
31. Jovanovic L, Pettit DJ. Gestational diabetes mellitus. JAMA. 2001;286:2516–2518.
32. Kim C, Newton KM, Knopp RH. Gestational diabetes and the incidence of type 2 diabetes: a systematic review. Diabetes Care. 2002;25:1862–1868.
33. Pietropaolo M, LeRoith D. Pathogenesis of diabetes: our current understanding. Clin Cornerstone. 2001;4:1–16.
34. Gu K, Cowie CC, Harris MI. Diabetes and decline in heart disease mortality in US adults. JAMA. 1999;281:1291–1297.
35. Downs JR, Clearfield M, Weis S. Primary prevention of acute coronary events with lovastatin in men and women with average cholesterol levels. JAMA. 1998;279:1615–1622.
36. Assmann G, Carmena R, Cullen P. Coronary heart disease: reducing the risk: a worldwide view. International Task Force for the Prevention of Coronary Disease. Circulation. 1999;100:1930–1938.
37. Wilson PW. Diabetes mellitus and coronary heart disease. Am J Kidney Dis. 1998:32:S89–S100.
38. Gaede P, Vedel P, Larsen N. Multifactorial intervention and cardiovascular disease in patients with type 2 diabetes. N Engl J Med. 2003;348:383–393.
39. UK Prospective Diabetes Study Group. Tight blood pressure control and risk of macrovascular and mcirovascular complications in type 2 diabetes: UKPDS 38. BMJ. 1998;317:703–713.
40. Vega Gl. Results of expert meetings: obesity and cardiovascular disease. Obesity, the metabolic syndrome and cardiovascular disease. Am Heart J. 2001;142:1108–1116.
41. Deen D. Metabolic syndrome: time for action. Am Fam Physician. 2004;69:2875–2882.
42. Wilson PW, Grundy SM. The metabolic syndrome: practical guide to origins and treatment. Circulation. 2003;108:1422–1424.
43. Knowler WC, Barnett-Conner E, Fowler SE, Diabetes Prevention Program Research Group. Reduction in the incidence of type 2 diabetes with lifestyle intervention or metformin. N Engl J Med. 2002;346:393–403.
44. Zinman B, Ruderman N, Campaigne BN, Devlin JT, Schneider SH, American Diabetes Association. Physical activity exercise and diabetes mellitus. Diabetes Care. 2003;26(suppl 1):S73–S77.
45. Rossouw JE, Anerson GL, Prentice RL. Risks and benefits of estrogen plus progestin in healthy postmenopausal women: principal results from the Women's Health Initiative randomized controlled trial. JAMA. 2002;288:321–333.
46. Hulley S, Grady D, Bush T. Randomized controlled trial of estrogen plus progestin for secondary prevention of coronary heart disease in postmenopausal women. Heart and Estrogen/progestin Replacement Study (HERS) Research Group. JAMA. 1998;280:605–613.
47. Manning P, Allum A, Jones S, Sutherland W, Williams S. The effect of hormone replacement therapy on cardiovascular risk factors in type 2 diabetes. Arch Intern Med. 2001;161:1772–1776.
48. Herrington DM, Vittinghoff E, Lin F. Statin therapy, cardiovascular events, and total mortality in the Heart and Estrogen/Progestin Replacement Study (HERS). Circulation. 2002;105:2962–2967.
49. Malmberg K. Prospective randomized study of intensive insulin treatment on long term survival after acute myocardial infarction in patients with diabetes mellitus. Diabetes Mellitus, Insulin Glucose Infusion in Acute Myocardial Infarction (DIGAMI) Study Group. BMJ. 1997;314:1512–1514.
50. Kjekshus J, Gilpin E, Cali G, Blackey AR, Henning H, Ross J. Diabetic patients and beta-blockers after acute myocardial infarction. Eur Heart J. 1990;11:43–50.
51. Chen J. Beta blockers in elderly diabetic patients post myocardial infarction. J Am Coll Cardiol. 1999;34:1388–1394.
52. Bakris G, Bell D, Fonseca V. GEMINI Investigators. The rationale and design of the glycemic effects in diabetes mellitus. JAMA. 2004;292(18):2227–2236.
53. Myers J, Prakash M, Froelicher V, Do D, Partington S, Atwood JE. Exercise mortality among men referred for exercise testing. N Engl J Med. 2001;346:793–801.
54. Vinik A, Flemmer M. Diabetes and macrovascular disease. J Diabetes Complications. 2002;16:235–245.
55. Patterson JE, Andriole VT. Bacterial urinary tract infections in diabetes. Infect Dis Clin North Am. 1995;9:25–51.
56. Patterson JE, Andriole V. Bacterial urinary tract infections in diabetes. Infect Dis Clin North Am. 1997;11(3):735–750.
57. Lunt H. Women and diabetes. Diabet Med. 1996;13(12):1009–1016.

58. Rayfield EJ, Ault MJ, Keusch GT. Infection and diabetes: the case for glucose control. Am J Med. 1982;72(3):439–450.

59. Addison WA, Livingood CH, Hill GB. Recurrent necrotizing fasciitis of vulvar origin in diabetic patients. Obstet Gynecol.1984;63(4):473–479.

60. Bohannon NJ. Treatment of vulvovaginal candidiasis in patients with diabetes. Diabetes Care. 1998;21(3):451–456.

61. Bell DS, Clements RS, Cutter GR, Whitey RJ. Condylomata acuminata in IDDM. Diabetes Care. 1988;11(3):295–296.

62. Stenchever MA, Herbst AL, Mishell DR (eds). Comprehensive Gynecology, 4th ed. St. Louis: Mosby; 2001.

63. Peer AK, Hoosen AA, Seedat MA. Vaginal yeast infections in diabetic women. S Afr Med J. 1993;83(10):727–729.

64. Tobin MJ. Vulvovaginal candidiasis: topical versus oral therapy. Am Fam Physician. 1995:51:1715–1720.

65. Coats AJ. Angiotensin receptor blockers – finally the evidence is coming in: IDNT and RENAAL. Int J Cardiol. 2001;79:99–102.

66. Heart Outcomes Prevention Evaluation Study Investigators. Effects of ramipril on cardiovascular and microvascular outcomes in people with diabetes mellitus: results of the HOPE study and MICRO-HOPE substudy. Lancet. 2000;355:253–259.

67. Spanheimer RG. Reducing cardiovascular risk in diabetes. Which factors to modify first? Postgrad Med. 2001;109:26–30; 33–36.

68. Adler AI, Stratton IM, Neil HA. Association of systolic blood pressure with macrovascular and microvascular complications of type 2 diabetes (UKPDS 36): prospective observational study. BMJ. 2000;321:412–419.

69. Colwell JA, American Diabetes Association. Aspirin therapy in diabetes. Diabetes Care. 2003;26(suppl 1):S87–S88.

70. Hansson L, Zanchetti A, Carruthers SG. Effects of intensive blood pressure lowering and low dose aspirin in patients with hypertension: principal results of the Hypertension Optimal Treatment (HOT) Randomized Trial (HOT Study Group). Lancet. 1998;351:1755–1762.

71. CAPRIE Steering Committee. Randomized, blinded trial of clopidogrel versus aspirin in patients at risk of ischemic events (CAPRIE). Lancet. 1996;348:1329–1339.

72. Gaede P, Vedel P, Larsen N, Jensen GV, Parving HH, Pedersen O. Multifactorial intervention and cardiovascular disease in patients with type 2 diabetes. N Engl J Med. 2003;348:383–393.

73. American Diabetes Association. Gestational diabetes mellitus. Diabetes Care. 2004;27(suppl 1):S88–S90.

74. Clapp IF. Exercise during pregnancy: a clinical update. Clin Sports Med. 2000;19:273–286.

75. Bertinin AM, Silva JC, Taborda W. Perinatal outcomes and the use of oral hypoglycemic agents. J Perinat Med. 2005;33(6):519–523.

76. Jacobson GF, Ramos GA, Ching JY, Kirby RS, Ferrara A, Field DR. Comparison of glyburide and insulin for the management of gestational diabetes in a large managed care population. Am J Obstet Gynecol. 2005;193(1):118–124.

77. Brody SC, Harris R, Lohr K. Screening for gestational diabetes: a summary of evidence for the U.S. Preventive Services task Force. Obstet Gynecol. 2003;101(2):380–392.

78. Kim C, Herman WH, Vijan S. Efficacy and cost of postpartum screening strategies for diabetes among women with histories of gestational diabetes mellitus. Diabets Care. 2007;30(5):1102–1106.

79. Rowan J, Hague W, Wanzhen G, Battin M, Moore P. Metformin versus insulin for the treatment of gestational diabetes. N Engl J Med. 2008;358:2003–2015.

80. Langer O, Brustman L, Anyaegbunam A, Mazze R. The significance of one abnormal glucose tolerance test value on adverse outcome in pregnancy. Am J Obstet Gynecol. 1987;157:758–763.

81. Landon MB, Vickers S. Fetal surveillance in pregnancy complicated by diabetes mellitus: is it necessary? J Matern Fetal Neonatal Med. 2002;12:413–416.

82. Meneilly GS, Tessier D. Diabetes in elderly adults. J Gerontol A Biol Sci Med Sci. 2001;56:M5–M13.

83. Franse LV, di Bari M, Shorr RI, Health, Aging, and Body Composition Study. Type 2 diabetes in older well functioning people. Data from the Health, Aging, and Body composition study. Diabetes Care. 2001;24:2065–2070. Diabetes Care. 2002;25:413.

84. Katakura M, Naka M, Kondo T, and the Nagano Elderly Diabetes Study Group. Normal mortality in the elderly with diabetes under strict glycemic and blood pressure control. Diabetes Res Clin Pract. 2007;78:108–114.

85. Johnston PS, Lebovitz HE, Coniff RF, Simonson DC, Raskin P, Munera CL. Advantages of alpha glucosidase inhibition as monotherapy in elderly type-2 diabetic patients. J Clin Endocrinol Metab. 1998;83(5):1515–1522.

86. Jain MK, Aragaki C, Fischbach L. Hepatitis C is associated with type 2 diabetes mellitus in HIV infected persons without traditional risk factors. HIV Med. 2007;8:491–497.

87. Brown TT, Cole SR, Li X. Antiretroviral therapy and the prevalence and incidence of diabetes. Arch Intern Med. 2005;165:2537.

88. Tebas P.Insulin resistance and diabetes mellitus associated with antiretroviral use in HIV infected patients. J Acquir Immune defic Syndr. 2008;49(suppl 2):S86–S92.

89. Saint-Marc T, Touraine JL. Effects of metformin on insulin resistance and central adiposity in patients receiving effective protease inhibitor therapy. AIDS. 1999;13:1000–1002.

90. National Institute of Diabetes and Digestive and Kidney Diseases. United States Renal Data System: USRDS 2005 Annual Data Report. Bethesda, MD: National Institutes of Health; 2005.

91. Snyder RW, Berns JS. Use of insulin and oral hypoglycemic medications in patients with diabetes mellitus and advanced kidney disease. Semin Dial. 2004;17:365–370.

92. Ahmed I, Goldstein B. Diabetes mellitus. Clin Dermatol. 2006;24:237–246.

93. Dittmar M, Kahaly GJ. Polyglandular autoimmune syndromes:immunogenetics and long term follow up. J Clin Endocrinol Metab. 2003;88:2893–2992.

94. Jennings AM, Millner PC, Ward JD. Hand abnormalities are associated with the complications of diabetes. Diabet Med. 1989;6:43–47.

95. Huntley AC. The cutaneous manifestations of diabetes mellitus. J Am Acad Dermatol. 1989;7:427–455.

96. Kono T, Hayami M, Kobayashi H, Ishii M, Taniguchi S. Acarbose induced generalized erythema multiforme. Lancet. 1999;354:396–397.

97. Blumer IR. Severe injection site reaction to insulin detimir. Diabetes Care. 2006;29:946.

98. Yang X, Hsu-Hage B, Zhang H, Zhang C, Zhang Y. Women with impaired glucose tolerance during pregnancy have significantly poor pregnancy outcomes. Diabetes Care. 2002;25:1619–1624.

99. American Diabetes Association. Standards of medical care for patients with diabetes mellitus. Diabetes Care. 2002;25(1):213–229.

SUPPLEMENTARY READINGS

Ahren B, Gomis R, Standl E. Twelve and fifty two week efficacy of the dipeptidyl peptidase IV inhibitor LAF237 in metformin-treated patients with type 2 diabetes. Diabetes Care. 2004;27:2874.

American Diabetes Association. Diabetic retinopathy. Diabetes Care. 2002;26(suppl 1):S99–S102.

American Diabetes Association. Diabetic nephropathy. Diabetes Care. 2003;26(suppl 1):S94–S98.

Aschner P, Kipnes MS, Lunjceford JK, Sanchez M, Mickel C, Williams-Herman DE. Effect of the dipeptidyl peptidase 4 inhibitor sitagliptin monotherapy on glycemic control in patients with type 2 diabetes. Diabetes Care. 2006;29:2632–2638.

Bakris GL, Williams M, Dworkin L. Preserving renal function in adults with hypertension and diabetes: a consensus approach. National Kidney Foundation Hypertension and Diabetes Executive Committees Working Gorup. Am J Kidney Dis. 2000;41(suppl 1):S22–S25.

Becker RH, Sha S, Frick AD, Fountaine RJ. The effect of smoking cessation and subsequent resumption on absorption of inhaled insulin. Diabetes Care. 2006;29:277–282.

Codario R. A guide to combination therapy in type 2 diabetes. Patient Care. 2003;5:16–24.

Codario R. Type 2 Diabetes, Pre-Diabetes, and the Metabolic Syndrome: The Primary Care Guide to Diagnosis and Management. Totowa: Humana; 2005, p. 14.

Codario R. Type 2 Diabetes, Pre-Diabetes, and the Metabolic Syndrome. The Primary Guide to Diagnosis and Management. Totowa: Humana; 2005, p. 101.

Codario R. Type 2 Diabetes, Pre-Diabetes, and the Metabolic Syndrome: The Primary Care Guide. Totowa: Humana; 2005, p. 17.

Dailey GE. Improving oral pharmacologic treatment and management of type 2 diabetes. Manag Care. 2004;13:41–47.

Davidson JA. Rationale for more aggressive guidelines for diabetes control. Endocr Pract. 2002;8 (suppl 1):13–14.

Davis MD, Fisher MR, Gangnon RE. Risk factors for high risk proliferative diabetic retinopathy and severe visual loss: Early Treatment Diabetic Retinopathy Report#18. Invest Ophthalmol Vis Sci. 1998;39:233–252.

DeFronzo RA. Pathogenesis of type 2 diabetes: metabolic and molecular implications for indentifying diabetes genes. Diabetes Rev. 1997;5:177–269.

DeFronzo RA. Pharmacologic therapy for type 2 diabetes mellitus. Ann Intern Med. 1999;133:73–74.

DeFronzo RA, Bergenstahl RM, Cefalu WT. Efficacy of inhaled insulin in patients with type 2 diabetes not controlled with diet and exercise. Diabetes Care. 2005;28:1922–1928.

Dressler A, Yki-Jarvinen H, Ziemen M. Less hypoglycemia and better post dinner glucose control with bedtime insulin glargine compared with bedtime NPH insulin during insulin combination therapy in type 2 diabetes. Diabetes Care. 2000;23:1130–1136.

Dungan KM, Buse JB. Glucagon-like peptide 1 based therapies for type 2 diabetes. Clin Diabetes. 2005;23:56.

Egan J, Rubin C, Mathisen A. Pioglitazone 027 Study Group: combination therapy with pioglitazone and metformin in patients with type 2 diabtetes. Diabetes. 1999;48:A117.

Genuth S, Alberti KG, Bennett P. Follow up report on the diagnosis of diabetes mellitus. Diabetes Care. 2003;26:3160–3167.

Grundy SM. Obesity, metabolic syndrome, and coronary atherosclerosis. Circulation. 2002;105:2696–2698.

Gominak S, Parry GJ. Diabetic neuropathy. Diabetic neuropathies, classification, clinical feautres and Pathological Basis. Adv Neurol. 2002;99:99–109.

Gulland J. Growing evidence supports role of chromium in prevention treatment of diabetes. Hollistic Primary Care. 2003;4:8.

Henry RR. Glucose control and insulin resistance in non-insulin dependent diabetes mellitus. Ann Intern Med. 1996;124:97–103.

Hoogwerf B. Exenatide and pramlintide: new glucose lowering agents for trating diabetes mellitus. Cleve Clin J Med. 2006;73(6):477–484.

Izucchi SE. Oral antihyperglycemic therapy for type 2 diabetes: scientific review. JAMA. 2002;287: 360–372.

LeRoith D. Beta cell dysfunction and insulin resistance in type 2 diabetes: role of metabolic and genetic abnormalities. Am J Med. 2002;113(suppl 6A):3S–11S.

McMahon G, Arky R. Inhaled insulin for diabetes mellitus. N Engl J Med. 2007;356:497–502.

Mogensen CE, Vestbo E, Poulsen PL. Micoralbuminuria and potential confounders. A review and some oservations on variability of urinary albumin excretion. Diabetes Care. 1995;18:572–581.

Moses R, Slobodniuk R, Boyages S. Effect of replaglinide addition to metformin monotherapy on glycemic control in patients with type 2 diabetes. Diabetes Care. 1999;22:119–124.

Nauck MA, Meininger G, Sheng D, Terranella L, Stein PP. Efficacy and safety of the dipeptidyl peptidase-4 inhibitor, sitagliptin, compared with the sulfonylurea, glipizide, in patients with type 2 diabetes inadequately controlled on metformin alone. Diabetes Obes Metab. 2007;9:194–205.

Nielsen LL, Baron AD. Pharmacology of exenatide for the treatment of type 2 diabetes. Curr Opin Investig Drugs. 2003;4:401–405.

Nielsen LL, Young AA, Parkes DG. Pharmacology of exenatide: a potential therapeutic for improved glycemic control of type 2 diabetes. Regul Pept. 2004;117:77–88.

Palumbo PJ. Glycemic control,mealtime glucose excursions and diabetic complications in type 2 diabetes mellitus. Mayo Clin Proc. 2001;76:609–618.

Parkes D, Jodka C, Smith P. Pharmacokinetic actions of exendin-4 in the rat: comparison with glucagon-like peptide-1. Drug Dev Res. 2001;53:260.

Patton JS, Bukar J, Nagarian S. Inhaled insulin. Adv Drug Deliv Rev. 1999;35:235–247.

Pierce NS. Diabetes and exercise. Br J Sports Med. 1999;33:161–173.

Ramlo-Halsted BA, Edelman SV. The natural history of type 2 diabetes. Implications for clinical practice. Prim Care. 1999;26:771–789.

Raskin P, McGill J, Hale P. Replaglinide/rosiglitazone combination therapy of type 2 diabetes. American Diabetes Association 61st Scientific Session. Diabetes. 2001;50(suppl 2):Abstract 516-P.

Ryan EA, Lakey JR, Paty BW, Imes S, Korbutt GS, Kneteman NM. Successful islet transplantation: continued insulin reserve provides long term glycemic control. Diabetes. 2002;51:2148–2157.

Salehi M, D'Alessio D. New therapies for type 2 diabetes based on glucagon-like peptide 1. Cleve Clin J Med. 2006;72(4):382–388.

Salehi M, D'Alessio D. New therapies for type 2 diabetes based on glucagon like peptide-1. Cleve Clin J Med. 2006;73(4):382–388.

Schmitz O, Rungby B. Amylin agaonists: a novel approach in the treatment of diabetes. Diabetes. 2004;53(suppl 3):S233.

Scott R, Herman G, Zhao P. Twelve week efficacy and tolerability of MK-0431, a dipeptidyl peptidase IV inhibitor, in the treatment of type 2 diabetes. Abstract Book. Diabetes Association 65th Scientific Sessions 2005; 41-O.

Simmons Z, Feldman EL. Update on diabetic neuropathy. Curr Opin Neurol. 2002;15:595–603.

Sinnreich M, Taylor BV, Dyck JB. Diabetic neuropathies, classification, clinical features and pathological basis. Neurologist. 2005;11:63–79.

The National Kidney Foundation Kidney Disease Outcome Quality Initiative. Clinical practice guidelines for chronic kidney disease: evaluation, classification, and stratification. Am J Kidney Dis. 2002;39(suppl 1):S1–S266.

Verne GN, Sninsky CA. Diabetes and the gastrointestinal tract. Gastroenterol Clin North Am. 1998;27:861–874.

Yki-Jarvinen H, Ryysy L, Nikkila K. Comparison of bedtime insulin regimens in patients with type 2 diabetes mellitus: a randomized controlled study. Ann Int Med. 1999;130:389–396.

Yeh GY, Eisenberg DM, Kaptchuk TJ, Philips RS. Systematic review of herbs and dietary supplements for glycemic control in diabetes. Diabetes Care. 2003;26:1277–1294.

Index

From: *Current Clinical Practice: Type 2 Diabetes, Pre-Diabetes, and the Metabolic Syndrome*,
Edited by: R.A. Codario, DOI 10.1007/978-1-60327-441-8
© Springer Science+Business Media, LLC 2011